Practice Nursi

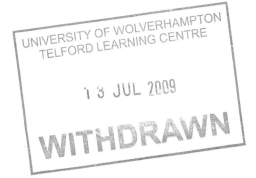

For Rachael

For Baillière Tindall:

Senior Commissioning Editor: Jacqueline Curthoys
Project Manager: Gail Murray
Project Development Manager: Karen Gilmour
Designer: George Ajayi

Practice Nursing

Edited by

Lynda Carey

BSc MSc(Nursing) RGN
Senior Lecturer, Department of Primary and Community Nursing,
University of Central Lancashire, Preston, UK

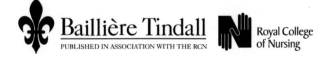

Baillière Tindall
PUBLISHED IN ASSOCIATION WITH THE RCN

Royal College
of Nursing

EDINBURGH ■ LONDON ■ NEW YORK ■ PHILADELPHIA ■ ST LOUIS ■ SYDNEY ■ TORONTO ■ 2000

BAILLIÈRE TINDALL
An imprint of Harcourt Publishers Limited

© Harcourt Publishers Limited 2000

♣ is a registered trademark of Harcourt Publishers Limited

First published 2000

ISBN 0 7020 2414 7

British Library Cataloguing in Publication Data
A catalogue record for this book is available from the British Library

Library of Congress Cataloging in Publication Data
A catalog record for this book is available from the Library of Congress

Note
Medical knowledge is constantly changing. As new information becomes available, changes in treatment, procedures, equipment and the use of drugs become necessary. The editor, contributors and the publishers have taken care to ensure that the information given in this text is accurate and up to date. However, readers are strongly advised to confirm that the information, especially with regard to drug usage, complies with the latest legislation and standards of practice.

The
publisher's
policy is to use
**paper manufactured
from sustainable forests**

Printed in China
NPCC/01

Contents

Contributors

Michelle Creed BA(Hons) ENG OTN RGN PN Cert Specialist Practitioner (GPN)
Practice Nurse, Riverside Centre for Health, Liverpool, UK

Sue Dobson RGN BA(Hons) MSc Nursing
Primary Care Nurse, North Mersey Community Trust, Merseyside, UK

Patsy Dodd BA(Hons) RGN Dip Asthma Dip Nursing Studies ENB 998 ENB Higher
Award, Specialist Practitioner (General Practice)
GP Specialist Practitioner, Liscard Group, Wallasey, Merseyside, UK

Pam Gastrell BA MPhil RGN RM RHVT DNT
Honorary Senior Lecturer, University of Southampton; formerly
Director of Studies, University of Southampton, Southampton, UK

Karen Gupta RGN DN ENB 998
Independent Practice Nurse, London; formerly Chair, RCN Practice
Nurse Association, London, UK

Roslyn Hope BA MSc CPsychol
Director of Corporate Development, Premier Health NHS Trust, St
Michael's Hospital, Lichfield, UK

Anne Jones MBA DMS RGN RM NDN RNT
Community Tutor, Emma Ferbrache Nurse Education Centre, St
Martin, Guernsey; formerly Professional Development Manager,
Chester and Halton NHS Community Trust, Chester, UK

Mark Jones BSc(Hons) MSc RN RHV
Primary Care Policy Advisor, Royal College of Nursing, London, UK

Daria McCusker BSc(Hons) DipHE RGN PN Cert Specialist Practitioner (GPN)
Practice Nurse, Riverside Centre for Health, Liverpool, UK

Mick McKeown BA(Hons) RGN RMN DPSN (Thorn)
Principle Lecturer, Mental Health Research, Department of Primary
and Community Nursing, University of Central Lancashire,
Preston, UK

Maureen Morgan MBA RGN RHV
Executive Director of Nursing, Premier Health NHS Trust, St Michael's Hospital, Lichfield, UK

Lyndsey Peacock BA MA RGN RM
Senior Lecturer, Faculty of Health, University of Central Lancashire, Preston, UK

Sylvina Tate BSc(Hons) MSc RGN Dip(N) PGDE RNT
Senior Lecturer, Centre for Community Care and Primary Health, University of Westminster, London, UK

Preface

Nursing is a living discipline that has continued to change in response to the demands of the population it serves (Baly 1995). This dynamic process is never more evident than in the development of the role of the nurse within the general practice setting, from its earliest beginnings as a support to the general practitioner to its present day purpose as an integrated member of the primary health care team.

What makes practice nursing different from other nursing disciplines is the speed with which the role has developed since the mid 1980s, both in its scope of practice and the recognition of the contribution of the nurse within this unique clinical environment. However, the recent changes in the policy and the introduction of practice nursing as an area of specialist practice have yet to fully impact upon existing practitioners and further challenge and shape the role. These recent developments will serve to offer practice nurses even greater opportunities for the growth of their sphere of practice.

The underlying belief of this text centres on the assumption that the role and function of nursing within general practice is undergoing fundamental change. This change has the potential to have a dramatic effect on the role of the nurse, particularly given the present situation and uncertainty about its future development. If nurses understand the factors and conceptual frameworks influencing practice, they are well placed to define their own future. This text therefore identifies and explores issues that are currently impacting upon role development.

The text is intended to enable nurses working within general practice to examine critical issues that impact not only upon their individual practice, but also the development of the profession. It is anticipated that through the exploration of the concepts, nurses will reflect and consider their own wider professional development needs. Readers are not expected to accept all of the issues raised and discussed at face value, but rather to question and at times challenge the ideas. Adoption of such an approach will facilitate readers to develop a greater understanding of professional and political issues as they impact upon everyday practice. For this reason the text includes Reflection Points, which aim to centre readers' attention on their own practice. To support the application of theory to practice, the authors are drawn from both practice and education backgrounds.

Reference

Baly M 1995 *Nursing and social change.* Routledge, London

Preston 2000   Lynda Carey

Structure and Organization of the Text

The text is structured into three distinct sections. The first section explores the current issues impacting upon nursing within general practice, moving from a historical perspective to examine the political, legal and organizational frameworks for care provision. This section will enable the reader to develop insight into the wider issues and developments that are shaping the context within which practice nursing is currently delivered.

The middle chapters of the text provide a critical review of the key areas impacting on the evolution of the role. In examining areas as diverse as nursing frameworks, mental health, clinical supervision, nurse prescribing and the promotion of health, this section intends to allow readers the opportunity to identify and explore issues that are shaping their role development from a practice level. The chapters within this section have been developed to facilitate readers to consider how the ideas can be implemented into their own practice, but have been chosen to encourage readers to consider practice on a wider level than merely completion of tasks and disease management.

The final chapters of the text are intended to assist readers in identifying a future for nursing within general practice. They are fundamentally concerned with offering an insight into how practice nursing can be shaped in the future. The chapters in this last section are intended to both challenge and inspire readers to explore the nature of their own individual practice and thereby realize their own potential.

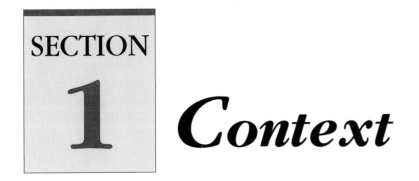

SECTION

1

Context

1 *Who is the Practice Nurse?*

Karen Gupta

INTRODUCTION

The discipline of practice nursing has grown directly out of a requirement for nurses to be employed in general practice, and is now accepted and respected as one of the specialist pathways of community nursing. This evolution of role has taken place against a background of wider developments in general practice and primary care, therefore it is necessary to look back over the past 30 years to gain a clear picture of who the practice nurse is. During this period, practice nurses have developed their role together with appropriate associated theory and skills to meet the diverse health needs of practice populations. The contribution that practice nurses have made to the delivery of quality primary care services has been considerable. Yet, despite this, it has been a hard struggle for recognition, not least among other nursing colleagues. Practice nurses have suffered from having no specialist qualification, and being disparagingly misrepresented as merely the 'handmaidens' of general practitioners.

In examining the development of practice nursing over the past century, and particularly the marked expansion of both quantity and role in the 1990s, it is fundamentally important to review the present position and role of the nurse. The description of the present role of the nurse will act as a springboard to a more detailed examination of the factors that have shaped the practice nurse's role to date.

Key Issues	
■ Historical developments	■ Influence of nurse education
■ Impact of government policy	■ Comparison with other nurses working in general practice

Who are Practice Nurses and What Do They Do?

In 1991 the Department of Health commissioned a national census of practice nurses to identify the characteristics and role of the nurse. Unsurprisingly, it concluded that practice nurses were predominantly female and predominantly white. In examining their readiness for the role they were undertaking, the survey concluded that 3% of practice nurses held a health visitor qualification, and 12% a district nursing qualification. Unconfirmed reports suggest that most practice nurses are recruited directly from hospital, with a number returning into employment after a break from nursing.

The picture emphasized by the study group (Atkin et al 1993) was of a strong professional group, confident in their identity and taking nursing forward by extending and expanding their role. At that time, the largest number had worked as a practice nurse for between 1 and 3 years. It is unlikely that such a major piece of research into the role will ever be carried out again; although now dated, it does effectively identify the diversity of the role. The survey confirmed that practice nurses undertake a wide variety of tasks, as well as being involved in running health promotion and minor surgery clinics. It highlighted that practice nurses undertook work that went beyond traditional nursing tasks, with 84% giving advice on common minor illness and some giving advice on welfare rights and identifying anxiety and depression in patients. Over 50% were also carrying out home visiting, mostly to undertake over-75 health assessments, although over 50% were also carrying out immunization and vaccination in the home. Nearly all were running health promotion clinics, over 50% were involved in minor surgery clinics and 26% were involved in running family planning clinics. There was evidently a need for more family planning trained nurses because, when asked to identify training needs, a significant proportion mentioned that they would like training in family planning. Approximately 80% were involved in running chronic disease management clinics, over half of which were asthma or diabetes clinics, and two-thirds ran hypertension clinics.

Working Environment of Practice Nurses

Practice nurses are unique in that not only do they work outside the NHS nursing structure, but also that they are directly employed by another professional group, namely GPs. This has directly impacted upon both their employment and financial status.

Most practice nurses stated one reason for leaving NHS employment as the wish to escape from nursing managerial control. The lack of a management structure undoubtedly enables practice nurses to be innovative in their practice, but does it leave them isolated and at risk? In 1996, the RCN published an assimilation of surveys of general practice nurses undertaken in 1994; one section covered preferred employment. The figures were unequivocal: 60–86% stated that they preferred to be directly employed by a GP practice, 3% preferred to be employed by a Trust, 5% by a 'practice nurse provider unit' and 5% preferred to be self-employed. In 1994 the majority of practice nurses therefore still wished to remain in GP employment.

However, the picture may be changing, and although a much smaller survey, the results of a questionnaire run by *Practice Nurse* journal among delegates at the National Practice Nurse Conference at York in 1998 gave a very different result. It reported that 37% wished to be self-employed, 33% to remain employed by GPs, and 29% preferred NHS Trust employment. It seems that practice nurses have a desire for independence, and if accurate, this survey reflects a drastic change in attitudes to employment, with a high number interested in the option of self-employment.

Employment status for practice nurses is a contentious issue, and undoubtedly some practice nurses have suffered by being employed in this way. General practitioners have not usually been trained in employment legislation and do not always prove to be 'good' employers (Bolden & Takle 1994). There are also fundamental concerns in relation to the impact of one professional being in a position to employ another, and whether this adversely affects what should be an equal relationship. Practice nurses found that in an employment dispute with the general practice, trade union recognition was not always accepted, and instead this was regarded by GPs as interference in their relationship with their employee.

Direct employment by general practitioners has directly impacted upon the financial remuneration received by practice nurses. This is best evidenced in the position surrounding their access to the NHS superannuation scheme. In 1996 the RCN Practice Nurse Association undertook a campaign to enable practice nurses to join the NHS superannuation scheme. This was despite the fact that there had been an 'agreement in principle' made by Virginia Bottomley in 1993 that this should be made possible. The RCN, together with the British Medical Association had continued to work for this to be implemented, but it was evident that the Department of Health was stalling. A strategy was developed to take this campaign forward, and achieve access to the NHS superannuation scheme for the 18 000 practice nurses in the United Kingdom.

The matter was raised by members of the Practice Nurse Association steering committee regionally and locally, and highlighted at meetings with the Department of Health. A flurry of articles and letters were sent to the nursing journals, and the issue was raised at conferences and meetings of practice nurses in an attempt to gain media coverage.

In response to this campaign, the government announced that practice nurses would be able to access the NHS superannuation scheme. Celebrations greeting this news however, were short-lived, when nurses realized that the regulations attached made the GP employer the 'gate-keeper' to access to the superannuation scheme. The Department of Health's original suggestion was that GPs should become 'employing authorities' under the NHS superannuating regulations and be able to choose whether to access the scheme for their practice staff. This was not acceptable to practice nurses who considered that they, not their employers, should be the ones to decide whether or not they join the NHS superannuation scheme. This severely disadvantaged practice nurses, who would have become the only nurses who could not have a pension by right, but only with the agreement of their employer. It was feared that other employing authorities would then be able to cite this as an argument to introduce the same restriction.

The campaign was continued to remove the 'employer's choice' clause, and finally the government announced that from September 1997 practice nurses, along with other practice staff, would be able to choose to access the NHS superannuation scheme as a right. This considerable and successful campaign, launched and taken forward by the RCN Practice Nurse Association and involving practice nurses across the United Kingdom, was a testament to the considerable power that practice nurses can have when working together to achieve a common aim.

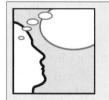

Reflection Points

■ Do you consider that employment of nurses by GPs has a positive or negative consequence for professional recognition?
■ What is your reasoning?

The significance of the practice nurse role over that of other community-based nurses is that its development has, to date, not been shaped by nurses but instead been moulded by other groups, in their attempt to reduce their contribution to the spiralling demands for health care within general practice. Central to the development of the role is the impact of changing government legislation and the needs of the GP. It is therefore necessary in examining the present day position of practice nurses to revisit the historical perspective and specifically examine the impact of legislation upon role development.

Historical Development of the Practice Nurse Role

The notion of nurses being employed in general practice is not necessarily confined to modern times; references to a nurse working alongside a GP in the community date back to 1913 (Jeffree 1996). For example, Hannah Mary Robson is recorded to have worked in Northumberland at the surgery of Dr Grant. She seemed to have a role not dissimilar to that of practice nurses of today – dispensing medicines, performing dressings and taking out of hours calls, deciding which could be dealt with by herself and which to refer to the doctor. She was evidently trusted and popular, both by the doctor and with the patients – enough to have operated what sounds like an early triage system, visiting the ambulance room at the local colliery, and undertaking home visits in neighbouring villages (Jeffree 1996).

Although the embryonic seeds of practice nursing were undoubtedly laid down by Robson, there is little documentary evidence of the development of the role after this date. However, the idea of a nurse working alongside the GP to provide nursing care to patients seems to be an attractive one – to nurses, doctors and patients, with a small number of nurses employed in general practice up until the 1960s. At this stage GPs generally worked alone, with little thought given to providing a nursing service for the practice population. It was only in the 1960s that the potential contribution of nursing was recognized, with the attachment of district nurses to general practice (Department of Health 1968) (Case Study 1.1). The benefits were clearly identified, although the relationship between the employing bodies of community nurses and general practice was not always easy. These troubled liaisons were central to the development of practice nursing.

By the late 1970s there were around 1500 practice nurses employed in general practice. In those early years, nurses were responsible for a variety of tasks, usually including immunization, women's health, dressings, giving routine injections such as hydroxocobalamin and increasingly depot neuroleptics, removal of sutures,

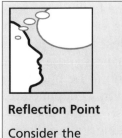

Reflection Point

Consider the description of early practice nursing. What are the similarities with current practice nursing?

Case Study 1.1

Practice Nursing in the 1960s

Mrs Reddington worked in Grimsby, Lincolnshire in 1969 undertaking six practice nursing hours per week. She had taken the post over from another nurse who had been coming into the surgery for a couple of hours a week for some years, and whose duties seemed to consist mainly of syringing ears. Mrs Reddington increased both the hours and the scope of the work by starting to undertake dressings and injections. From ear syringing, dressing, routine injections such as hydroxocobalamin, travel and childhood immunization, the role expanded to include cervical cytology and, increasingly, the care of people who had chronic conditions.

During busy periods Mrs Reddington was also expected to help staff the reception desk and help with filing and other clerical duties, when her own work allowed. No appointment system was operated. At that time pay and conditions did not correspond to national guidelines, but Mrs Reddington saw the potential for practice nursing, expanding her own role and taking a leading part in setting up a local practice nurse association.

collection of blood and other samples, recording electrocardiograms and ear syringing (Reedy 1980). By 1980 the Medical Research Council identified the need to examine the role of this growing number of nurses (Reedy 1980). In analysing the distribution and function of both attached and directly employed nurses in general practice, they concluded that there were considerable differences in the roles. Their findings noted that district nurses were more often likely to be carrying out traditional nursing roles whether in the home or the health centre, such as dressings, urinalysis and removal of sutures. Practice nurses, in contrast, were found to be undertaking a more extended role – including immunization, venepuncture, carrying out ECGs and cervical cytology, and also seeing undifferentiated self-referred people (i.e. they were providing a minor illness service; Reedy 1980). It was highlighted that district nurses were more limited in the work they were prepared to carry out, and did not see immunization, venepuncture, and other tasks as within their remit. This contrasted with the practice nurses who, not constrained by a nursing management structure, felt able to adopt an extended role, although this caused some anxiety to nurses who sometimes worried about where their professional responsibilities lay. The key factor in role differentiation was time, with the district nurses not having sufficient time to fulfill the growing nursing needs of the surgery. This lack of time and reluctance to take on new roles meant that practice nurses found themselves in an ideal position to exploit the new opportunities that were opening up in general practice.

During the 1970s and 1980s nurses began to concentrate their knowledge and practice in areas such as women's health, asthma and diabetes. However, most practice nurses still maintained their generalist role, providing care for a wide range of people, ages and conditions. In single-handed practices with a male GP, the role of the nurse in providing a service for women was especially important and appreciated (Greenfield, Stilwell & Drury 1987).

Government Policy – Impact Upon Practice Nurse Development

The development of the practice nurse's role cannot be discussed without a wider analysis of the impact of government policy. This has been crucial in defining both the historical working environment of practice nurses, the relationship with GPs and expected clinical duties. The key pieces of government legislation are discussed below.

1966 – Family Doctor Charter

The 1966 Family Doctor Charter facilitated the first real growth in the number of practice nurses employed by GPs as the Treasury sought to provide new money for the development of general practice (Gillie 1963). It now became possible for GPs to claim reimbursement from the Department of Health and Social Security for 70% of any salary paid to ancillary staff, including nurses.

The Charter formed a distinct initiative to improve and expand the service provided by general practice, with finance made available to GPs to improve or rebuild their premises, and encouragement for purpose-built health centres complete with treatment rooms. It led to a dramatic change for general practice, and ushered in a period when the morale of general practice was improved, and advanced the service from what had been described in 1963 by the Central Health Services Council working group chaired by Gillie as 'a cottage industry' towards the general practice of today (Gillie 1963).

1968 – Health Service and Public Health Act

The Health Service and Public Health Act signalled to GPs the potential of nurses within a community setting, specifically highlighting the potential for nurses within the surgery setting. District nurses at this point were employed by either the district or area health authorities, and a few were attached to general practice surgeries. Most district nurses rarely worked in the surgery alongside the GP, perceiving their primary role as providing a service in the patient's home. However, attempts were made in response to the demands of the 1968 Act for closer collaboration and for district nurses to have discreet clinical sessions within the surgeries. The work mostly involved ear syringing, urinalysis, dressings and assisting in child immunization clinics.

Although in some cases this worked well, and provided the service that general practice was asking for, there were problems. The GP still had no choice in the appointment of the district nurse, who continued to be employed by the health authority. The health authority frequently omitted to provide cover for holidays or sickness, leaving the surgery without a nursing service, thereby demonstrating an unconvincing commitment to the service. District nurses felt that their responsibility lay not with the surgery, but with their work on the district, and that they were not accountable to the practice, but to the health authority. Surgery sessions were frequently regarded as something to be fitted in if possible – the service was not regarded as a priority so time-keeping was erratic. General practitioners were understandably not happy with this arrangement and felt that it did not provide the service they and their patients required. The result of this dissatisfaction was that they turned in ever increasing numbers to the option of employing a nurse in the surgery (Davidson 1998).

1986 – The Cumberlege Report

In 1986, the Department of Health and Social Security published the Community Nursing Review – *Neighbourhood Nursing – a Focus for Care* – under the chairmanship of Julia Cumberlege (Department of Health and Social Security 1986). The review carried a number of recommendations, but one proposal in it caught the attention of practice nurses everywhere. It proposed that practice nurses should be phased out, with the withdrawal of the 70% reimbursement, and replaced by health authority-employed 'community nurse practitioners'. This proposal caused an outcry from practice nurses, who made it quite clear that they wished to continue to be employed by general practice directly, and that they had no wish to be directly employed by the NHS, with its hierarchical nurse management structures (Crawford 1991).

The RCN, which had expressed support for the Cumberlege report, faced a considerable campaign by its practice nurse members to change its position. The powerful campaign launched by practice nurses to resist this proposal impacted upon its failure to be implemented at any level. The review, however, did impact upon practice nursing as a discipline, forming a catalysis for practice nurses to organize themselves and gain a political voice in the national nursing arena (Allen 1991).

1990 – The New General Practitioner Contract

The new GP contract was a critical piece of legislation and led to the biggest ever expansion of both the role and numbers of nurses employed in general practice. The legislation, implemented in April 1990, introduced major reforms in the way in which general practice would deliver the service (Department of Health 1990). The impetus for such a change was unequivocally the spiralling costs of providing health care at both a primary and secondary care level (Loudon, Horder & Webster 1998). The mechanism to contain costs was identified by the Conservative Government as the introduction of market forces into the NHS.

The introduction of the new GP contract was not universally welcomed by GPs (Morrell 1998). It contained requirements for them to provide specified services, such as new patient checks, over-75 health assessments, health promotion and minor surgery clinics, and included payments for reaching set targets for cervical cytology and child immunization. It did, however, give formal recognition to the value of health promotion in general practice, and importantly, it provided funding for the provision of health promotion clinics.

The new GP contract created radical changes in the underlying philosophy of health care provision – from a focus on illness to a focus on maintaining health. This was taken on board enthusiastically by practice nurses, who rose to the challenge and established a role in providing health promotion clinics, leading group sessions and increasing their involvement in educating and motivating patients to improve and take control of their own health. Chronic disease management became an important part of primary care services, and practice nurses demonstrated their adaptability in the provision of care, providing education in asthma, diabetes and family planning (Jeffree 1998). It provided practice nurses with the chance to demonstrate yet again their versatility and innovative skills. It changed the face of general practice, and led to the wide scale introduction of nurses into this setting. By 1992, 15 123 practice nurses were employed in England and Wales, representing 9500 whole-time equivalents. (Atkin et al 1993).

The requirements of the contract were soon delegated to the nurse. The role of the nurse was now to include the following.

Health Checks

All patients within the age range of 16–74 years who had not been seen within 3 years, were to be offered a consultation to undertake a health check. The aim was to identify undiagnosed conditions such as diabetes, hypertension and drug or alcohol problems (Department of Health 1990). The check had to include measurement of height, weight, blood pressure and urinalysis.

Over-75 Assessment

General practices were obliged to offer all patients aged 75 and over (in writing and recorded in the notes, including whether accepted or not) an annual consultation or domiciliary visit to assess whether any personal medical services were required. The assessment would include sensory functions, mobility, mental condition, physical condition including continence, social environment and use of medicines (Department of Health 1990).

New Patient Medical

All new patients over 5 years of age registering with the practice were to be offered a medical. A fee was payable if carried out within 3 months of acceptance. It took the form of a routine health check, but additionally identified past personal medical history and current medication and provided the opportunity to check on uptake of vaccination and cervical screening. It provided the new patient with an introduction to the nursing staff and information on the services the practice offered.

Target Payments

Item of service payments for cervical cytology or childhood immunization were abolished and replaced by a system of target

> **Box 1.1**
>
> **Target Payments and Levels of Uptake**
>
> Target payments related to:
>
> ■ cervical screening for women within the age band 25–64 years (21–60 years in Scotland)
> ■ immunization for children aged 2 years and under
> ■ pre-school booster immunization for children aged 5 years and under
>
> Levels of uptake were defined as:
>
> ■ cervical screening – target population percentage levels (lower: 50%; higher: 80%)
> ■ child immunization all under 2 years of age (lower: 70%; higher: 90%)
> ■ pre-school booster all children aged 5 years (lower: 70%; higher: 90%)

payments based on specific levels of uptake (Box 1.1). Each doctor's list was assessed individually, and payment made according to the level of the target reached.

Payments were also offered for minor surgery to be carried out by GPs within the surgery, child surveillance services and changes to night visit fees and deprivation payments.

Health Promotion Clinics

The underlying philosophy of the new GP contract identified the need for general practice to positively promote health rather than maintain its traditional role of managing illness. This was to be achieved through the establishment of specific health promotion clinics aimed at disease management and the promotion of health. Payment was made for each clinic that successfully attracted ten patients per session. These sessions were almost exclusively delivered and managed by the practice nurse. They proved a major source of income generation for general practitioners and the number of practices employing a practice nurse rose dramatically. However, although admirable in its intention, this process proved difficult to monitor or to identify any clear outcomes of the health promotion clinics.

Impact of the Contract on Role Development

The demands made on general practice by the 1990 contract meant that a practice nurse became an essential member of staff instead of a luxury. Practices wishing to offer a good service to their patients complying with the terms of the contract, and in aiming to maximize the practice income, had to employ practice nurses (Pyne 1993). It provided a vehicle for nurses to expand their practice, taking on new skills, with nurses becoming experienced in chronic disease management for asthma and diabetes, in travel health, women's health and monitoring conditions such as hypertension and coronary heart disease (Hibble 1995). The initiatives introduced by practice nurses offered an effective and valuable service to the practice population, but they proved expensive and administratively difficult to audit and monitor. They were abandoned in 1993 in favour of a new system of payment – health promotion banding.

Case Study 1.2

The New Practice Nurse (1990) – A Personal Account

Louise Andrews had been working as a staff nurse on the district, and in 1990 was offered the opportunity to undertake the District Nurse Diploma. She had, however, reservations about this, feeling that going 'higher up the ladder' may mean more of a management role, taking her away from hands-on nursing.

> 'I was looking around for a job where I would be able to continue to use my nursing skills directly with the patients. Practice nursing was one of the options, and I "sat in" with a local practice nurse, and I liked what I saw. I was not worried about being directly employed by the GP – in fact, I was relieved to be leaving NHS employment, with its hierarchical nursing structures. I wanted to be able to work as part of a team, and to continue to give hands-on patient care. My present post was the second job I applied for. The job had come about directly as a consequence of the new GP contract. I was actually employed at first to undertake the over-75 assessment, and my previous district experience was seen as an advantage because initially these were all domiciliary visits. I was lucky in that we had a mentor system in my area, one of the first such schemes in the country – I had 2 weeks working with my mentor in her practice before I started in my own. I felt that I had found what I wanted, I loved the work, but soon felt constrained by the restriction to elderly assessment only, and wanted to branch out to other aspects of the role. My employers were very supportive about this, allowing plenty of time for study and further training, and I was never asked to do anything that I did not feel comfortable with. We were a nonfundholding practice, and so there was not so much pressure to run health promotion and chronic disease management clinics. In fact, our work changed most when the clinic system went and we had to submit proposals for health promotion banding. Then we found that we started to provide a much more structured approach to the service we offered, particularly in chronic disease management, where we had for the first time to produce and maintain asthma, diabetes and coronary heart disease registers, and to undertake health checks at regular intervals.
>   I have never regretted leaving the district for practice nursing, although I have concerns now about the introduction of integrated nursing teams and skill mix.'

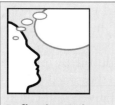

Reflection Point

How does the account in case study 1.2 compare with your own experiences of practice nursing?

1991 – General Practice Fundholding

In 1991 the government dramatically implemented a new approach to the funding of primary health care provision – offering GPs who met given criteria the opportunity to purchase a defined range of health services directly for their patients. This change in the funding arrangements complemented wider changes in social and health care provision, with the introduction of internal markets and direct competition by service providers. Specifically for general practice, financial resources were offered to offset the cost of setting up and management of the necessary elaborate systems. The practice was able to retain any surplus funds for health-related projects in the practice, approved by the regional health authority (Department of Health 1991).

The first wave of fundholding came in on 1st April 1991, and between 1991 and 1995, 2000 general practices joined the scheme. Fundholders' budgets from 1994 to 1995 totalled £2800 million (approximately 9% of all NHS resources). In April 1993, the scheme was extended to encompass the purchase of community health services, including community nursing and health visiting, dietetics and chiropody.

The introduction of an element of competition between practices impacted upon practice nurses and their work. Some practices sought to discourage nurses from cooperating and sharing information with other practices, presumably feeling that such activity threatened the viability of their own practice. The major effect was an increase in equipment and computerization of the practice. Better systems for information and the recording of patient care were required. Practice nurses learned to make use of the computer – using it to record consultations, prescriptions and clinic sessions (Loudon, Horder & Webster 1998).

1992 – The Health of the Nation

In 1992 the government published the white paper *The Health of the Nation* (Department of Health 1992). Continuing the drive towards improving health, the white paper set targets for health professionals based on the recommendations of the World Health Organization (WHO 1978). These targets related to the specific areas listed in Box 1.2.

Impact upon the Role of the Practice Nurse

The Health of the Nation was an important piece of legislation for practice nursing, highlighting as it did the increasing move away from an illness approach towards a service based upon meeting health needs. In this respect the legislation strengthened the role of the practice nurse, moving it increasingly away from a treatment room perspective towards that of a health promoter. However, on a

Box 1.2

The Health of the Nation Targets

■ Coronary heart disease and stroke
  — to reduce death rates for both in people under 65 years of age by at least 40%
  — to reduce the death rate for coronary heart disease in people aged 65–74 years by at least 30%
  — to reduce the death rate from stroke in people aged 65–74 years by at least 40%
■ Cancers
  — to reduce the death rate for breast cancer in the population invited for screening by at least 25%
  — to reduce the incidence of invasive cervical cancer by at least 20%
  — to reduce the death rate for lung cancer in people under 75 years of age by at least 30% in men and 15% in women by the year 2010
  — to halt the year-on-year increase of skin cancer by 2005
■ Mental illness
  — to improve significantly the health and social functioning of mentally ill people
  — to reduce the suicide rate by at least 15%
  — to reduce the suicide rate of severely mentally ill people by at least 33%
■ HIV/AIDS and sexual health
  — to reduce the incidence of gonorrhoea by at least 20% by 1995 (as an indicator of HIV/AIDS trends)
  — to reduce by at least 50% the rate of conceptions among the under-16s by the year 2000
■ Accidents
  — to reduce the death rate for accidents among children aged under 15 years by at least 33% by 2005
  — to reduce the death rate for accidents by at least 25% by 2005
  — to reduce the death rate for accidents among people aged 65 years and over by at least 33% by 2000

more negative note the medical model approach adopted in *The Health of the Nation* targets has served only to limit the true potential of the nurse in the promotion of health, emphasizing individualistic health education rather than wider population-based approaches to care provision.

1993 – Health Promotion Banding

In the face of continued criticism of payment for health promotion clinics, the government was compelled to change the system of payment introduced in the 1990 GP contract (Jones 1993). Therefore, in 1993 'health promotion banding' (Box 1.3) was introduced, and payment for

Box 1.3

Health Promotion Banding

The bands were as follows:

■ Band 1 – programme to identity smokers and reduce smoking
■ Band 2 – to minimize mortality rates and morbidity of patients at risk from hypertension or who had established coronary heart disease (this was in addition to Band 1)
■ Band 3 – full programme offering primary prevention of coronary heart disease and stroke (this was additional to successfully demonstrating Band 1 and 2 outcomes)

clinics was discontinued. This new structure for health promotion funding required the practice to submit proposals for the provision of a health promotion and chronic disease management service for the practice population (Department of Health 1993). Instead of the original piecemeal approach, the practice would be paid a fixed annual fee according to which band they achieved. The highest payment was available for those practices achieving band 3. The pressure to reach attendance figures of ten at each clinic, and the insistence by some practices on strict time adherence was removed. This move was supported by practice nurses who had complained that these constraints had restricted their nursing skills by forcing them to work in a 'sausage machine' approach to health promotion (Jones 1993). With this removed, they now had the opportunity to plan and implement a more comprehensive health promotion strategy for the practice population. The new system meant that audit, a requirement of payment by the Family Health Services Authority (FHSA), became more widely used.

Impact upon the Role of the Practice Nurse

The loss of income the practice suffered from the abandonment of the clinic payment system caused fears and dire predictions that this would mean the wholesale loss of practice nurse employment (Zuckerman 1992). However, the predictions did not materialize, and to the author's knowledge only one job was lost as a result of the change; most practices found that they still needed practice nurses to carry out the work required by health banding. Moreover, practice nurses had proved their worth as part of the primary health care team. The role of the practice nurse remained important because the requirement for health promotion remained, and was strengthened by the continued development of chronic disease management. However, health promotion banding required considerable administration. Returns detailing all figures were required to be completed regularly, and consumed time and effort because this was increasingly coordinated by practice nurses.

Case Study 1.3

Implementing Health Promotion Banding – A Practice Nurse Account

'My practice ran a wide range of successful health promotion clinics that were popular with the patients and brought in a not inconsiderable income for the practice. When health promotion banding came in, it was necessary to change how we organized our workload. We had to submit a proposal to the health authority giving details of our health promotion work, with figures saying what we were doing and how many patients we saw. We had to compile and maintain registers for patients who had asthma, diabetes and coronary heart disease, and this entailed a lot of work. My practice was fundholding and computerized – it would have been much more difficult to have done this without computer records. As the senior practice nurse, I wrote the proposals for the practice for submission to the FHSA. Our proposal was accepted as Band 3. Each year thereafter we had to complete a report on what had been achieved in the previous year – we had to reach certain targets within a percentage of the practice population for how many patients had their blood pressure measured, and so on. Administrative work increased. I was generally in favour of the changes, because they removed the strict requirements to see an agreed number of patients within a certain time, and to run as many clinics as possible. This had resulted in pressure that could have been detrimental to the care patients received. The practice was less happy to allow us to continue to run some group clinics – for example, the smoking cessation or the popular menopause clinic. However, it did help us to implement a more comprehensive and seamless system of health promotion for our patients.'

Nurse Education and its Influence on the Practice Nurse Role

As well as the inevitable impact of government legislation on practice nurse role development, the role has also been influenced, both positively and negatively, by nurses' access and uptake of education opportunities.

Informal Education – The Practice Nurse Interest Groups and Commercial Sponsorship

In the past education was rarely provided specifically for practice nurses. Practice nurses either accessed training and development provided for other branches of nursing, or shared experience and knowledge among themselves in a fairly informal way (Jeffree 1998). One source of informal education was unquestionably the local practice nurse interest group. These interest groups were often the initiative of one or two local nurses, who aimed to gain alliances with other nurses and so reduce the inevitable isolation, and

> **Case Study 1.4**
>
> **Developing Local Education – The Yorkshire Practice Nurses**
>
> In 1986 a group was formed consisting of GP trainers and leaders of local practice nurse groups from across the region, who formed the Yorkshire Practice Nurse Professional Development Committee, dedicated to the provision of nurse-organized and nurse-led education for practice nurses. From an initial 2–3-day course, several study days were run over the course of a year, each focusing on an area of educational need for nurses. These were very successful, and led ultimately to the setting up of a regional association, which took over the provision of study days and professional development for practice nurses in the region.

occasional antagonism from community nurse colleagues. Practice nurse groups sprang up in many areas, and the first National Practice Nurse Conference was held in Durham in 1984. Organized, planned and run by local practice nurses, it was a resounding success, and from this event came the commitment to run a national conference every year in a different part of the country. These conferences have, uniquely, always been organized and run by different regional practice nurse groups and coordinated and supported by the RCN Practice Nurse Association. They enabled networking and consolidation, and encouraged the emergence of a distinct and empowered group of nurses. Frequently run successfully on a shoestring budget, they were vital in giving the newly emerging group a professional focus and identity.

In conjunction with peer support, practice nurses also gained support for their development from the pharmaceutical industry. Keen to establish networks into general practice and influence prescribing patterns, the drug companies where quick in their sponsorship of both individual study days and longer courses for nurses. Although raising a number of ethical considerations for nurses themselves, who were reluctant to advocate one product over another, this sponsorship did provide a key opportunity for nurses to update their knowledge. This in part resulted in a situation where the major educational development of a number of nurses was met by commercial sponsorship. This phenomenon did little to increase the status of the practice nurse among other community nurses or nursing as a whole.

Formal Education

The questionable system of professional development, which evolved from an informal unstructured approach, was highlighted by practice nurses who felt disadvantaged in comparison with other community nurses. This was particularly evident in the 1980s with the resultant situation of practice nurses accessing courses set up for other groups, although the content of the courses was frequently not appropriate to their role. This lack of formal education galvanized nurses to force for the provision of training and education that would meet their needs (Davidson 1998).

The first initiative was a training programme for practice nurses organized in 1971 by the Thames Valley faculty of the Royal College of General Practitioners (RCGP; Jeffree 1998). This was a 10-day course for treatment room and practice nurses. The need for this was quickly recognized in other areas, although it was not until 1988 that the RCGP set up a working party to help practice nurses to identify their training needs (Jeffree 1998).

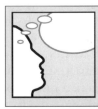

Reflection Points

■ What contribution do you feel the RCGP could have made to practice nurse education?
■ What would you have liked practice nurses to do?

The key issue for practice nurses in accessing formal education was funding (Slaughter 1991). Some funding was available through the FHSA, and joint initiatives took place between FHSAs and local education institutions to provide the ongoing education and training that practice nurses needed. However, it varied considerably from area to area: for example, in my own and other nurses' personal experience, the provision of funding to access education and development further afield (namely, away from the FHSA locality) was frequently denied.

Practice nurses also faced difficulty in persuading their employers of the value and necessity of continuing education and training (Damant 1990). Although most practices fully recognized the value of continuing professional development for staff, a number perceived the nurse as a source of income and service provision and too valuable to be released for more than an absolute minimum of time. Therefore obtaining sufficient time to undertake further education has been problem for some practice nurses. This was partially overcome when in 1989 the Department of Health provided funding for practice nurse education for some approved educational courses. Part of the sum was set aside to develop a distance learning pack for practice nurses, which covered areas including cervical cytology and health promotion – topics considered to be central to the practice nurse's role. This also provided a source of education for those nurses for whom it was difficult to obtain study leave from the practice, and was popular for this reason.

By 1990, with expansion in the numbers of practice nurses, many of whom were recruited from hospitals, it became necessary to provide rapid induction and training for large numbers of nurses working in a totally new field, and in an environment very different to the one they had been used to. This was achieved through recognition by the English National Board (ENB) in 1989, when it validated its first programme. The 20-day course provided a basic training to meet the variety of learning needs of practice nurses who had usually been in post for 1 year or more. The course covered topics such as professional role development, procedures and techniques used in the health centre or treatment room, and management roles. A certificate of attendance was issued, and successful completion depended upon full attendance, completion of projects and course work, satisfactory performance of essential techniques and evaluation undertaken after each course.

Although this course went some way to satisfying the training needs of practice nurses, it was frequently judged to be inadequate and was largely taught by district nurse tutors who were not always fully conversant with the practice nurse role and training needs.

Recognizing other educational needs practice nurses accessed other ENB courses relevant to their role, such as the ENB 928 – Diabetes, the Asthma Diploma, the ENB 901 (Family Planning) and the ENB 998 (Teaching and Assessing in Practice). This led to a variable standard of education for practice nurses. In response to this and the ever increasing number of nurses working in this area, in 1990, the ENB, in collaboration with the UKCC, and the National Boards for Scotland, Wales and Northern Ireland, commissioned an exploration of practice nurse education. Chaired by Margaret Damant, the review group consisted of educationalists and practice nurses, as well as GPs, and its remit was to look at practice nurse education and training, and included an evaluation of courses provided by the National Boards.

Among several important and key recommendations of the subsequent report was the adoption of a recordable qualification for practice nurses, the suggestion being that this should be modular and in line with the education provided for health visitors and district nurses. For the first time, an ongoing professional profile was suggested, and there was a recommendation that practice nurses should be encouraged to take on the role of lecturer/practitioner so that relevant training could be offered. This report was influential and had a far-reaching effect on subsequent developments in practice nurse education and the training and professional development of all nurses. This was ultimately to be achieved in 1994 as the UKCC introduced post-registration education and practice (PREP; UKCC 1994).

1994 – UKCC and PREP

During 1989 the UKCC set up a working party to consider PREP (UKCC 1994). Five years later in 1994, the UKCC finalized its review

Reflection Point

Did this initial course undermine practice nursing in failing to introduce a programme of study comparable with that for other community nurse education?

and set standards for the new recordable qualification for all community nurses, including practice nurses. The report set out clear standards for:

■ preceptorship
■ maintaining registration
■ professional and specialist level practice

The main purpose of PREP was to facilitate nurses to continue to undertake further training and education to improve the standards and knowledge and competence that they achieved at registration, which in turn would improve quality of patient care. This was acceptable to nurses given the changing clinical environment with advances in treatment and care. The requirements made by the UKCC stated that every nurse had to undertake the equivalent of 5 days relevant study every 3 years to maintain registration (UKCC 1994).

In line with continuing professional development, the UKCC also introduced specialist practitioner status, with a separate area for community-based nurses. The UKCC identified eight areas of nursing suitable for specialist community level qualification, one of which was general practice nursing. At last practice nurses had a recordable qualification. Nurses qualified to practise at specialist level would be able to record their name with the UKCC as specialist practitioners. This was a welcome recognition of practice nursing, and a considerable triumph for practice nurses to have gained one of the community pathways, enabling them to achieve a specialist professional status on a par with that of their community colleagues. However, it had not been without a considerable campaign by practice nurses, who in the initial consultation document had been included with district nursing, under a category of 'nursing care of the adult' (UKCC 1992). Outraged, practice nurses lobbied to persuade the UKCC to recognize practice nursing as a separate branch of community nursing, and accord them a specialist qualification.

The success of the practice nurse lobby was a hard-won achievement. In introducing their new standards for practice, the UKCC announced a period of transition from April 1995 to October 1998. The final arrangements, in response to the practice nurse lobby, offered the first real opportunity for practice nurses to achieve equal recognition to other community nurses.

Transitional Arrangements
Within the 3-year period of transition, the UKCC accepted that nurses who had a specialist qualification could record their names on the register without having to first undergo the specialist community qualification at degree course if they had completed a programme longer than 16 weeks' full-time education. This meant that health visitors and

district and school nurses could gain a specialist level qualification on the register, but practice nurses, who had not had a recordable qualification in the past, would be unable to do so.

The practice nurse lobby was extremely aggrieved at this, arguing that they would be seriously disadvantaged in relation to other community nurses, who were able to claim specialist qualification without undertaking more study. They argued that practice nurses, although not having a recordable qualification to aim for, had nonetheless taken the initiative in examining their practice, identifying specific educational needs and accessing education to develop their practice for the benefit of their client group. It was unjust for them to be penalized by having to undertake a full-time degree level course to achieve specialist practitioner status.

A campaign was launched by the RCN Practice Nurse Association to persuade the UKCC and the ENB of the injustice of their initial decision. In 1996 the ENB and UKCC accepted that practice nurses who could demonstrate through a portfolio of previous certificated learning that the outcomes of these combined to meet the outcomes of the ENB A51 could register their names as specialist practitioners on the UKCC register. Educational establishments were accredited by the ENB to validate portfolios. This was a valuable route to a specialist practitioner title, allowing practice nurses a level playing field with community colleagues, and many nurses took advantage of this to record their name on the UKCC register as a specialist practitioner – general practice nurse. Other nurses chose to undertake the ENB A51 – Practice Nurse Diploma programme as a means to gaining the specialist title. Some nurses felt that on completing the ENB A51 course their role did not alter from that of practice nurse, whereas others considered that confusion between the title and qualification led to pressure being put on them to undertake tasks that they were not adequately trained in. However, the transitional arrangements did allow practice nurses to have equal status with other community nurses.

Integrating the Practice Nurse into the Wider Primary Health Care Team

The changes in government policy since the 1990s have been instrumental in the establishment of integrated nursing teams, with health visitors, district nurses, community psychiatric nurses and practice nurses coming together to plan a more integrated approach to the provision of the nursing service for the practice population. Initiatives along these lines had been happening in general practice for some time, but were encouraged by GPs and their practice managers with the introduction of fundholding. The practice was 'buying in' the services of community nurses, and expected to have some control over the service.

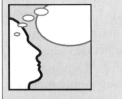

Reflection Point

Has the specialist community practitioner qualification ensured equity with other community nurses?

Where integrated nursing teams happened with the full involvement and control of the nurses involved, it was both empowering and successful (Young 1997). However, there were some problems when the nurses themselves were not in the driving seat and were not allowed to control the nursing budget. Nurses expressed concerns when the work of the team was seen to be strongly influenced by decisions made by management and GPs, and there were considerable worries over the blurring of professional boundaries and the suggestion of a generic community nurse (Practice Nurse Conference 1997). This proposal was and continues to be perceived as threatening to professional specialties by many nurses working in primary care, despite the following published policy of the UKCC:

> The term 'community health care nurse' will be used in future ... to describe a registered nurse who has completed a specific post-registration preparation, which meets the Council's standards, in order to provide specialist nursing care in the community. This is not a proposal for a 'generic nurse', as a specialist preparation will be required for specific areas of practice, to reflect the diversity of need within the community. (UKCC 1992)

The need to work collaboratively is important for practice nurses as the demands of practice increase further (Jenkins-Clarke, Carr-Hill & Dixon 1998). This approach, however, has not always been evident, as witnessed by the introduction of newer nursing roles into general practice. Indeed, the introduction of 'new' groups of nurses in general practice, employed with the title of nurse practitioner, has proved contentious for many practice nurses, with nurse practitioners being promoted as being different from practice nurses, in some way a new type of nurse altogether. Although not all nurses using this title have undertaken specific education courses, the educational opportunities for this group are varied (similar to early practice nurse courses). The description of the key elements of the nurse practitioner role have been given as:

- has undertaken first degree level study
- makes autonomous decisions
- assesses patients with undifferentiated problems
- screens patients for disease risk and early signs of illness
- provides counselling and health education
- develops care plans with patients with an emphasis on preventative measures
- admits, discharges and refers patients as appropriate (RCN 1997)

The major dispute arises because general practice nurses argue that these roles can be carried out by specialist practitioners because they provide the service that general practice needs, the standard of nursing care that patients need and the ability to continue to expand and develop practice nursing.

It seems that the need for a separate nursing role in general practice remains contentious. Although the research by Stilwell, Restall & Burke-Masters (1988) and a further survey by Coopers & Lyband (Paniagua 1997) highlighted that this group of nurses proved a valuable asset to general practice, there is little research to compare their role with that of general practice nurses. The difficulty in comparing the roles is compounded by the great variance in practice, within both professional groupings. The issue is further clouded by the continued expansion and extension of the practice nurse's role.

Historically, nurse practitioner courses offered a way for motivated and enthusiastic nurses to undertake education not otherwise available. With the introduction of the specialist practitioner – general practice nurse degree level qualification, this is no longer the case. Practice nurses, who have for many years expanded and extended the role, can now, as specialist practitioners, continue to do so. The UKCC acknowledged the lack of a clear common understanding or agreement about the role, responsibilities or preparation of nurse practitioners or clinical nurse specialists, and recognized the need to develop a means of assessing what it has called a higher level of practice through assessment of clinical practice, as it is practice centred, as well as post-registration qualification. This work will address the problems and difficulties in employment practice that exist around the adoption of titles that cause confusion to nurses, patients and medical colleagues. Practice nurses voice considerable support for one pathway in general practice nursing, with the accepted qualification to work in general practice nursing to be that of specialist practitioner – general practice nurse. Assessment and recording a higher level of practice should resolve some of the problems that concern practice nurses. What remains important for nursing is the significance of working together in general practice to improve patient care.

Conclusion

Practice nurses have proved in the past that they can and do overcome obstacles and take nursing practice forward, and will continue to do so. It seems that the role of the practice nurse today is as vital to the provision of nursing care in the community as over the past 30 years. The role that has been developed is unique and must be recognized as contributing significantly to the health care of the population. Although it may once have been true to say that the role could be described as an employment status, practice nurses have shown that this is no longer the case, and that they have themselves taken an important place within primary health care, and as such are a distinct group of community nurses.

References

Allen M 1991 Practice nursing profile: Meradin Peachey. Practice Nursing, January

Atkin K, Lunt N, Parker G, Hirst M 1993 Nurses count: a national census of practice nurses. Social Policy Research Unit, The University of York

Bolden K, Takle B 1989 Practice nurse handbook, 2nd edn. Blackwell, London

British Medical Association 1990 Survival guide to the new contractual arrangements, part 2. General Medical Services Council, London

British Medical Association 1993 The new health promotion package. General Medical Services Council, London

Crawford M 1991 Practice nursing profile: Ruth Cheery. Practice Nursing, October

Damant M 1990 Report of the review group for the education and training for practice nursing: the challenges of primary health care in the 1990s. ENB, London

Davidson Y 1998 The rise and rise of practice nursing. Practice Nurse 15:449–450

Department of Health 1968 Health service and public health act. HMSO, London

Department of Health and Social Security 1986 Neighbourhood nursing – a focus for care. Report of the community nursing review (the Cumberlege report). HMSO, London

Department of Health 1990 General medical service council – new GP contract. HMSO, London

Department of Health 1991 General practice fund holding. HMSO, London

Department of Health 1992 The health of the nation. HMSO, London

Gillie A 1963 Report of the sub-committee of the central health services council: the work of the family doctor (the GP's charter). HMSO, London

Greenfield S, Stilwell B, Drury M 1987 Practice nurses: social and occupational characteristics. Journal of the Royal College of General Practitioners 37:341–345

Hibble A 1995 Practice nurse workload before and after the introduction of the 1990 contract. British Journal of General Practice 45:35–37

Jeffree P 1996 Education and training needs of practice nurses. Unpublished PhD thesis

Jeffree P 1998 A high profile career opportunity. Practice Nurse 15:461–467

Jenkins-Clarke S, Carr-Hill R, Dixon P 1998 Teams and seams: skill mix in primary care. Journal of Advanced Nursing 28(5):1120–1126

Jones M 1993 Working with the new banding. Primary Health Care 3(7):4–8

Loudon I, Horder J, Webster C 1998 General practice under the National Health Service 1948–1997. Clarendon Press, Oxford

Morrell D 1998 The NHS's 50th anniversary. Something to celebrate. As I recall. British Medical Journal 317:40–45

Paniagua H 1997 Are nurse practitioners a viable option? British Journal of Nursing 6(5):245

Practice Nurse Conference 1997 Integrated nursing. Practice Nurse 13(6):308–311

Pyne R 1993 Frameworks. Practice Nurse, September 21, 4–15

Reedy B 1980 Nurses and nursing in primary care in England. Journal of the Royal College of General Practitioners 30:483–489

RCN 1996 The lucky ones: an assimilation of three current surveys of GP practice nurses. Royal College of Nursing, London

RCN 1997 Nurse practitioners – your questions answered. Royal College of Nursing, London

Slaughter S 1991 Practice nursing profile: Susan Slaughter. Practice Nursing 5:15

Stilwell B, Restall D, Burke-Masters B 1988 Nurse practitioners in British general practice. In: Bowling, A, Stilwell B (eds) The nurse in family practice. Scutari Press, London

UKCC 1992 Registrar's letter – proposals for the future of community education and practice – the Council's policy following consultation. UKCC, London

UKCC 1994 The future of professional practice – the Council's standards for education and practice following registration. UKCC, London

WHO 1978 Health for all: European targets for health. WHO, Geneva

Young L 1997 Improved primary health care through integrated nursing. Primary Health Care 7(6):8–11

Zuckerman C 1992 Jobs may be under threat. Practice Nursing 5:200

2 *Managing Nursing Care in General Practice*

Anne Jones

INTRODUCTION

To achieve its goals and objectives the work of an organization has to be divided among its members. General practice, however large or small, is no exception. Some structure is necessary to allow the effective performance of key activities and support the efforts of its staff. Mullins (1996) argues that the structure provides the framework of an organization. He states that it is by means of structure that the purpose and the work of the organization is carried out. Set in this context nurses in general practice who intend to develop and change their role to shape their future, need to understand the effect of organization structure and systems to sustain success, impact on care and achieve results.

Nursing care in general practice, now more than ever before, has enormous potential to become nurse led, and move away from the medical model, with its necessary emphasis on treatment rather than patient needs. Nurse-led initiatives in general practice offer a great opportunity for the future in primary care. The scope for practice nurses to develop their role in the changing climate of care delivery is very promising. The challenge for nurses is whether they are ready to grasp this opportunity and move practice forward. A major strategic issue for all nurses in primary care is inevitably the set-up and implementation of primary care groups (PCGs) and their potential development towards primary care trusts as laid down in the government white paper *New NHS Modern Dependable* (Department of Health 1997). This is a new structure within which nurses face a challenge and an opportunity to develop nurses and nursing in general practice. This chapter provides a framework within which nurses may consider ways for nursing care to be managed proactively in general practice.

Key Issues

- Future challenges facing health care delivery
- Organizational structure
- Process of health care delivery
- Managing change in an organization

Future Challenges Facing Nursing in the Delivery of Health Care

In 1996 the English National Board described their predictions for health care in the year 2010 and its subsequent impact upon nursing care in *Shaping the Future* (English National Board 1996a). They identify the main challenges outlined below.

Health Need
New diseases will emerge. The declining resistance of many viruses to many antibiotics will lead to new strains of already known diseases for which no current treatment is available. Attention now needs to be paid to the implications of major changes in research priorities on an international scale. Available resources will have to be pooled.

Health Preference
Tastes will change in health care. In the developed world, at least for the relatively affluent population protected from the emergence of adverse diseases, attention and concern will shift towards ways of reducing pain in long-term conditions, such as rheumatism and arthritis, that will improve the quality of life for affected people.

Ethics
Voluntary euthanasia will be commonplace. It will be insisted upon by consumers. Coalitions of religious groups opposed to this will engage in low-intensity conflict like pro-life groups have done in the past for example.

Demography
By 2010 the numbers in work are predicted to be at an historic low. In turn the ageing population will increase the demand for services.

Technological Change
A number of crucial innovations will become available. They will raise expectations of standards of health attainable, and some will increase people's control over their own health, so reducing medical control. Examples include keyhole surgery, robotic surgery, chemotherapeutic advances, non-invasive laser surgery and neutral net and expert system diagnoses.

Public Health
Prevention will be the centre of public attention. Efforts will focus on the poor, whereas curative work will continue to focus on the rich.

In summary health care in the United Kingdom in 2010 will be:

- more conflict ridden
- more expensive
- more clearly divided between rich and poor
- under more pressure to demonstrate value for money
- more effective
- more internationally focused in provision, research, financing and regulation
- more clearly and transparently regulated

This vision for the next decade stimulates serious thought and consideration. Although the prediction is for 10 years hence, there are lessons to be learnt, in terms of developing nursing strategy that will provide nurses with a framework against which they can develop nursing services in general practice. The time to start that process is now. This is best achieved through an exploration of the organization of care in general practice.

Organizational Structure of General Practice

Organization structure is concerned with the pattern of relationships among both members and their respective positions within an organization (Mullins 1996). In managerial terms, the structure defines the tasks and responsibilities, work roles and relationships, and channels of communication (Woodward 1980). The concept of organization can, in principle, be applied to those organizations that make up general practices. Although the tasks and responsibilities are dictated by the professional roles and expertise of clinicians to a greater extent, general practice is nonetheless a business organization operating within a finite resource. The purpose of structure is the division of work among members so that their activities are directed towards the organization's goals.

In general practice the members include a variety of staff from receptionists and practice managers, doctors, nurses and ancillary staff. This list is by no means exhaustive and the skill mix will differ the bigger the practice. The structure, however, makes it possible to apply the management process in the organization of care. Mullins (1996) maintains that it is the structure that creates a framework of order and command through which the activities can be planned, organized, directed and controlled. He further suggests that in small organizations there will be few problems with structure; this is questionable in general practice! As in small organizations the definition of authority, the distribution of work and responsibility, and the relationships between members can be established on a personal and informal basis. Illes (1997) supports this, believing that the small organization has greater ability to communicate effectively because everyone can talk to each other. In fact she argues that there does not need to be an organizational structure. In general practice where there is just one doctor this would be the case. However, the caveat to note is that with increasing size, and certainly in the larger group practices already established, there is a need for a carefully designed and purposeful structure.

Having contextualized general practice as an organizational structure it is pertinent to examine the assertion that the workplace as an organization is a complex social system and the sum of many parts. Organizations need to achieve a set of goals and objectives. The structure provides a framework for this, but the work of individuals must be linked into coherent patterns of activities and relationships. It is perhaps worth reflecting here on conflicts encountered at work. Personal reflection indicates that most conflict actually arises from problems with relationships to a greater or lesser extent.

Roles and Relationships

A further issue for consideration in the organizational structure is the development of new roles and relationships. The traditional role of the nurse was developed to treat and care for people who were ill or incapacitated by disease. In the future, it is anticipated that the role of nurses will focus on how they can better inform individuals to make their own informed choices about their own life and health (Oakley 1984). This is due to the inevitable wider societal changes and changing attitudes towards health in general. The approaches to be developed will by necessity be based on partnership with patients and clients, in which nurses assist rather than advise or direct. If the United Kingdom is to retain a health care system funded through general taxation, and so be free at the point of need, it seems clear that nursing will be required to accommodate changed circumstances alongside other health care professionals. It is anticipated that there will be increased opportunity for care to be provided in the community with more self care and care supported by a range of agencies. This will offer the chance for nurses to become involved in initiatives that will facilitate a refocus, as the shift away from institutional care is reduced even further. Essentially the context of care in the future will be different.

For practice nursing, an examination of new roles and relationships requires nurses to explore partnerships, not only with clients, but also with other community nurses, whose role has a focus in general practice. These may include, for example, district nurses and health visitors as well as newer nursing roles, such as the nurse practitioner. In exploring partnerships there is a necessity to understand the wider concept of role structure and how it relates to practice nursing.

Role Structure

Coherent patterns of activity and relationships are achieved through what is described as role structure. A 'role' is generally described as the expected pattern of behaviours associated with members occupying a particular position within the organization structure (Goffman 1969). The description also includes the way individuals perceive their own situation. The concept of role is important to the functioning of groups and for an understanding of group processes and behaviour at work. It would be futile to talk about developing roles and developing nursing practice without drawing attention, albeit briefly, to some fundamental problems in role and perceptions of role.

Role Conflict

Role conflict occurs when a person faces a situation in which simultaneous, different or contradictory expectations create inconsistency. Compliance with one set of expectations makes it difficult or impossible to comply with other expectations (Mullins 1996).

A typical example in general practice would be if the GP's perception of the nurse's role and responsibility is not consistent with that of the other partners in the practice, thereby resulting in a discrepancy in their expectations of the nurse's capability and subsequent (perceived) effectiveness. The nurse would experience conflict in having to modify practice to suit the demands of two (if not more) GP partners.

Role Ambiguity

Role ambiguity occurs when there is lack of clarity about the precise requirements of the role and the person is unsure what to do. The person's own perceptions of the role may differ from the expectations of others (Mullins 1996). The corollary to this is that the role is inadequately performed because of a lack of information. A suggested example to illustrate this would be if a nurse was required to carry out a procedure or provide a service outside the boundaries of nursing practice or that was contradictory to safe nursing practice. The ambiguity would arise as the role became more unclear to all parties.

These cited examples of conflict and ambiguity in role are intentionally simplistic. They highlight that in any attempt to change and manage innovation that entails role change and development, it is important to involve all those who will be affected. Furthermore, the perceptions and personal constructs from nurses concerning nursing must also be taken into account.

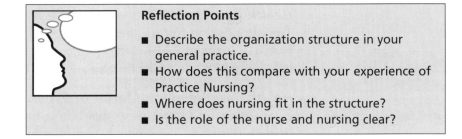

Reflection Points

■ Describe the organization structure in your
  general practice.
■ How does this compare with your experience of
  Practice Nursing?
■ Where does nursing fit in the structure?
■ Is the role of the nurse and nursing clear?

Process of Health Care Delivery

Identifying Need

The NHS exists to meet health care needs (Seedhouse 1994), yet it is
often unclear what is meant by the term 'health care need', or indeed
what health care need would be met appropriately in the NHS.

Need is a relative concept and therefore a practical concern. Need
and needs assessment are controversial issues in today's health service. Different professional groups define need in different ways and
different people in the same profession may define need in different
ways (Runciman 1989, Watson & Taylor 1996). Furthermore, definitions of need vary according to the context in which it is being
assessed (Bergen et al 1996). Yet health needs assessment is crucial
to the effective management of care, in enabling the organization to:

■ plan service development
■ identify where services exist that do not meet need
■ evaluate the effectiveness of service provision
■ compare and contrast different types of service
  provision
■ be able to indicate an order of priority

Yet, as identified, the concept of need is complex, with practitioners
uncertain of identifying need with any degree of confidence. If, as
Seedhouse (1994) argues, there are at least three official versions of
a 'health care need' employed in the NHS it is perhaps not surprising that practitioners encounter problems at the point of identifying
the needs of individual patients and clients. The three definitions of
need, as suggested by Seedhouse (1994), commonly used in the
NHS are as follows.

Health Care Need

This is 'the ability to benefit from health care' (Seedhouse 1994). It
is a service-led rather than a needs-led definition, implying that if
there is no cure or treatment then there is no health care need. The
corollary to this is that if there are fewer services there will be less
need and, conversely, if there are more services there will be more
need.

Health Care Need Exists when there is 'Ill-health'

This supposition restricts health care needs to the scope of medical practice. It therefore excludes other health care practitioners from meeting patient and client needs.

Health Care Need is a Matter of Expert Judgement

In Seedhouse's (1994) view this is the most commonly employed definition in day to day practice and is problematic because 'expert' opinion may vary, be wrong or may not accord with the patient's or client's view.

In examining the factors affecting the varying definitions of need in the NHS, this section discusses the following two approaches to needs identification:

- Bradshaw's (1972) taxonomy of need
- Seedhouse's (1994) philosophical inquiry into the nature of need

Both Seedhouse (1994) and Bradshaw (1972) argue that a lack of something may result in a need, but there will always be situations when this will not be the case. Seedhouse actually proposes that if needs are a means to an end, it is the duty of practitioners to work in partnership with patients and clients to identify their needs and how to meet them. The corollary to this then, is that within this relationship honesty must prevail so that the level of input and availability of resource are discussed.

Bradshaw's Taxonomy of Need

As the concept of health care need is inherent in the idea of health service so the concept of social need is inherent in the idea of social service. Bradshaw (1972) identified four definitions of social need which can be usefully applied to the health care context.

Normative Need

This is in line with the 'need is a matter of expert judgement' from the Seedhouse perspective cited above, and is therefore dependent upon subjective assessment. A GP may define a man who has diabetes mellitus as having a primary need for hypoglycaemic agents, such as insulin. A nurse may define his primary needs as understanding his condition and being able to administer his drugs safely. A health educator may believe that that the man has a primary need to understand that a programme of weight control can lead to better control of blood sugar levels, reducing further illness and perhaps avoiding the need for medication altogether.

Although the three professionals may agree on the extent of needs associated with diabetes mellitus as a condition, they will each seek to address different needs as a matter of priority. Expert judgements about needs can vary a great deal (Runciman 1989) and their validity can therefore be questioned.

Felt Need

This is often equated with want. In this context the definition of need is limited by the perceptions of the individual patient or client who is asked if they feel they have a need by the professional. This is service led and essentially a top-down approach to needs assessment. Health checks, for example, may be offered to someone in a well person's clinic. The patient or client may be given advice and a treatment plan to follow, but may choose to ignore the advice and abandon the programme altogether.

Expressed Need

This is a felt need turned into action (i.e. a demand). Patients who have diabetes mellitus who are not satisfied with waiting times in a hospital outpatient's clinic may demand that the clinic is relocated to the community. The caveat to note is that not all felt needs become expressed needs and expressed needs may not always fully represent the range of felt needs.

Comparative Need

This is a measure of need often used to assess eligibility for selective services. A frail 76-year-old lady living alone with osteoporosis would be in more 'comparative' need than one of the same age who is symptom-free and mobile if both apply to be housed in sheltered accommodation. Every day, multidisciplinary groups are involved in discussions based on comparative need before mobilizing or accessing services for people. The problem with this form of need identification is in establishing which characteristics of the case are significant when deciding upon who should and who should not receive care.

Seedhouse's Philosophy of Need

Seedhouse (1994) suggests that an open-minded inquiry into the nature of need is required if needs are to be properly understood, better defined and therefore better addressed by the NHS. Seedhouse's definition of need allows for needs and wants and is categorized as follows.

Wanted Only

Here there is a want, but not a need. Essentially something is wanted for no real reason. If this want is met there would be no beneficial outcome. A patient requesting prescription-only medication for treatment of the influenza virus is an example encounted in general practice.

Needed Only

This is when there is an identified need, but the means to meet the need is not wanted. In effect, the patient or client does not recognize the need. For example, patients may be advised to reduce their dietary fat intake to lower cholesterol levels, but choose to ignore it.

Wanted and Needed

This is clear. The need is identified and recognized as such.

Needed and Not Wanted

Here there is a recognition of a need, but the means to address it is rejected. This explains, in some part, the least successful health education campaigns.

Identifying Need at an Individual Level

Practice nurses are in a key position to be able to assess needs in a one-to-one or group relationship with patients or clients. This is fundamental to the role. As they are often the first contact for patients or clients with health care needs, they can, within their relationship, make a systematic assessment of need when the patient or client has accessed the service for specific nurse-led management of a problem, for example, asthma. In addition, because of the context in which practice nursing is set, there is the capacity to deliver opportunistic health care and thereby maximize the ability to assess health at one-off encounters with people attending the surgery.

Identifying Need at a Population Level

Government legislation and social policy propose that care is provided for distinct population groups. Although different definitions of need are used The NHS Community Care Act (1990), The Children's Act (1989), The Disabled Person's Act (1986) and The Carer's (Recognition & Services) Act (1995) all assume that the needs of a given population will be assessed by health and social services. Based on this assessment, care services can be planned to meet identified needs.

Health needs assessment is the basis of a population health profile. A health profile is a record of the health, demographic and socio-economic status of a community and will enable practitioners to plan their work according to local needs (Blackburn 1992, Robinson & Elkan 1996, Twinn et al 1990). Health and social profiling is an attempt to identify the level and distribution of health and social needs within a defined geographical area or population. Following the implementation of the NHS Community Care Act (Department of Health 1990), community practitioners have been encouraged to complete a comprehensive record or profile of the local health and social needs and the resources currently provided in their general practice population.

Compiling a Community Profile

Compiling a community profile must be regarded as an ongoing process of developing more responsive services for patients and clients and their families. Essentially there are five stages (Box 2.1).

> **Box 2.1**
>
> **Compling a Community Profile – The Key Stages**
>
> - Data collection
> - Data analysis
> - Data collation
> - Action planning
> - Evaluation

Data Collection

Information that would be gathered for the profile would reflect:

- age and sex structure
- social class
- child health statistics
- ethnic groups and minorities
- trends in family life (e.g. single parents, elderly people, etc.)
- mortality and morbidity data
- disease prevalence
- accidents on the roads and in the home
- numbers of children on the child protection register
- poverty levels – indicated by the number of people in receipt of means tested benefits
- housing situation
- unhealthy environments, such as overcrowding
- specific health issues, for example, drug and alcohol misuse, employment status of the adult population
- the environment – as in local facilities, transport provision, mobility, industrial emissions, isolation and home ownership

The source of this information is varied but includes:

- the annual report of the Director of Public Health
- census figures
- public data sources, such as the employment, housing and education departments
- child health statistics, including the child protection register and immunization and vaccination uptake
- GP annual reports
- Community Health Council reports
- local crime statistics
- community action groups
- annual reports of health authorities and social service departments
- data collected on health status by health care practitioners
- personal caseload and activity analysis
- 'soft' information known to practitioners about the local culture, attitudes and way of life

- practice-held information, for example data from chronic disease management clinics

Data Analysis

Having collected the data, the next step is to place it in a semblance of order. It needs to be compiled as a document to provide a comprehensive survey of the population. An important point to make here is that the reliability of the information and its accuracy must be checked. Information collected for a population profile does become outdated fairly quickly. It is therefore necessary to update it on a regular basis. A population profile is essentially dynamic if it is to be useful in identifying and meeting the local population's health care needs.

Data Collation

The next stage in the process is data collation. Having gathered and analysed the information it will be possible to identify patterns and trends. The information should be presented so that relationships between factors are made clear. Significant links can be made between, for example, pregnancy and teenagers, poor nutrition and unemployment, and so on.

The information presented at this stage will inform the action plan.

Action Planning

To ensure that the population profile is meaningful it is necessary that practitioners use the evidence it provides to target health care activities at specific groups in priority order. This will provide a rationale for activity with agreed targets for action. Targets are central to the development of local primary health care strategies. It is therefore essential that they are realistic, understandable, measurable and achievable within the primary care team.

Evaluation

As a retrospective exercise, and in keeping with the move towards outcome-based care, the profile should be reviewed on an annual basis. This provides the opportunity for identifying success factors and reseting goals and priorities.

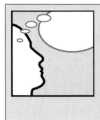

Reflection Points

- What is the status of your population profile?
- Think about its use in making an impact on health and health care activity in your practice
- How much more target oriented and innovative could you become in your work area?

The organization structure within general practice, the practice profile and health needs assessment provide a framework for the process of managing the provision of nursing care.

Resource Management

Effective resource management is a management process rather than a discrete programme of activity. In any health care setting it is crucial that decision making takes place as closely as possible to clinical services. This is to ensure that resources are where they are most needed and that patients' and clients' needs are being met. Indeed, health care practitioners make important resource allocation decisions through their clinical and managerial judgements about the provision of service (Jones & McDonnell 1993).

Resource management is an important concept in the provision of care because it provides an opportunity to integrate quality of care thinking and dialogue with the management process. It also creates communication channels that cut across traditional management boundaries and professional tribalism, enabling accountability for both the management of resources and the quality of care to be held at the nearest point of care delivery. In order for this to happen, clear processes must be established for the planning, organization and control of resources so that care services can respond to the demands placed upon them. This is achieved in the operationalization of health care delivery.

The operational structure of health care delivery is comprised of input, process and output. In terms of input, human, material and financial resources are available to support health care delivery. The amount or availability of these resources and the demand for health care will continually change. It is the responsibility of the organization and its professionals to work together to predict and plan for change and also make informed judgements about how resources are allocated to meet the demand. These inputs are combined in different ways to produce the processes of health care. The processes (a series of health care activities) describe the mechanisms through which the allocation and subsequent use of resources takes place. A process translates the inputs into outputs or outcomes. It is at this point that the issues of efficiency and effectiveness are mainly focused.

The outputs of health care delivery, although not obviously concerned with resources and their management, relate to the efficiency and the effectiveness of their use. Efficiency may determine a measure of the output, for example high throughput because of a robust appointments system. Outcome is an evaluation of the output and indicates the effectiveness or otherwise of health care.

To assist practitioners in understanding the process of health care delivery, the essence of the resource management approach is to provide better information to support both clinical and managerial decisions. Improving health care information is focused at three very different levels:

- first for the patient, this information must enable informed judgements to be made on the benefits or risks involved in choosing a certain treatment or course of action
- second, for the practitioner to advise patients and clients and to record, monitor and evaluate their own practice
- third, for society as a whole, to develop a responsible attitude to health and to work with the health service to determine priorities for deploying whatever resources are available for health care.

Information

Clinicians need credible information to support meaningful dialogue with other professionals when setting resource priorities. Information is a message. It is composed of data that can be described as the raw material from which information is extracted, analysed and then supplied in a suitable form for a specific purpose, for example, decision and intelligence material (research or background data). Data need to be processed to become information and in the same way, information needs to be processed to become meaningful and useful.

Information provides a powerful tool to analyse a situation, and enable the user to form an opinion and ultimately support the decision process. Information is used to support many professional and managerial functions (Box 2.2).

Box 2.2

Use of Information for Planning and Management

- Planning – the bringing together of information in order to formulate strategic and operational plans
- Control – information is essential to monitor the work of the organization and evaluate its efficiency and effectiveness
- Research and audit – information to identify wide variation in practice and to measure the effectiveness or otherwise of clinical interventions – analysis into the content and delivery of health care is necessary
- Intelligence gathering – this is a necessary technique in determining a whole range of information related to the internal and the external environment, for example, market research, patient satisfaction and audit
- Decision making – information will be reviewed by the professional/manager and choices made on the basis of the information received

---

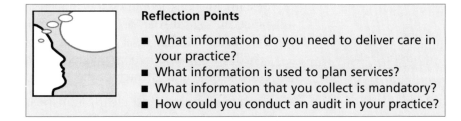

Reflection Points

- What information do you need to deliver care in your practice?
- What information is used to plan services?
- What information that you collect is mandatory?
- How could you conduct an audit in your practice?

Human Resource

Drucker (1989) says of the human resource 'that the whole man is, of all the resources entrusted to man, the most productive, the most versatile and the most resourceful'. Skilled professional time is a crucial but expensive investment, and as manpower is one of the most costly items for any employer, therefore, it is necessary that considerable focus is placed on its use and effectiveness. As clinical accountability for resource management develops, the responsibility for determining an optimal skill mix is paramount.

What is Skill?

Skill is difficult to define. It may be described as an expertness or a practised ability. Similarly, it may be separated into two components – mental skill (abilities required to interact socially, calculation, etc.) and action skill (abilities to carry out activity). Skill is often described in the context of work productivity, categorizing it into the following four components:

- technical skill: this identifies the practitioner's knowledge of and proficiency in activities involving methods processes and procedures
- human skill: this identifies the practitioner's ability to work with people to communicate effectively and to function in a team and relate comfortably with other team members – it is particularly the human skills that reflect the traditional role of health care professionals (i.e. the caring for others and the development of the practitioner/patient relationship)
- conceptual skill: this identifies the practitioner's ability to see the 'big picture', for example, to understand health in its wider context of physical, mental and social wellbeing rather than to continue to perpetuate a disease focus, and to understand that the clinical service is but one part of a whole range of support processes that the patient may need; conceptual skill also encompasses a recognition of significant elements in a situation and to understand the relationships among the elements, for example, to understand that what might be beneficial for the professional might not be beneficial for the patient or the organization; it recognizes the ability to work towards reconciling differences

■ design skill: this identifies the practitioner's ability to work out a practical, logical solution to a problem in a way that will enhance the situation. This is of particular importance as responsibilities are devolved and where judgements relating to the feasibility, effectiveness and efficacy of the service have to be made

These categorizations are clearly transposable to health care practitioners and their work. Yet, health care professionals are often unaware of the diversity and flexibility of their skills, and managers, either through ignorance or self interest, restrict skills development in their staff. This results in what many practitioners perceive as the confines of the 'natural role' of their own profession, which in turn has resulted in their becoming trapped in narrow stereotyped roles rather than being able to expand their personal and professional development more creatively. This is a particularly salient point for many nurses working within the confines of general practice. Individuals must take ownership and responsibility for their role and career development within the infrastructure of their work practice.

It is important at this stage to make it clear that skill does not necessarily equate to grade or qualification. Practitioners have many skills, but it is the identification of the appropriate skills necessary to meet specific demands at the required quality that is needed to determine the right nursing skill mix. In general practice where there is only one nurse, skill mix will not be an issue because such individuals will practise within the confines of their own professional competence. However, in larger practices where there are more nurses operating as a team, skill mix will be important in the division and delegation of nursing workload. Skill mix is described as the necessary proportion of staff, qualifications, levels of competence, abilities, knowledge and expertise to achieve an agreed level of demand (Jones & McDonnell 1993). A nursing skill mix therefore consists of a group of nurses working and interacting together with common goals. Much about managing the human resource is about managing people at work, understanding their needs, supporting them in using the skills they have and maximizing their potential – an important sentiment as practice nursing considers the potential of skill mix to professional development – indeed one may define this as collaborative working.

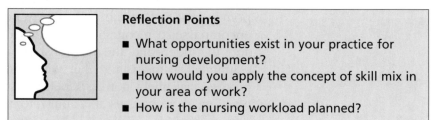

Reflection Points

■ What opportunities exist in your practice for nursing development?
■ How would you apply the concept of skill mix in your area of work?
■ How is the nursing workload planned?

Resource Management and Ethical Considerations

There are undoubtedly ethical and personal dilemmas in considering the allocation of resources for patient and client care. Mooney (1992) identifies three principal theories of ethics: the ethics of virtue, of duty and of the common good. The first two are essentially individualistic ethics and the last a social ethic. Medical ethics deals in the main with the theories of virtue and duty, but the nature of contemporary medicine and health service management philosophy increasingly demands that these be complemented by the third theory – the common good. It is suggested that constructive dialogue between such forums as the local medical committees, health authorities and public health specialists will serve to develop a more realistic appraisal of service development, consumer need and common good.

At the macro level (Department of Health and the health authority) the emphasis of resource allocation will increasingly be driven through a social ethical base, primarily because of the government public health philosophy. However, at the micro level (the patient and client and the practitioner) consideration must be given to the individual ethical base where conflicts will undoubtedly arise if resources are diverted away from the individual to serve the common good.

The resource management approach serves to highlight the ethical considerations that must be made when allocating resources from one group to another or from one intervention to another. Judgements about what is ethical will necessitate a professional view supported by comprehensive audit information and clinical group discussion. There can be no real debate about identifying and choosing between resource allocation priorities until more is known about the costs and benefits of many existing clinical practices. Until such robust information is available it will be extremely difficult to address the more sensitive task of choosing between them. Ethical considerations until that time will be governed by medical rather than social ethics. The extent to which individual practitioners allow resource constraints to influence their behaviour will remain a matter for their own clinical and professional judgement.

Collaborative Working

It is a feature of the history of mankind that people have always organized themselves into ingroups and outgroups (Jones 1994). Health care professional groups are not an exception. It is useful to acknowledge this in attempting to understand the causes of communication failure, to help ensure that relationships between our own ingroup and other's outgroups do not degenerate into hostility. This in turn will help individuals to take responsibility across professional boundaries and to accept charitably the attempts of others to do so, for the benefit of patients and clients.

Illes (1997) argues that fundamentally our ability and desire to take responsibility for others is dependent up on our ability to take responsibility for ourselves. It is only when we decide to choose how to behave, rather than reacting to circumstances, that we can choose to exercise care for others. To illustrate his point Peck (1990) defines love as 'the will to extend one's self for the purpose of nurturing one's own or another's spiritual growth'. This definition makes reference not to feelings but to intent. Most nurses would not argue with the idea that care and respecting other's contributions involves work. The work includes all the years of work and study required to develop the skills and knowledge to care for patients. It encompasses the direct care undertaken. It also includes, for example, the effort required to communicate effectively with other disciplines and the time it takes to ensure that resources are deployed to best effect.

Considering the role of nurses as managers of care in this way gives them, among other benefits, some criteria for many of the decisions they are called to take that are not clinical or technical. One example here would be a concern for a colleague's clinical performance. If the colleague's patients are to be cared for, then it is the role of the nurse to have a duty to remove the obstacles in the way of development.

It can therefore be suggested that the keys to working well with others are self discipline and generosity. The discipline is to take the time and effort to understand the needs of colleagues and to choose to behave towards them in a constructive way. The generosity is to interpret their motives and behaviours positively. Both discipline and generosity are easy to sustain if you are clear about what it is you are trying to achieve or contribute. Achievement of one's own goals requires the involvement of others. A goal clearly stated and agreed can help direct more energy into the building of good relationships with others. This is an important, although difficult issue for a number of nurses working within general practice, given that their relationship with their employing GP may not be built upon the principles of generosity and discipline. Instead, the unequal power relationship of employee and employer status, and the current funding of general practice may mean that GPs identify the setting of organizational priorities as their sole responsibility. This can be a troublesome situation and will necessitate practice nurses re-examining their remit and working positively towards and endorsing a collaborative approach to the setting of organizational goals.

Managing Care and Effecting Change

This section examines some of the key issues that nurses might address in their thinking. The challenge is to develop a mind-set that guides the gaze towards appropriate action to enable nurses to influence and shape nursing practice over the coming years and meet the needs of those who access nursing care.

Evolutionary history teaches us that all organisms must adapt with their environment or die, and that organisms developing a feature that helps them to succeed in their environment prosper at the expense of those who do not (Handy 1989). The lesson to all work organizations, large and small, is that change is essential when there are changes in their environment. They are also necessary if a change in the organization will help it to be more successful even when there are no changes in the environment. In essence, necessary change can be prompted externally or internally. It must always take account of the environment, the resources of the organization and what the organization deems success to be. Handy (1989) describes this as discontinuous change.

The thought processes necessary when considering intervening with a service or organizational change are comparable with those considered when intervening clinically with a patient. They require a similar evaluation of condition, prognosis, options, costs, benefits and risks. Just as '*primum non nocere*' (at least do no harm) is an important value in the health care professions, so it is when managing change. It has to be remembered that all interventions in changing work organizations and practice incur costs and risks, and the anticipated benefits should always outweigh them.

The Change Process

The planned process of change in any organization is achieved through the use of behavioural science technology and theory. Many models provide a guiding frame of reference for any change effort (Robbin 1997). However, although they are not mutually exclusive, they all stem from the original thinking of Kurt Lewin (1958). According to Lewin, 'unfreezing' the present level of behaviour is the key factor in engendering change within an organization. This Lewin suggests involves identifying the change, planning the activity to follow and gaining the commitment of all those to be affected. The second phase of the change cycle is 'movement'. This is identified as taking action that will change the social system from its original level of behaviour or operation to a new level. 'Refreezing' is the third step in the cycle and involves establishing a process that will make a new level of behaviour 'relatively secure against change'. The refreezing process may include different conforming patterns such as collaboration rather than competition.

> **Box 2.2**
>
> **Lewin's Cycle of Change – An example**
>
> The demarcation line that exists between the roles of community nurses is quite clearly defined. To change this to foster maximum collaborative approaches to delivering nursing in primary care according to Lewin means unlocking or unfreezing the social system. This requires a programme of education because behavioural movement must occur in the direction of the desired change.

Table 2.1 *Turrill's Approach to Change*

Strategy	Devise an overall strategy
Plan	Turn the strategy into a plan
Implementation	Seek sanction from those in authority
Change behaviour	Implement the plan

Lewin's three step approach is simple to state. The implementation of this model is rather more difficult. Yet despite the difficulties, general practice presents many challenges and opportunities to work in new ways and provide services for patients that meet their needs effectively.

In contrast to Lewin's approach, Turrill (1990) describes a logical approach to change (Table 2.1). This process is questionable because it wrongly assumes that man is rational and will accept a well-reasoned well-presented argument. If he resists, opposition can be overcome by the use of authority. Again wrongly, the assumption might be that the organization has the competence and the capacity to carry out the new arrangements.

Resistance to Change

Changes do not always go according to plan. Indeed, some changes do not go through at all. Change can meet resistance of a kind that stops it completely or, more frequently, diverts it in a direction other than anticipated. Some theorists imply that resistance to proposed change is irrational, that it arises from personality structures that are rigid, biased, authoritarian and insecure (Hall 1987). This can be true, but there are instances when it is not. Some proposed changes are poor ideas and not in the interests of the organization. In such cases, irrationality is on the side of the resistors. Change for its own sake has no inherent value; only change that contributes to the organization's goals is organizationally rational.

Who are the Resistors of Change?

Pym (1996) identifies individuals who resist change as those who:

- are concerned for safety and security
- preoccupied primarily with means rather than ends
- have a belief in 'a one best way'
- aspire to regularity, order, financial security and prestige
- view managers as experts on the work of subordinates
- are submissive with superiors and directive with subordinates
- assume that old solutions once successful can be applied to new problems as well

In contrast those who embrace change are classified as:

- having a desire for new experiences and some risk
- pay greater attention to ends rather than means
- are open to alternative courses of action
- aspire to achievement, interesting work, freedom and personal responsibility
- view managers as generalists and not experts in all areas they supervize
- emphasize authority appropriate to an individual's contribution
- place less emphasis on previous solutions and more concern with evidence related to the specific problem at hand

It is through the change process that any organization is responsive to need and prepares its future with the intention of achieving success and the effective delivery of care. The critical factor in successfully managing change is to recognize the complex nature of change management and the people – organization relationship. In the general practice setting this will involve an exploration of relationships, in particular, that of the GP with other members of the team. This is important because divergent visions for care provision in any team will make it difficult (not to say frustrating) in aiming to change practice.

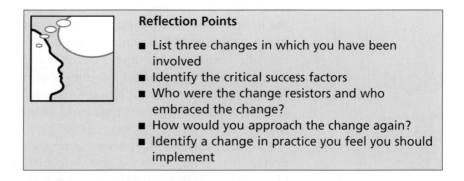

Reflection Points

- List three changes in which you have been involved
- Identify the critical success factors
- Who were the change resistors and who embraced the change?
- How would you approach the change again?
- Identify a change in practice you feel you should implement

Evaluation of Care Provision

The essential purpose of all management in the NHS is to ensure effective and efficient use of the resources that have been made

> **Box 2.3**
>
> **Key Activities to Support Clinically Effective Practice (NHS Executive 1998)**
>
> - Select a particular aspect of practice to examine or question
> - Conduct a literature search to review and critique examples of best practice
> - Implement best-known clinical practice
> - Change practice to improve standards of care

available for health care. There is now more than ever a central need for the evaluation of care and the requirement for robust information to support it. Clinical effectiveness in relation to the clinical governance agenda is a high priority for all health care practitioners. The RCN, in 1996, defined clinical effectiveness as 'doing the right thing, in the right way, at the right time and for the right patient'.

It is therefore reasonable to assume that in the wider context, evaluation will receive increasing attention in terms of dedicated research, evaluation and implementation strategies. The development of evidence-based practice will continue to underpin clinical decision making in practice. In addressing this the NHS Executive (1998) highlights the key activities to support clinically effective practice as listed in Box 2.3.

In addressing the issues it is necessary to explore some of the evaluation tools appropriate for evaluating care provision in general practice.

Quantifying Nursing in General Practice

Practice nurses have always been required to record basic information about nursing intervention. This information has been useful for measuring the nursing workload in the practice. In aggregated form the information would then be used to develop the rationale for the nurse staffing establishment as activity levels increased or decreased. For this reason nurses increasingly became involved in recording information about specific activities such as 'the number of homes visited' or the 'numbers of immunizations and vaccinations achieved' or 'the number of newly registered families seen in the previous month'.

Manual information systems were used and subsequently supported or even replaced by information technology systems. However, what happened to the information once collected was not always known. Hicks (1976) reported that one shrewd observer of primary health care commented that collecting data in this way 'was a bit like counting rivets in the Queen Mary – interesting, but would tell us nothing about how well the ship functions'. This comment

Figure 2.1   *The Audit Cycle*

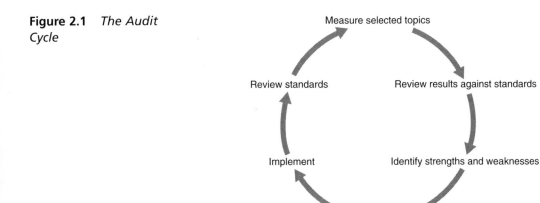

suggests a distinct difference between collecting information that has statistical value and collecting information for a meaningful purpose. In collecting meaningful data it is therefore necessary for the practice nurse to examine both the issues of audit and peer review.

Audit

Audit is described as a cycle of activity (Tugwell & Mongonelli 1986). This cycle (Fig. 2.1) involves a systematic review of practice, identification of problems, development of possible solutions, implementation of the change and review again. Given this process, audit can be described as a form of peer review, although Shaw (1990) suggests that it differs from medical review in that it uses measurement rather than judgements. He argues that an effective system of audit contains three elements:

- agreed criteria for 'good' practice
- methods of measuring performance against these criteria
- mechanisms for implementing appropriate change in practice

Agreement on criteria for 'good' practice leads quite naturally to the establishment of clinical protocols for specific medical diagnoses or standards for universal practices (e.g. the treatment of hyperlipidaemia or the management of asthma in primary care).

Audit as a method of scrutiny has its roots in the world of finance where the review of accounts and organization performance is undertaken by an external assessor. This concept of external review has been used within medicine as a method of audit, but nursing has opted for specific quality measuring packages, for example Monitor (Goldstone, Ball & Collier 1983). These packages have relied heavily on a Donabedian (1986) approach to standard setting: that of structure, process and outcome.

Nursing Audit

Nursing audit is defined as:

> 'Part of the cycle of quality assurance. It incorporates the systematic and critical analysis by nurses, midwives and health visitors in conjunction with other staff, of the planning, delivery and evaluation of nursing and midwifery care, in terms of their use of resources and outcomes for patients/clients, and introduces appropriate change in response to that analysis' (NHS Management Executive 1991)

Accepting this definition of nursing audit incorporates all aspects of supply and delivery of service, not only those directly related to the delivery of care to patients. The general principles of nursing audit are similar to all forms of audit (Box 2.4).

In considering the scope of nursing audit, it may be useful to consider the Framework of Audit for Nursing Services (NHS Management Executive 1991). This document provides a framework within which nursing audit may be considered, an indication of the areas which may be suitable for audit, a distillation of current audit practices, and importantly practical advice on what to consider when establishing an audit plan.

Organizational Audit

On a wider issue, practice nurses may also be involved in the process of organizational audit. In contrast to specific nursing interventions, organizational audit reflects the mission statement and specific goals of the general practice as a work organization (Box 2.5).

Box 2.4

General Principles of Nursing Audit

- Define the objectives
- Set the standards to meet the objectives
- Implement the standards
- Measure and record the standards set
- Monitor new standards and change as appropriate

Box 2.5

Example of Organizational Goals

- All patients will be treated with confidentiality, dignity and courtesy
- All staff will be prepared through appropriate training and education for their responsibilities in providing a high-quality service.

The standards set will succinctly express the intentions of the organization in relation to the service provided.

Using Peer Review in the Audit Process

A key issue in the audit process is the question of who sets the standards and evaluates the practice. This is particularly pertinent because there is an increasing move towards multidisciplinary audit and standard setting. The collaborative approach to quality has raised the issue of whether one profession can really examine the quality of care given by another profession. This problem has raised an awareness of peer review as part of the bigger audit process. Peer review is identified by Passos (1973, cited in Pearson, 1987) as a hallmark of professionalism, a view supported by Maas & Jacox (1977), who identify it as a necessity in the demonstration of accountability for practice.

Reflection Points

- What is the potential to evaluate your practice through audit?
- How has audit been used in your practice to evaluate care?
- What changes in care were implemented?

Conclusion

This chapter has set out the key issues pertinent to the management of nursing care in general practice. General practice as a contextual setting was the backcloth for the application of the management theory in describing some concepts related to organization structure. All organizations are complex social systems and the sum of many parts, not least because the work of organizations involves people. The need for the nurse in managing care to understand the nature of organizations and the main features that affect the structure, management and the functioning of the work organization has been thematic throughout. The management process offers a timely insight into the relationships and skills that are central to effective working. Indeed, the rise of resource management based on efficient and economical allocation and service delivery in health care delivery clearly illustrates the point.

The concept of needs-based care was developed using the assessment models of Bradshaw (1972) and Seedhouse (1992). This framework was used to underpin a proposed methodology for health needs assessment. The purpose was to present a rationale on which to base the emphasis on the requirement to consider the economic climate and the ethical and personal dilemmas that may be involved in resource allocation. Finally some consideration of change theory was made upon which the process of change management could be planned and carried out.

The early assertion is now reiterated. That is, nursing in general practice is entering a period of opportunity as the organization of general practice changes to meet its new challenges. The question remains – are nurses ready to meet the challenges and seize the opportunity?

Further Reading

■ Rowe A, Mitchinson S, Morgan M, Carey L 1996 Health profiling – all you need to know. Liverpool John Moores University and Premier Health NHS Trust

References

Bergen A, Cowley S, Young K, Kavanagh A 1996 An investigation into the changing education needs of Community Nurses with regard to needs assessment and quality of care in the context of the NHS and Community Care Act 1990. Final report to the ENB for Nursing, Midwifery and Health Visiting. ENB, London

Blackburn C 1992 Improving health and welfare work with families in poverty. Open University Press, Buckingham

Bradshaw J 1972 The concept of human need. New Society 19:640–643

Department of Health 1986 The disabled person's act. HMSO, London

Department of Health 1989 The children's act. HMSO, London

Department of Health 1990 The NHS community care act. HMSO, London

Department of Health 1995 The carer's (recognition & services) act. HMSO, London

Department of Health 1997 New NHS, modern dependable. HMSO, London

Donabedian A 1986 Criteria and standards for quality monitoring. Quality Review Bulletin: 12(3):99–100

Drucker P 1989 The practice of management. Pan Business Management, London

English National Board 1996 Offprint 1 visions of health care in 2010: the pressures for change. English National Board, London

Goffman E 1969 The presentation of self in everyday life. Penguin, Harmondsworth

Goldstone L, Ball J, Collier M 1983 Monitor: an index of the quality of nursing care for acute medical and surgical wards. Newcastle upon Tyne Polytechnic Products, Newcastle upon Tyne

Hall RH 1987 Organisations: structure, processes and outcomes, 4th edn. Prentice Hall, New Jersey

Handy C 1989 The age of unreason. Arrowe Books, London

Hicks D 1976 Primary health care review. HMSO, London

Illes V 1997 Really managing health care. Open University Press, Buckingham

Jones A, McDonnell U 1993 Managing the clinical resource: an action guide for health care professionals. Baillière Tindall, London

Jones S 1994 The language of genes. Flamingo, London

Lewin K 1958 Group decision and social changes: readings in social psychology. Holt, Rinehart & Winston, New York

Maas M, Jacox A 1977 Guidelines for nurse autonomy/patient welfare. Appleton-Century Crofts, New York

Mooney G 1992 Economics, medicine and health care, 2nd edn. Harvester Wheatsheaf, London

Mullins LJ 1996 Management and organisation behaviour, 4th edn. Pitman Publishing, London

NHS Management Executive 1991 A framework for audit of nursing services. HMSO, London

NHS Executive 1998 Achieving effective practice, a clinical effectiveness and research information pack for nurses, midwives and health visitors. HMSO, London

Oakley A 1984 What price professionalism? The importance of being a nurse. Nursing Times 80(50):24–27

Pearson A (ed) 1987 Nursing quality measurement: quality assurance methods for peer review. John Wiley & Sons, Chichester

Peck M Scott 1990 The road less travelled. Arrow Books, London, p. 85

Pym D 1996 Effective managerial performance in organisational changes. Journal of Managerial Studies, February.

RCN 1996 Clinical effectiveness. A Royal College of Nursing guide. RCN, London

Robbin SP 1997 Essentials of organisational behaviour, 5th edn. Prentice Hall, New Jersey

Robinson J, Elkan R 1996 Health needs assessment: theory and practice. Churchill Livingstone, London

Runciman P 1989 Health assessment of the elderly at home: the case for shared learning. Journal of Advanced Nursing 14:111–119

Seedhouse D 1994 Fortress NHS: a philosophical view of the National Health Service. John Wiley & Sons, Chichester

Shaw C 1990 Criterion based audit. British Medical Journal 300:649

Tugwell P, Mongonelli E 1986 The clinical audit cycle. Australian Clinical Review June: 101–105

Turrill A 1990 Resource management – changing the culture. Occasional papers. NHS Training Authority, London

Twinn S, Dauncy J, Carnell J 1990 The process of health profiling. Health Visitors Association, London

Watson J, Taylor J 1996 Carer assessments: standard practice. Community Care 8–14 Feb, 7–9

Woodward J 1980 Industrial organisation: theory and practice, 2nd edn. Oxford University Press, Oxford

3 *Legal Issues Pertinent to Role Development in General Practice*

Lyndsey Peacock

INTRODUCTION

The expanding role undertaken by the nurse and specifically that of the role of the practice nurse has led to the position in which they are far more aware of the consequences of legal issues within their practice. Although overall knowledge levels remain limited, this is certainly a subject that has captured interest (Young 1995). In particular, practice nurses are now regularly adopting duties that used to be the sole responsibility of the GP and these duties are often performed in isolation and without the potential advice of colleagues.

It is this combination of our evolving role and the isolated nature of nursing in general practice that acts as a key factor in the need to address the legal implications of nursing care provision in this context. This chapter will focus on a number of key principles relevant to both practice nursing and nursing in general. It aims to examine the principles in relation to practice nursing and offer insight into the legal and professional obligations of the nurse.

Key Issues

- Accountability
- Duty of care
- Vicarious liability

- Record keeping
- Use of clinical protocols

Accountability and Duty of Care

Accountability is one of the fundamental issues concerning many nurses in general practice. There is often a doubt raised over whether the nurse is accountable or whether the GP is accountable through delegation. In response to this Dimond (1997) clearly states that practice nurses are accountable to themselves, their patients and the GPs for whom they work. This statement appears relatively straightforward, but unfortunately the delineation of accountability is more complex and relates directly to issues surrounding duty of care.

Duty of Care

As with many legal terms, duty of care was not defined from first principles, but through the process of legal action resulting in case law. Specifically, the principle that identifies a duty of care was laid down by Lord Atkin, in the case of Donoghue v Stevenson (1932). He stated that:

> 'you must take reasonable care to avoid acts or omissions which you can reasonably foresee would be likely to injure your neighbour. Who, then, in law is my neighbour? The answer seems to be persons who are so directly affected by my acts that I ought reasonably to have them in contemplation as being so affected when I am directing my mind to the acts or omissions that are called in question.'

In considering the role undertaken by nurses within their clinical practice, it is evident that this statement is influential (and indeed potentially the key underpinning belief of nursing practice) in shaping the boundaries of practice. Given that the client or patient is someone 'who is so closely affected by their acts that he or she ought reasonably to have them in contemplation', all practice nurses have a duty of care to every person on their employing GP's list and any other person, who undertakes treatment on a voluntary basis, who is not on the list but visiting the area temporarily (Korgaonkar & Tribe 1995).

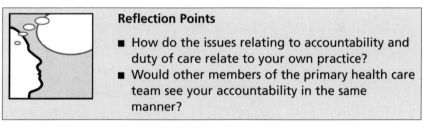

Reflection Points

- How do the issues relating to accountability and duty of care relate to your own practice?
- Would other members of the primary health care team see your accountability in the same manner?

Defining the Boundaries of Duty of Care

The principle laid down by Lord Atkin highlights the relative ease in demonstrating that a client or patient is owed a duty of care by the practice nurse; however, the important question is when does this duty come into existence? (This is particularly relevant in that it is not uncommon to have practice lists of up to 10 000 patients.) Is it when the patient registers with the GP, enters the doors of the surgery, 'books in' at the reception desk or first receives treatment from the clinical staff? Although there is no case law specifically relating to general practice, the relevant case law is exemplified in the case of Barnett v Chelsea and Kensington Hospital Management Committee ([1968] 1 All ER 1068). Specifically, the issue arose as to whether a duty of care was owed to three nightwatchmen who had attended a local accident and emergency department after drinking tea and consequently vomiting. They reported their symptoms to an attending nurse who informed the casualty officer by telephone. The casualty officer did not see or treat the men, but suggested that they go home and visit their own GPs. One of the men later died from arsenic poisoning.

In the discussions surrounding the issue of a duty of care that followed this case it was stated that:

> 'this is not a case of a casualty department which closes its doors and says that no patients can be received ... In my judgement there was such a close and direct relationship between the hospital and the watchmen that there was imposed on the hospital a duty of care which they owed to the watchmen'.

This particular judgment indicates that a duty of care arises when clients make their presence known in the surgery to the appropriate clinical staff (Korgaonkar & Tribe 1995). This is especially true of patients who attend a surgery as an emergency. However, in cases of nonemergencies the obligation to treat only arises when the client is registered with the GP and/or has consulted with the GP on the occasion in question (NHS [General Medical Services] Regulations 1992 cited in McHale, Fox & Murphy 1992). The existence of a duty of care in this instance depends upon the presence of an express or implied undertaking that the client will be treated (Cassidy v Ministry of Health [1951] 2 KB 343).

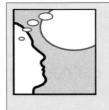

Reflection Point

Consider the potential situation of a patient attending the surgery out of normal consulting hours. There is no doctor on the premises, but the receptionist asks you to see them. What obligations do you have in relation to a duty of care?

Breach of the Duty of Care

The above reflection point highlights the need for further clarity concerning what is a duty of care and when this is breached. To establish that a breach has occurred with regard to the legal duty of care, the plaintiff (the person bringing the action) must prove negligence against the defendant (the nurse or the nurse's employer). It must also be ascertained that a duty of care existed in the first instance.

This at first appears relatively clear. However, the nature of nursing and individual interactions with patients and clients means that it is not always possible to identify and define specific nursing actions. This individuality of nursing interventions, although on the one hand meeting individual patients needs, must not be detrimental to their care and impact upon whether they are able to demonstrate a breach of care has occurred. It therefore follows that a standard needs to be confirmed against which the action of the defendant may be judged. In cases that are nonmedical in their nature the dictum from Blyth v Birmingham Waterworks Co. ([1856] 11 Exch. 781 26) is often used as a definition for negligence:

> 'Negligence is the omission to do something which a
> reasonable man guided by those considerations which
> ordinarily regulate the conduct of human affairs would do
> or doing something which a prudent and reasonable man
> would not do.'

However, in the case of the nurse this definition is too vague because the 'prudent and reasonable man' does not hold himself out to possess any of the essential skills of professional nursing practice (Korgaonkar & Tribe 1995). This lack of clarity has necessitated further exploration from case law, resulting in the principles of negligence being laid down in the case of Bolam v Friern Hospital Management Committee ([1957] 2 All ER 118) commonly referred to as the 'Bolam test'. This case identified the standard as that of the reasonably competent practitioner in the same speciality. In this case McNair J stated that:

> 'The test is the standard of the ordinary skilled man
> exercising and professing to have that special skill. A man
> need not possess the highest expert skill; it is well
> established law that it is sufficient if he exercises the
> ordinary skill of an ordinary competent man exercising
> that particular art ...'

McNair J then further stated that a professional would not be held to be negligent:

> '... if he has acted in accordance with a practice accepted
> as proper by a reasonable body of medical men skilled in
> that particular art ... Putting it the other way round, a
> man is not negligent, if he is acting in accordance with
> such a practice, merely because there is a body of
> opinion who would take a contrary view'.

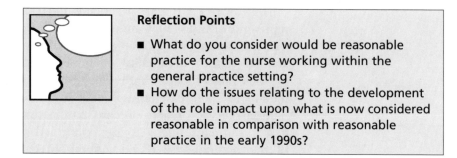

Reflection Points

- What do you consider would be reasonable practice for the nurse working within the general practice setting?
- How do the issues relating to the development of the role impact upon what is now considered reasonable in comparison with reasonable practice in the early 1990s?

The issues highlighted by the Bolam test are particularly relevant to practice nurses because they often work in isolation. For this reason, to exempt them from any liability with regard to negligence it is important that if nurses are unsure of their competence in the performance of any clinical skill, they seek the advice of a more experienced practitioner (Wilsher v Essex Area Health Authority [1988] 1 All ER 871). In support of this, Dimond (1997) suggests that 'one of the major concerns of practice nurses has always been in defining their role and competence'. Even though the UKCC (1996) has attempted to resolve this issue with regards to their directions on 'extended role', it is evident that practice nurses remain concerned about taking on aspects of patient care that used to be the sole responsibility of the GP.

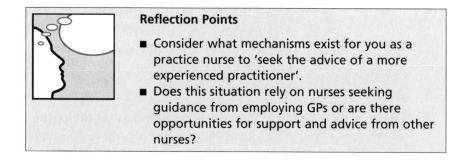

Reflection Points

- Consider what mechanisms exist for you as a practice nurse to 'seek the advice of a more experienced practitioner'.
- Does this situation rely on nurses seeking guidance from employing GPs or are there opportunities for support and advice from other nurses?

Difficulty, however, may arise in certain situations where there are differences of opinion about what constitutes reasonable clinical practice. In cases of litigation, this is often resolved through the use of expert witnesses advising lawyers and the courts about what constituted acceptable practice at the time when the alleged negligence occurred. However, at times, professional opinion may differ. This fact was considered in the House of Lords in a case that involved a nurse as the plaintiff (Maynard v West Midlands Regional Health Authority [1984] 1 WLR 634). In this case Lord Scarman stated that:

'A case which is based on an allegation that a fully considered decision of two consultants in the field of their special skill was negligent clearly presents certain difficulties of proof. It is not enough to show that there is a body of competent professional opinion which considers that theirs was a wrong decision, if there also exists a body of professional opinion, equally competent, which supports the decision as reasonable in the circumstances. It is not enough to show that subsequent events show that the operation need never have been performed, if at the time the decision to operate was taken it was reasonable in the sense that a responsible body of medical opinion would have accepted it as proper ... Differences of opinion and practice exist, and will always exist, in the medical as in other professions. There is seldom any one answer exclusive of all others to problems of professional judgement.'

The impact of this ruling by Lord Scarman on nursing, means that the nurse may not be deemed to have been negligent if there is a departure from accepted nursing practice if the departure can be justified. This raises the important issue for all nurses, of learning to carefully critique new research papers before adopting any highlighted changes to current practice (Tingle 1998). It also raises questions about whether nurses read peer reviews of research relevant to practice, for example, research available on the Cochrane database.

Likewise, if the practice nurse is given an instruction from the GP to perform a specific task and the nurse perceives this instruction to be wrong, but after consultation the doctor still considers this to be the correct course of action and the nurse then goes ahead and carries out the task, if harm results the nurse may not be liable because she was merely carrying out the doctor's instructions (Gold v Essex County Council [1942] 2 All ER 237). It is important to note here that although the judgment in this case perhaps 'flies in the face' of what nurses have always been led to believe about carrying out a doctor's instructions when they are deemed to be potentially harmful, it must be remembered that in most instances of this nature if a claim results then an important factor for an expert to determine would be whether the nurse was correct in the assessment of the situation or not (Tingle 1998).

The above scenario differs from the instance when a practice nurse takes and acts on mistaken advice from a more senior nursing colleague because it is considered that a junior member of the same profession should be able to recognize gross errors in nursing practice (Montgomery 1995).

These rulings highlight the imperative for practice nurses (and for that matter medical practitioners) to keep themselves up to date with critical developments in nursing practice because if they do not they may be in breach of the legal duty of care. This factor is highlighted by the UKCC (1992a) where it is stated that:

> 'As a registered nurse, midwife or health visitor, you are personally accountable for your practice and in exercise of your professional accountability, must ... maintain and improve your professional knowledge and competence.'

Maintaining Clinical Competence

The need for continual professional development to ensure the maintenance of standards of nursing care was clearly set out with the introduction of both clinical supervision, in the *Vision for the Future* document (Department of Health 1994) and the post registration education and practice project (UKCC 1996). However, the issue of professional updating was considered by the court in Crawford v Board of Governors of Charing Cross Hospital (1953, The Times, 8 December 1953) where it was held that although practitioners cannot be expected to read all the professional articles that appear in the countless journals, there is an expectation that they keep abreast of important developments on the subject of their speciality. If a practitioner fails to do this it may lead to a finding of negligence if harm occurs to a client (McHale, Fox & Murphy 1997). This decision has recently been upheld by the courts in Gascoine v Ian Shendan and Co. and Latham ([1994] 5 Med LR 437), and for this reason it is imperative that the practice nurse 'remembers the professional and legal duty to keep up to date with the developments in nursing practice' (Tingle 1998, p. 23).

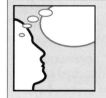

Reflection Points

- What mechanisms do you use to ensure that you are professionally up to date?
- Are there any barriers which hinder this development?

One method of maintaining one's professional knowledge is to undertake continuing formal education. This is an important issue for practice nurses both in developing their own learning, but increasingly as they participate in training other nurses. In relation to the issues surrounding negligence, if the practice nurse is acting as a 'trainee' then she will be held to the same standard as that of a competent practitioner (Nettleship v Weston [1971] 2 QB 691). In particular the Nettleship v Weston (1971) case held that a learner driver would be liable in negligence if an inability to drive as a competent qualified driver was not demonstrated. Although this judgment may appear severe its appropriateness to nursing lies in the fact that all clients are entitled to receive an appropriate standard of care (Montgomery 1995).

Having addressed the broader issue of breach of duty of care, it is necessary to further examine the concepts that relate to the crux of the issue. Namely, the question of damage, causation, remoteness of damage and *res ipsa loquitor* as related to breach of duty.

Damage

Within the legal process it is the responsibility of the client to prove that the nurse's breach of duty led or materially contributed to the harm caused. It is essential that a direct link is established between the breach and damage caused. Clients must prove that negligent acts make a difference and adversely affect their condition in some way. The first step in this process is to prove factual causation (Tingle 1998).

Causation

The traditional approach to the establishment of causation is often referred to as the 'but for test'. Within this context the question is asked 'But for the defendant's action, would the plaintiff have sustained the injury?' If the answer to this question is 'no' then it is inevitable that the defendant can be found to have caused the harm in question. However, if the answer is 'yes' then it is evident that the harm would have occurred anyway and in this instance the defendant cannot be held to be liable. The 'but for test' is an important abstraction, because it acts as a filter to exclude events that do not affect the outcome of the act. However, it is important to realise that this test cannot resolve all of the problems of factual causation (Korgaonkar & Tribe 1995).

The application of this principle in law can be demonstrated in the case of Barnett v Chelsea and Kensington Hospital Management Committee ([1968] 1 All ER 1068), the facts of which have already been discussed within this chapter. In this instance it was up to the plaintiff to prove that the acts or omissions of the defendant (in this case the doctor) caused or materially contributed to the death of the nightwatchman. This can be difficult to establish in both medical and nursing negligence cases because biological and other factors may have contributed to the resultant harm. However, the burden of proof remains on the plaintiff to establish that the breach in the duty of care was a material contribution to the harm caused (Wilsher v Essex Area Health Authority [1986] 3 All ER 801).

Similarly, in the case of Kay v Ayrshire and Arran Health Board ([1987] 2 All ER 417) a 2-year-old infant who had meningitis was administered an overdose of penicillin. The child was later found to be deaf. His parents brought an action for negligence. However, the action failed because material contribution could not be established; it could not be proven that the overdose of penicillin and not the meningitis had caused the resultant harm.

Both these cases highlight the difficulties that can occur in the plaintiff identifying that damage was caused through the negligent act of the professional. However, it must be remembered that these are still highly traumatic experiences for all those involved irrespective of the outcome of the final verdict. This is further demonstrated in considering the concept of remoteness of damage.

Remoteness of Damage

This concept specifically relates to occasions when although the defendant's negligent act has been proved to have been the cause of the harm complained of, liability for that harm may be excluded on the grounds that it was too remote – that is, that the damage:

- was more extensive
- was of a different type
- occurred in a different manner than would normally have been foreseen

This is best illustrated through the two cases of Re (Korgaonkar & Tribe 1995) Polemis ([1921] 3 KB 560) and The Wagon Mound (No 1 [1961] AC 388 PC). These cases denote that the damage complained of must be a direct and reasonably foreseeable consequence of the defendant's act. It is, however, evident from the case law that the requirement of foreseeability is not dependent upon proof that the exact extent of the damage was envisioned (Korgaonkar & Tribe 1995).

There is, however, one exception to the foreseeability rule and this is the notion that the defendant must 'take his victim as he finds him'. This principle is often referred to as the 'thin skull rule'. In the case of Robinson v Post Office ([1974] 2 All ER 737) the plaintiff was injured as a result of the defendant's negligence. He suffered a serious anaphylactic reaction to a tetanus injection given to him by a doctor. The Court of Appeal held that the doctor was liable for the injury, and stated that 'a person who could reasonably foresee that the victim of his negligence may require medical treatment is liable for the consequences of the treatment although he could not reasonably foresee those consequences or that they could be serious'.

Res ipsa loquitur

This principle relates to those occasions when the plaintiff is not required to establish proof of negligence, but instead will be prepared

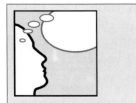

Reflection Point

Take this opportunity to reflect upon your own practice. Can you identify potential situations where the 'remoteness of damage' principle may apply?

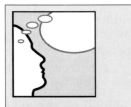

Reflection Point

Are there any potential consequences of the ruling of this case for your own practice?

to infer from the facts of the case that the defendant was negligent. It therefore follows that this principle will apply only where it is obvious that there has been negligence. However, this principle is rebuttable and under this process the rule of the burden of proof is not reversed in any formal sense; instead the legal process is that of a 'rule of evidence'.

This process may undoubtedly appear confusing, although it is an important concept to understand, particularly with regard to medical negligence claims. An example of this principle was highlighted in the case of Cassidy v Ministry of Health ([1951] 1 All ER 574). Ruling on this case Lord Denning LJ stated that:

> 'If the patient had to prove that some particular doctor or nurse was negligent, he would not be able to do it, but he was not put to that impossible task. He says: "I went into hospital to be cured of two stiff fingers. I have come out with four stiff fingers and my hand is useless. That should not have happened if due care had been used. Explain it if you can". I am quite clearly of the opinion that that raises a prima facie case against the hospital authorities.'

However, it is only in the most obvious of negligence claims that the principle of *res ipsa loquitur* will apply and a number of conditions must be satisfied first:

- first, the incident when it occurred must have been under the direct supervision of the defendant
- secondly, the incident would not under normal circumstances have happened unless there was negligence
- lastly, the defendant must not have offered any reasonable explanation about why the negligence occurred (McHale, Tingle & Peysner 1998)

Vicarious Liability

If accountability is a key concern for many practice nurses, then it is closely followed by doubts over the concept of vicarious liability. Specifically, nurses are often concerned about who pays the compensation if they have been found to have performed a negligent act or omission with regards to client care. This issue is addressed within the basic common law principle that the employer (in this case the GP) is liable for the negligent acts or omissions of his employees acting in the course of employment. This is known as 'vicarious liability'. It is a form of strict liability because it originates from the employer–employee relationship without reference to any fault of the employer (Jones 1997).

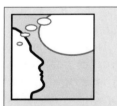

Reflection Point

Reflect upon your current working practices. Are there any issues that you need to address in ensuring that you are delivering appropriate care to the practice population?

Several reasons have been articulated about the introduction of 'vicarious liability', but perhaps the most appropriate is that the employer has the 'deepest pockets' and in cases of negligence claims, which emphasize the compensation function of the law of tort, the overall wealth of the defendant or one that has access to resources by means of insurance has gone some way to influence the development of legal principles (Jones 1997).

However, it must be noted that the whole issue of vicarious liability does not relieve the employee of liability to the plaintiff because the plaintiff may seek compensation from either or both parties. But it could be difficult for the client to identify exactly which member of the team caused the harm and therefore an opportunity to sue the employer becomes an attractive alternative (Korgaonkar & Tribe 1995). With regards to the practice nurse all are vicariously covered by their employers – the GPs. Therefore a GP would be vicariously liable for the negligent acts or omissions of the practice nurse as long as it could be proved that the negligent act or omission had actually occurred during the course of employment and had caused the harm complained of by the client.

The concept of vicarious liability does not mean that the nurse is not accountable. In all instances the practice nurse who commits a negligent act remains professionally and personally responsible and accountable for that action and it is potentially possible that an employer could attempt to recover any costs paid out on the nurse's behalf. However, guidelines from the NHS (1996) suggest that employers should not strive to recover costs in this fashion although the nurse may have breached an implied clause in the contract of employment, that being she will use all reasonable skill and care (Martin 1996).

Nevertheless, problems may arise for the practice nurse if it can be proved that the resultant harm occurred while the nurse was practising outside the course of her employment. In these instances a lawyer may attempt to sue an individual nurse. However, generally it is considered that the nurse would not have the finances to settle the compensation claim and therefore such an action would be highly unlikely. Still, in all instances, because practice nurses are perhaps more vulnerable than some of their professional counterparts they should ensure that they are appropriately covered against any negligence claim as it would appear to be the most sensible thing to do.

Having addressed the major issues of accountability and vicarious liability this chapter will now examine the more practical issues of both record keeping and use of clinical protocols. These issues have been specifically included within the text in recognition of the potential difficulties experienced by some practice nurses within this area. Consideration of these issues within this chapter should facilitate the adoption of good practice within the clinical setting.

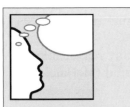

Reflection Point

Discuss the issues raised concerning vicarious liability and insurance cover with your employing GP. Are you satisfied with your insurance cover? (Note that insurance is usually provided by your professional body or trade union.)

Record Keeping

Record keeping is one of the most important aspects of a practice nurse's role given that the maintenance of accurate patient records is critical should a case of negligence be brought against the nurse. The maintenance of accurate records of care is an important factor in demonstrating high standards of client care (Dimond 1997). Within the legal process, it is the records that demonstrate what care was given; it is not acceptable to say care was given if it was not documented.

This issue was highlighted by the UKCC (1998), in the revised guidelines for record keeping. Specifically, they state that 'good record keeping helps to protect the welfare of patients and clients by promoting:

- high standards of clinical care
- continuity of care
- better communication and dissemination of information between members of the interprofessional health care team
- an accurate account of treatment and care planning and delivery
- the ability to detect problems, such as changes in the client's condition, at an early stage'

In developing the argument further the UKCC asserts that the overall quality of a nurse's record keeping is a reflection of the professional's standard of practice.

> 'Good record keeping is a mark of the skilled and safe practitioner, whilst careless or incomplete record keeping often highlights wider problems with the individual's practice' (UKCC 1998, p.7)

Therefore it is imperative that all practice nurses must be constantly aware of the importance of accurate record keeping because instances do arise when nursing records may be called in evidence before a court of law or by the Health Service Commissioner so that a complaint can be investigated at a local level.

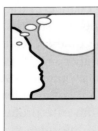

Reflection Points

- What level of record keeping is maintained by practice nurses within your practice?
- Are records sufficiently detailed to be presented in a court of law?
- If not what issues need to addressed to ensure that your record keeping is adequate?

> **Box 3.1**
>
> **Record Keeping Features in Practice Nurse Records to Uphold their Legal Duty of Care (UKCC 1998)**
>
> ■ A full account of any nursing assessment and the subsequent care that has been planned and implemented
> ■ Relevant information pertaining to the client's condition at any given time and the measures adopted to respond to their needs
> ■ Evidence that the nurse has understood and honoured the duty of care, and that all reasonable steps have been taken to care for the client and that any acts or omissions on the part of the nurse have not jeopardized the client's safety or wellbeing in any way

Although the importance of detailed accurate record keeping cannot be stressed enough, it is necessary to recognize that written records are merely hearsay evidence, in that it is often difficult to ascertain whether something that is written down actually provides proof of the truth. Inaccuracies, misleading statements and possible exaggerations can all be recorded. However, if records are called into evidence the writer of the entries will be cross-examined and the weight that may be afforded to those entries will be ascertained. It therefore follows that practice nurses who are subpoenaed to court with their written records will almost certainly be questioned and cross-examined to determine the accuracy of the records in question (Dimond 1997).

In ensuring that as professionals practice nurses uphold their legal duty of care, all records should demonstrate the features listed in Box 3.1.

These comprehensive points recommended by the UKCC are at times difficult if not impossible to implement, particularly if the general practice still uses only the Lloyd George record system. This is problematic because if litigation does arise it is apparent that the courts tend to adopt the opinion that if care has not been recorded, then it has not been done. It is therefore essential that practice nurses use their professional judgement in determining relevant information for inclusion in the nursing records. This might be of particular importance when a certain aspect of client care has remained unchanged for an appreciable period of time because there has been no apparent change in the client's overall condition. It may be appropriate in these instances to develop local clinical guidelines so that acceptable time lapses between all record entries in these cases can be determined.

Good record keeping is not only important in cases of litigation, but also in addressing wider communication issues between the practice nurse and other health care professionals. It is possible that colleagues will rely upon the information that has been recorded.

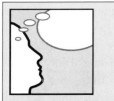

Reflection Point

What does the scenario depicted in Case Study 3.1 highlight in relation to the issues of both duty of care and record keeping?

Case Study 3.1

A Case of Poor Record Keeping

A mother attends the surgery requesting that her child receives her third set of injections.

The child is now 6 months old and the nurse is aware that they are overdue. However, the family are newly registered and the patient's notes have only just been received. The nurse examines the records and reads the following statement: '*Immunizations given*'. There is no signature by the individual who administered the immunizations.

The nurse is in a quandary about whether to give the immunizations and this is aggravated by the mother persisting that she wants them done. She (the nurse) decides to give the immunizations, at which point the mother is surprised because she now thinks that the immunizations were given.

Box 3.2

Examples of Deficiencies in Record Keeping (Dimond 1997)

- A failure to note times and dates
- Illegible writing
- Use of abbreviations
- Errors covered in Tippex
- Omission of a signature or use of initials
- Omission of relevant client information
- Omission of follow-up dates for review by the GP
- Delays in writing up the client record
- Allowing someone else to complete the record
- Inaccuracies in name, date of birth or address
- Use of unprofessional terminology

The issue of comprehensive record keeping does not, however, only apply to the individual nurse's working practice. If the practice nurse is working as the supervisor of a 'trainee' any entry made into the client records by that trainee must be countersigned by the supervisor who remains professionally accountable for the consequences of any such entry (UKCC 1998). It therefore follows that the practice nurse must ensure that all entries made into any client record are of a good standard and contain no deficiencies, such as those listed in Box 3.2

It is important that any deficiencies concerning the above are addressed in practice because if litigation does occur the records of all those involved will be examined. If it is evident that there is disparity between the health care professionals involved, it is up to the judge to decide upon the credibility of each of the individuals involved and to note how they have withstood any cross-examination. The practice nurse must therefore on the rare occasions that conflict may arise ensure that all client records are appropriately kept in the first instance. Such an approach will ensure that in the event that litigation does arise then more weight will be afforded to her credibility.

The need for accurate record keeping is particularly necessary where records are shared, for example the Lloyd George files. Within shared notes it is necessary, in terms of the practice nurse's own professional accountability, for the nurse to clearly detail the assessment, planning, implementation and evaluation of any provided care. This is a universal concept, and as such applies not only to written records, but also information recorded on any computer system (UKCC 1998). The need for accurate documentation, however, does not require the nurse or health care professional to duplicate their records, but instead adhere to the principles highlighted.

As well as maintaining accurate records, there is also the need to subject record keeping to the same quality assurance mechanisms as the nurse would for any other aspect of care provision. For this reason, records should be audited on a regular basis so that areas for improvement and staff development may be identified. The length of time that records are kept depends upon both Department of Health recommendations and local guidelines. Local protocols generally ensure that all records are kept for a period of at least 8 years and in the case of a child all records should be kept until the child reaches the age of 21 years.

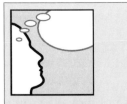

Reflection Point

Consider contacting the records and information department at your local health authority to identify any local protocol for the retention of patient records.

Maintaining Confidentiality

The recording of detailed information manually, but particularly on a computer system, highlights the need to protect patient confidentiality. It is therefore the duty of the nurse to ensure that no unauthorized access is gained to records held on a computer and any unauthorized access may constitute a criminal offence under the Computer Misuse Act (1990). Although stringent in its approach, the Act does, however, make provision for any incidents where the information was obtained through an accident, extortion and blackmail (UKCC 1996). Developing the principles highlighted within the Act the UKCC (1996) further emphasizes the need for confidentiality with regards to computer-held records by stating that:

'As far as computer-held records are concerned, you must be satisfied that as far as possible, the methods you use for recording information are secure. You must also find out which categories of staff have access to records to which they are expected to contribute important personal and confidential information. Local procedures must include ways of checking whether a record is authentic when there is no written signature. All records must clearly indicate the identity of the person who made that record.'

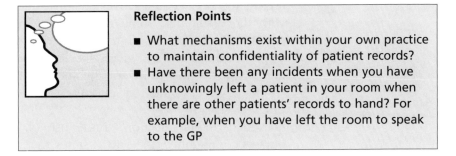

Reflection Points

- What mechanisms exist within your own practice to maintain confidentiality of patient records?
- Have there been any incidents when you have unknowingly left a patient in your room when there are other patients' records to hand? For example, when you have left the room to speak to the GP

Patient Access to Their Own Records

Following implementation of the Data Protection Act (1984), Access Modification (Health) Order (1987) and the Access to Health Records Act (1990) patients have a legal right to request to view their own records, whether these are manually written or held on a computer. Although heralded as a victory and well publicized the 1990 Access to Health Records Act does not state that patients have an absolute right to access their records. Specifically, information may be withheld if it is considered that it may cause serious harm to either the patient's physical or mental state or even cause harm to another person. Even withstanding this issue, the access to health care records needs to be exercised with caution and sensitivity if the patient's rights are to be protected (McHale et al 1998).

Clinical Guidelines and Protocols

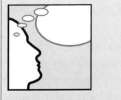

Reflection Point

What procedures exist within your practice to enable patients to view their records?

For many practice nurses the legal position of clinical guidelines and protocols is fundamental to their practice. Indeed, the increasing interest in the legality of protocols has arisen as a direct response to the evolving role of the practice nurse, and in particular the acquisition by the nurse of tasks that were previously the sole responsibility of the doctor (Tingle 1998). This may in part be due to nurses' heightening demands to be recognized as more independent practitioners or the UKCC's desire to move away from the traditional approach of competency certificates and rejection of the term 'extended role' (Standing Medical Advisory Committee and the Standing Nursing and Midwifery Advisory Committee 1989). The UKCC (1992b) was particularly hostile to the term stating that 'the terms "extended" or "extending roles" are no longer favoured as they … limit rather than extend the parameters of practice'.

Although a potentially liberating statement by the UKCC, there still remains some controversy about the overall position that should be adopted within clinical nursing practice. At present it would appear that the whole concept of role definition differs from region to region and between GPs. This has provided uncertainty and conflict, with the result that some nurses perceive care as becoming less patient centred and far too technical in its origins (Healey 1996). This is particularly relevant given the increasing importance currently placed on the autonomy of the individual nurse to decide if and when they feel competent enough to undertake a particular aspect of client care.

Indeed, in its rejection of the use of certification to 'prove' a nurse's competence, the UKCC states that:

> 'In order to bring into proper focus the professional responsibility and consequent accountability of individual practitioners, it is the Council's principles for practice rather than certificates for tasks which should form the basis for adjustments to the scope of practice.' (UKCC 1992b)

Furthermore, Tingle (1998) suggests that by giving a nurse a certificate of competence a situation may develop where the nurse feels a false sense of security where it is considered that accountability for their actions has shifted to the initial assessor. As previously noted, it is important that the practice nurse keeps up to date with relevant clinical developments. Without a heavy reliance on competency certificates, the development of clinical guidelines and protocols is increasingly perceived as a potential means to ensure a safe environment for client care, particularly where duties are devolved from the GP to the practice nurse.

Similarly, with an ever increasing emphasis on the need to demonstrate the quality of health care delivered, clinical guidelines and protocols are being developed within the realms of evidence-based practice for both medical and nursing resources. Tingle (1998) specifically highlights the specific value of clinical protocols as 'at the very least demonstrating that there is a controlled environment of care'. However, with the advent of such initiatives it is almost certain that there will be an increase in the amount of litigation arising from their use (Tingle 1993). It is therefore essential that all practice nurses are aware of the potential legal problems that may ensue if and when these guidelines are adopted.

To be perceived in a legal context it is essential that all clinical guidelines and protocols mirror a responsible body of professional knowledge. This falls in line with the whole concept of the Bolam test, that is, would all practitioners working within the same specialty have formulated and used the guidelines or protocols in a uniform way? The Department of Health (1996) defines clinical guidelines as 'systematically developed statements which assist the individual clinician and patient in making decisions about appropriate health care for specific conditions'. It therefore follows that if a clinical guideline or protocol has been formulated by the GP and the practice nurse, and the nurse has subsequently not adhered to the agreed guideline, then there is a distinct possibility that this will be taken into account by a court if harm occurs to a client. However, this does not necessarily mean that a court will accept the guideline without question; it may be considered that it goes against the practice of an ordinary skilled practitioner working within the same specialism (Tingle 1998).

In relation to case law the case of Early v Newham Health Authority ([1994] 5 Med LR 214) clearly identifies the use of clinical guidelines and protocols within practice. In this particular case a 13-year-old child was to undergo an appendectomy. The anaesthetist was to follow the health authority's guidelines on intubation. Unfortunately, the adolescent was unsuccessfully intubated and awoke to find herself partially paralysed due to the effects of intravenously administered suxamethonium. The plaintiff claimed negligence because the anaesthetist had failed to intubate her appropriately and she further argued that the health authority's clinical guidelines on intubation were unsound. The judge, however, found the guidelines to be reasonable and no negligence was found in the procedure. It was decided that the guidelines themselves were based on a responsible body of medical knowledge and that the legal principles of the Bolam test were satisfied.

Drawing on the inferences of this case, it is important that, to satisfy legal requirements with regards to duty of care, any practice nurse involved in the formulation of clinical guidelines and protocols ensures that these are all based on a responsible body of nursing knowledge and that any ordinary skilled practitioner working in the same specialty would act in the same way.

However, it is imperative that the practice nurse does not disregard other forms of care simply because a clinical guideline or protocol is in existence. Tingle (1993) argues that clients may request a different type of treatment themselves and in some cases this might be an acceptable course of action. Further, on these occasions it is important that the treatment is discussed with other members of the multidisciplinary team because there may be medical, nursing or other resource implications. Practice nurses should never standardize care; it should remain holistic and individual in its nature. Clients' autonomy and choice should to a large degree govern the ways in which care is prescribed and administered and therefore the appropriateness of clinical guidelines and protocols must always be ascertained. In situations where the nurse is faced with contradiction or uncertainty, then it is necessary to exercise discretion and be vigilant in ensuring that all relevant issues are well documented and clarified. This is vital because in these cases the nurse is not automatically liable, but it is essential that clear and accurate documentation is kept to make it clear why this particular variance in care has occurred. Indeed, the courts acknowledge that differences in clinical practice do exist, but a judge would seek to ascertain the facts about why this departure had come about and the rationale behind the decision will undoubtedly be sought (Tingle 1993).

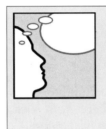

Reflection Points

■ What protocols do you currently use in practice?
■ Are these evidence based? Where was your evidence drawn from? Is this evidence kept with the protocol to inform other practitioners?
■ Has your practice changed due to new knowledge, but the protocols remain the same?

Reviewing Protocols

There may be times when situations change within the surgery; perhaps there might be a reallocation of resources or appointment of new staff. At this point it is imperative that if clinical guidelines and protocols are in use that they are re-evaluated, because they may at this time no longer be pertinent for client care and they may need to be withdrawn. If this re-evaluation does not occur then the nurse may be viewed as being negligent if harm results. As previously stated it is imperative that nurses keep themselves up to date to fulfil the requirements of their 'scope of professional practice' (Tingle 1998). It is therefore argued that the content of clinical guidelines and protocols should be reviewed on a regular basis, as should the processes under which they are written, to ensure that the concepts of risk management and quality assurance are properly addressed.

Conclusion

The rapidly changing nature of practice nursing, and the increasing demands currently being placed upon general practice will undoubtedly result in a growth and expansion in the role presently undertaken by the practice nurse. These changes offer a great opportunity for nurses; however, there will, as a result of this, be an increase in the level of responsibility and an increase in awareness of the accountability. It is therefore important for practice nurses to reaffirm to whom they are accountable – most importantly the patient.

It is this issue, and the central belief in 'doing no harm' that underpins nursing practice and will ensure that nurses act in an appropriate manner within their role. This important tenet needs to be considered by all practice nurses, even when faced with pressure to undertake inappropriate tasks from both the patient and at times the GP.

References

Department of Health 1996 Promoting clinical effectiveness: a framework for action in and through the NHS. Department of Health, London

Department of Health 1994 A vision for the future. The nursing, midwifery and health visiting contribution to health and social care. HMSO, London

Dimond B 1997 Legal aspects of care in the community. Macmillan, London

Healey P 1996 Nurses doing junior doctors work are safe claims unions. Nursing Standard 10(34):5

Jones MA 1997 Textbook on torts, 5th edn. Blackstone Press, London

Korgaonkar G, Tribe D 1995 Law for nurses. Cavendish Publishing, London

McHale J, Fox M, Murphy J 1997 Health care law: text, cases and materials. Sweet & Maxwell, London

McHale J, Tingle J, Peysner J 1998 Law and nursing. Butterworth Heinemann, Oxford

Martin J 1996 Law of negligence. Primary Health Care 6(2):18–19

Montgomery J 1995 Negligence: the legal perspective. In: Tingle J, Crib A (eds) Nursing law and ethics. Blackwell Science, Oxford

NHS Executive 1996 NHS indemnity arrangements for clinical negligence claims in the NHS. Department of Health, Leeds

Tingle J 1993 The extended role of the nurse; legal implications. Care of the Critically Ill 9(1):30–34

Tingle J 1998 In: McHale J, Tingle J, Peysner J (eds) Law and nursing. Butterworth Heinemann, London

UKCC 1992a Code of professional conduct. United Kingdom Central Council for Nursing, Midwifery and Health Visiting, London

UKCC 1992b The scope of professional practice. United Kingdom Central Council for Nursing, Midwifery and Health Visiting, London

UKCC 1996 Guidelines for professional practice. United Kingdom Central Council for Nursing, Midwifery and Health Visiting, London

UKCC 1998 Guidelines for records and record keeping. United Kingdom Central Council for Nursing, Midwifery and Health Visiting, London

Young A 1995 The legal dimension. In: Tingle J, Cribb A (eds) Nursing law and ethics. Blackwell Science, Oxford

4 *The Political Framework of Practice*

Pam Gastrell

INTRODUCTION

This chapter will examine the changing structure of health care provision and the impact of recent policy changes on the organizational shift towards a primary care-led NHS. The discussion will open with a consideration of the changing patterns of health care provision and a brief review of some of the policies influencing this shift. The NHS remains the subject of much public comment and media scrutiny as to whether or not the reforms set in place by the last Conservative Government are working. Of particular interest in the context of this debate are the Labour Government's proposals for the strengthening of primary care through the establishment of primary care groups (Department of Health 1997). Issues of specific importance to primary health care will be discussed in relation to prevailing government ideology and opportunities for development. These proposals will be explored alongside a consideration of perspectives of primary care as outlined and envisaged by the World Health Organization. This will lead into a discussion of definitions of primary care. The impact of *The Health of the Nation* strategy' (Department of Health 1992) on the definition of health and health promotion will also be explored.

If practice nurses are to take advantage of the opportunities created by the shift from secondary to primary care, nurses working in primary health care settings need to work in new ways and in close collaboration with GPs and others. To illustrate this, the chapter concludes with a discussion of a triage scheme for nurses working in primary health care settings and a brief review of the new NHS direct nurse-led 24-hour telephone health advice line.

Primary Care Moves Centre Stage

It has been argued by some that the key concerns about primary care emanated from the Conservative Government's desire to control overall spending on the NHS. In particular they sought to control access to expensive acute-based health care, with concern over the lack of ability to control the demand-led expenditure of general practice. The

Key Issues

- A primary care-led NHS – primary care moves centre stage
- Changing policies, practice or rhetoric – the NHS and Community Care Act
- Definitions of primary care – health for all

- *The Health of the Nation* strategy – health and health promotion redefined
- How did the Conservative Government do?
- The new NHS – what does the future hold?
- Implications of policy changes for practice nursing

Box 4.1

Reasons why the Government Shifted Resources from Secondary to Community Care

- Issues relating to the inappropriate use of hospital facilities
- To enhance the scope and standards of primary care

Government was critical of the quality of management and coordination in primary care and frustrated by the independence of the GPs and by the inability of the family practitioner committees to influence their performance. There is no doubt that primary care issues came under close political scrutiny in the 1980s. The initial approach to reforming primary care was, according to Baggott (1994), rather piecemeal, although the shift towards an outcome-driven needs-led, primary care service began to gather pace.

The reasons why the Government considered it useful to shift resources from secondary to community care are summarized in Box 4.1.

The Government's overriding desire to control costs and to provide more cost-effective care is encompassed in both of these goals. The main issues in terms of enhancing primary care according to Taylor (1991) quoted in Peckham (1996) are as listed in Box 4.2.

Although there can be little doubt that financial considerations provided a clear incentive for shifting health care into the primary sector, this development should be considered against the continuing movement in hospital care. Secondary care consumes twice as much resources as primary care, but it treats only one-tenth of the episodes of ill health that are treated within primary care settings. A clear incentive for change! It should also be borne in mind that progressively throughout the 1980s and into the 1990s, more high-cost, high-technology care involving shorter hospital stays and an increase in day surgery was becoming the norm. It was no surprise to nurses working within general practice to know that, by 1991, a paper published by the then Wessex Regional Health Authority pointed out that 90% of health care was already provided within primary health care settings!

Box 4.2

Main Issues to Enhance Primary Care (Taylor [1991] quoted in Peckham [1996])

1. Opportunities to improve patient's access to care in the context of
   - Initial contact with the GP
   - Other services in the community obtained via the GP
   - Hospital care following GP contact
   - GP and other community service care received after discharge from hospital
2. Opportunities to improve cooperation and the 'effective sharing of care' between doctors and other service providers including consultants, nurses working in community and hospital liaison posts, health visitors, midwives, community psychiatric nurses and social staff
3. Opportunities to raise clinical and patient support standards in the context of conditions and services such as diabetes mellitus, epilepsy, childhood asthma, depression and antenatal care
4. Opportunities to promote an enhanced sense of confidence, self-esteem, control and ownership among individuals involved in primary care, whether patients or service providers

A Primary Health Care-led NHS

All these factors have in their own right been driving forces in the shift towards a primary care-led NHS, but what do we mean by this term? According to government policy the overall objective of a primary care-led NHS is to improve the health of the nation and the efficiency and effectiveness of NHS care.

The implementation of this strategy requires both:

- a specific focus on the needs of the individual
- a population perspective on the needs of the whole community

Against this backdrop, the government recognized that general practice is most people's first and indeed main point of contact with the NHS, and should by definition be the natural place where patients', clients' and carers' voices can be heard and respected. Hence, a primary health care-led NHS gives GPs and primary care teams greater influence in the purchasing and provision of health care within agreed priorities.

By this definition, a primary care-led NHS is about:

- making decisions about health and health care as close to patients as possible – these decisions being informed by an assessment of need and public health priorities
- general practice being the focus for the purchasing and delivery of services to meet the health needs of the majority of the population

Indeed, it has been argued that the policy shift to primary care has been expressed almost entirely in terms of GP purchasing and controlling mechanisms for hospital referrals and assessment (Gordon & Hadley 1996). The introduction of contracts for GPs specified precisely the services GPs were required to provide for their patients and also spelt out the terms and conditions of service for GPs. Despite fierce opposition the new contract was imposed by the government, and as a result of continued scrutiny and debate, brought many of these issues to the fore, which over time can be seen to have provided a focus for moving forward the debate. Certainly, the purchaser/provider split and the introduction of GP fundholding have had a significant impact on the way primary care services have developed and been organized and delivered.

Funding

The reasons for this shift in the organization and delivery of care are open to debate, but a discussion such as this needs to focus on the prevailing political ideology, which during the late 1980s was responsible for seeking to shift the focus of care away from the acute sector into primary care.

Throughout the 1980s the Conservative Government placed the need for a strong economy before issues of social welfare. It also publicly stated its distrust of certain professional groups and public bureaucrats in general. In particular the NHS was seen as a vast and growing consumer of public funds; a body which, if not controlled, it was argued, would consume more than its fair share of public funds to the detriment of others. This claim was a constant cry of politicians. Yet, from the nurses and other professionals working in the health service and from the public at large, questions of funding and claims of under-resourcing of the NHS were constantly in the media. The dispute rumbled on with claims and counterclaims on both sides until 1987, when a survey undertaken by the National Association of Health Authorities of 106 health authorities showed that most were experiencing some degree of financial crisis.

At this time the NHS was constantly under media scrutiny, yet across a range of services, including education and housing, the Conservative Government had begun a gradual but relentless process of creeping privatization by both slowing down and in some instances reversing the growth in public spending. As for the NHS, Holliday (1992) argues that at this time 'all aspects of NHS spending were under scrutiny and efficiency savings were being sought at every opportunity'. Given the fact that government ministers were keen to develop a new style business-like health service the introduction of general management principles was a necessary prerequisite for subsequent changes. Hence, under the chairmanship of Roy Griffiths a working group was established to look at the management arrangements in the NHS in England. Baggott (1994) suggests that the Government already knew what it wanted to hear from the team of inquiry, namely, a management structure that facilitated greater control, particularly over the costs of the service.

Introduction of General Management

The suspicion was proved right and the report of the NHS Management Inquiry Team was published in 1983. The report proposed a series of changes aimed at making the existing organization more efficient. Their recommendations were accepted reluctantly on the part of some professional groups including nurses, who considered the Inquiry Team's commercial approach to management to be inappropriate for the NHS. There is no doubt that battle lines were drawn and the Government was concerned with trying to balance the escalating demands from professional providers of the NHS for more resources and the need to centrally control the overall budget. The political temperature was raised and media attention on all aspects of the organization and delivery of health care was intense.

The Government, realizing the weight of public pressure, rather unexpectedly announced a review of the NHS, the first for 40 years. In the late 1980s a Government working party was established to determine how to improve efficiency in the NHS given that there would be no new money available. From the outset the context of this debate centred on the need for efficiency and improved performance. Ministers remained convinced that increased efficiency rather than increased spending was the way forward (Peckham 1996). Not everyone shared this view, however, some arguing that a new structure was needed because the changes to date had been largely ineffectual. Political commentators suggested that the idea of an internal market, where cash would follow the patient, would result in better quality, more cost-effective care.

These events, however, were not happening in isolation; at the time the review group was meeting key changes were beginning to take place in parts of the NHS. London teaching hospitals began to charge for out-of-district work, and following a pilot study in East Anglia, Enthoven was advocating for a market in health care to be introduced in the United Kingdom. He proposed the separation of purchasers and providers (Enthoven 1985), an opinion that fitted well with the government's view that the health service was bureaucratic and inefficient and that private markets were more efficient. Although acknowledging that there were a number of concurrent and interweaving political pressures influencing the government's deliberations at this time, there is no doubt that the idea of the internal market in health care had arrived – a political stance, which over time was to allow GPs to hold their own budgets and to begin the shift towards a primary care-led NHS. This fundamental change in NHS philosophy was long overdue, but as some commentators identified, came about in a curious way: critics argued that the review's findings presented a limited view of the concept of health, and the document itself was perceived by some as lacking in detail. However, after fierce public debate, *Working for Patients* (Department of Health 1989a) and recommendation for community care (Department of Health 1989b) were implemented and ultimately led to the enactment of the NHS and Community Care Act in June 1990 (Department of Health 1990b).

The NHS and Community Care Act

The Government claimed that these reforms, designed to bring about change in structure, organization and management of the NHS, would enable the Government and the public 'to focus on health as much as health care'. However, critics such as Harrison & Schulz (1989) argued that the review's diagnosis was mainly about ill health, focusing on hospitals, general practice and ill people. There was scant mention of a positive health agenda, persistent inequalities in health and the level of preventable illness, and issues of underfunding were completely ignored. Many voices were raised in protest at the review's findings and recommended solutions. The Association of Community Health Councils argued that the white paper concentrated almost entirely on the acute sector, and that whole sections of the NHS were either dealt with in a cursory way or overlooked. Community care was not discussed and wider public health issues were referred to briefly. Perhaps the most contentious issue for some was the fact that the review appeared to equate the NHS with hospital and general practice.

However, the failure to specifically focus in depth on issues relating to community care did not stop the flow of government directives and advice. In relation to general practice and community care, the NHS Management Executive (1992) published a book of guidance for general practice which sought to spell out the implications of the white paper *Caring for People* and the NHS Community Care Act 1990. The booklet highlighted the central role that GPs were expected to play in implementing these policies. It also acknowledged the contribution made by community nurses and practice-employed staff and the importance of collaborative working and a team approach to care was emphasized. Although continuing to emphasize the medical and curative aspects of care to the detriment of health and wellness, the role of general practice as the first point of contact was acknowledged.

General Practitioner Fundholding

The proposal for GP fundholding stemmed from the white paper on the future of the NHS *Working for Patients* (Department of

Health 1989a). The proposals set out in this report represented some radical changes to the NHS. For whatever reason, whether economic or political, the government recognized that GPs were uniquely placed to improve patients' choice and quality of service and GPs were perceived as having a crucial role in:

■ advising patients
■ ensuring that it was the patient who benefitted from the NHS reforms

It was argued that the introduction GP fundholding would offer GPs a new freedom of activity to secure better value for money, to improve standards of care, to offer greater consumer choice and to improve waiting lists. In short, GP fundholders would be encouraged to shop around for the best services and to employ the right sort of staff to meet the assessed need of their practice population. GPs were also to be allowed to advertise and develop available practice expertise and services which would help to attract more patients and bring more money into the practice. Any savings made, it was argued, would be ploughed back into the practice, thus raising the standard of patient care and at the same time enriching the potential work of general practice for all involved, including practice nurses (Fatchet 1994).

At the time of its inception, GP fundholding was seen as one of the key forces for change within the reformed NHS. What was seen by some as a last-minute ploy to provide a more radical edge to government reforms, not only took on a life of its own but also fundamentally changed patterns of service delivery in some areas of health care (Glennerster et al 1994). During 1993, fundholding practices were able to purchase community services including district nursing, health visiting and community psychiatric nursing. Although these services had to be purchased from existing community units, GPs not being given the resources to employ directly community nurses, GPs were able via the 'contract' to specify conditions about the nursing service they wished to purchase.

In some parts of the country this resulted in changing relationships within primary care teams as tensions developed between area base approaches to care, envisaged by Cumberlege (Department of Health 1986), and the focus on the practice list. One positive move to arise from these developments was an increase in the direct employment, growth and status of practice nurses. While some welcomed these developments and viewed the emerging influence and power of general practice in a positive light, seizing the opportunity for innovation, others, including some community nurses, viewed the developments as a threat (Mackenzie & Ross 1997). However one views these developments, there is no doubt that the introduction of GP fundholding has had a significant influence on the reshaping of primary care and the development of practice nursing. What is debatable is to what extent the introduction of fundholding met government objectives.

Defining Primary Care

For some the meaning of primary health care also came under increasing scrutiny throughout this period. Fatchet (1994) argues that the opportunity for community nurses, including practice nurses, to undertake a truly primary health care approach was rejected by the Government. With the GP as the first point of contact, Fatchet believes that health interventions invariably became secondary and tertiary, a view not shared by everyone. Some GPs and practice nurses claim that the increased emphasis on general practice, resulting in the introduction of the GP contract, allowed the practice nurse new and unlimited opportunities for developing new and innovative ways of working (Smail 1996).

How an individual interprets and interacts with these issues is in part dependent upon their working definition of primary care. Mackenzie & Ross (1997) suggest that there has always been some debate about the meaning of primary care. One of the most commonly used definitions relates to general practice; indeed, some of the rhetoric behind government policy assumes that primary care is synonymous with general practice. Others widen this rather narrow view to define it on the basis of first contact, continuous and coordinated care provided to individuals or populations undifferentiated by age, gender and disease (NHS Management Executive 1993). However, for some this is still too prescriptive a definition: Gordon & Plampling (1996) describe it as a community-based health service linked to a much wider social network. This definition fits well with the Labour Government's agenda for health which was spelt out in a consultative green paper on public health called *Our Healthier Nation* (Department of Health 1998), and also with the World Health Organization's concept of primary care.

Health for All

In 1978 the World Health Organization conference on primary health care in Alma-Ata, Russia agreed the need for a global effort to achieve health for all people. The WHO European Regional Office subsequently worked with its 33 member states to translate these general aims into a European regional strategy and in 1984 38 targets to be achieved by the year 2000 were set and agreed. They are contained in the document *Regional Targets in Support of the Regional Strategy for Health for All* (WHO Regional Office for Europe 1984).

The six major themes run through this document are:

1. *Health for All implies: equity.* This means that the present inequalities in health between countries and within countries should be reduced as far as possible.
2. *Health for All implies: health promotion.* The aim is to give people a positive sense of health so that they can make full use of their physical, mental and emotional capacities.
3. *Health for All implies: community participation.* Health for all can be attained only with the active participation of the whole community. This means giving people the skills and knowledge to empower them to take control over decisions affecting their own health. A well-informed, well-motivated and actively involved community is essential for the attainment of this goal.
4. *Health for All implies: multisectoral cooperation.* Health authorities can deal with only part of the problem to be solved. A coordinated action on the part of all sectors concerned is required: between government, business, academia, and voluntary and community organizations.
5. *Health for All implies: primary health care.* The focus of the health care system should be on meeting the basic health needs of the community as fully as possible through services provided as close as possible to where people live and work, and which are readily accessible and acceptable to all.
6. *Health for All implies: international cooperation.* Health problems transcend national frontiers – for example AIDS, pollution and trade in health-damaging goods – and their resolution requires international cooperation.

The document refers first to the prerequisites for health: a Europe free from the fear of war, equal opportunity for all, and the satisfaction of people's basic needs for food, basic education, water and sanitation, decent housing, secure employment and a useful role in society. It acknowledges that the achievement of these goals requires both political will and public support. In essence, it identifies health promotion and public health issues as the key strategies underpinning 'Health for All'. The United Kingdom formally stated its commitment to the World Health Organization's 'Health for All' initiative and agreed the objectives to be achieved by the year 2000.

During the 1980s the European Community also began to take an interest in tackling health problems, for example by seeking to implement measures designed to impose a common set of health warnings on tobacco products in member countries – moves which were vigorously and unsuccessfully opposed by the United Kingdom. So where did the Government stand on these issues? Although acknowledging these international developments and, indeed, being a signatory to the Health for All initiative, the Conservative Government failed to formulate a national policy designed to translate WHO goals into meaningful policy. Commenting on this, Dooris (1988) argued that throughout most of the early and mid-1980s the Government was complacent and self-satisfied when it came to debating issues concerned with the nation's health. When ministers reported on health matters they used highly selective material focusing almost entirely on the role of the NHS. Interrelated issues affecting health, such as poverty and unemployment, were ignored or glossed over.

Maybe this lack of action and commitment on behalf of the Government could have been expected. For sure, many of the targets of Health for All were over-ambitious and almost impossible to achieve: the abolition of war in Europe is a case in point! However, as Ranade (1994) points out, the importance of the strategy was that it caused governments throughout Europe to think about, understand and make decisions about health. The vision at the heart of the strategy has, over time, inspired many thousands of ordinary people, public and political activists to view health as a state of 'complete wellbeing', a wholeness in individuals, communities and society. Certainly, the Health for All initiative has generated a lot of interest and activity both in the statutory and voluntary sector.

Baggott (1994) suggests that as the NHS dragged its feet, many local authorities bypassed central government and set up their own strategies for health. By the late 1980s the 'Healthy City' movement was in full swing with some parts of the country endeavouring to work in a truly multisectorial collaborative way. The Healthy City programme sought to improve the health of local people in a comprehensive, coordinated way. In the early days the programme was targeted at inner city areas but by 1990 around three-quarters of all health authorities had established local priorities in line with Health for All (Disken 1990). But the prospect for future development and a truly coordinated approach as envisaged by the WHO was constrained by political manoeuvring. In England less than a third of health authorities had specifically allocated resources to Health for All and very few had appointed an individual to take responsibility for the initiative.

However, this was about to change. The NHS reforms through the new strategic role given to health authorities and the separation of purchasing and providing functions created a window of opportunity for the re-emergence of public health. Acknowledging that while health authorities can lead, coordinate and support change, most action involves multisectoral working across a range of other agencies, some health authorities seized the opportunity and, in cooperation with a range of statutory and voluntary organizations, devised imaginative programmes designed to meet the assessed need of local people.

For many community nurses this was an exciting yet challenging time. For the first time since the inception of the NHS, health policy seemed set to refocus the service away from a merely illness-related service. Talk of health promotion and positive health began to appear in government rhetoric, culminating in the publication of the white paper *The Health of the Nation* (Department of Health 1992). Ranade (1994) and others suggest that the publication of this paper could be seen as the Government's first attempt to adopt a national strategy for health.

The Health of the Nation: A Change of Direction?

Having pressed ahead with its somewhat controversial health service reforms, the Government published *The Health of the Nation* white paper in July 1992. This was heralded as a landmark for the NHS and according to the then Secretary of State for Health, Virginia Bottomly, 'the next logical step in health care reforms'.

However, while some professionals and members of the public welcomed the new emphasis on promoting health, a number of people were disappointed that the emphasis on ill health, rather than health and wellness, remained central to the discussion. For some this was to be expected, given the Government's past track record and the focus of the health service reforms. Indeed, critics including Fatchet (1994) went so far as to suggest that the Government's main objective in publishing this strategy was to divert attention away from the health service reforms towards more positive debate. From the wide-ranging discussion that followed the publication of this strategy, it was clear that for some this was the long-awaited chance to redress the balance in health care, away from an illness-focused service towards a positive health agenda. Others were cynical, questioning the Government's real intention given the lack of extra resources and its apparent unwillingess to acknowledge the interrelated importance of factors such as poverty and unemployment. Despite the fact that the Government was a signatory to the WHO's Health for All initiative, the document failed to acknowledge the role of government departments other than the Department of Health. This was seen by some as particularly significant, as over time many people had come to recognize the inability of the health service to resolve health issues alone. Yet, at the time of the launch the Government claimed to support the idea of multi-sectoral working. Indeed, when the earlier green paper was published in 1991, the then Secretary of State for Health claimed that the approach envisaged by the Health of the Nation strategy had been endorsed in warm terms by the World Health Organization.

By inviting comment and discussion the Government appeared to be adopting a consensual approach but criticism and comment continued unabated. The Health Visitor Association, for example, cited various studies that demonstrated clear links between poverty and infant morbidity. Others centred their criticism around the document's emphasis on individual lifestyle at the expense of collective political action on the part of the Government, arguing that in reality the emphasis remained focused on the medical–illness aspect of care. A significant group of others including Fatchet (1994) argued that the very concept of health, and by implication health promotion, had been redefined in so far as the health promotion strategy outlined in the white paper was focused on targets which were illness-related. However, this trend had been set earlier with the introduction of the GP contract (Department of Health 1990a) which not only set out the terms and conditions of service for GPs but also introduced the controversial health promotion banding scheme. Some health promotion activities, initiated in general practice as a result of the GP contract, according to Smail (1996) were not set up in response to the assessed health needs of the practice population. While the Government responded quickly to such criticism, the fact remains that local intervention to promote health in its fullest sense needs a collaborative, multiprofessional approach which can be difficult to achieve in general practice. A team approach is essential.

How did the Conservative Government do?

In summary, throughout the last 20 years all of the previous government's reforms appear to have emphasized the medical–illness aspect of care, rather than focusing on health in its widest sense. The health promotion targets outlined in *The Health of the Nation* focused on specific diseases and individual habits. As a result, the set targets related to the prevention of disease rather than the promotion of positive health. Inequalities in health were largely overlooked and true collaborative working with other central and local government agencies was not high on the agenda. Baggott (1994) suggests that given the competitive nature of the purchaser/provider split, this was inevitable as the development of a health strategy is at odds with the concept of the internal market in health care. Indeed, it was claimed by some that the internal market, which was designed to create competition for patients and hence an improved service, in itself created an unfair system which advantaged some groups at the expense of others.

GP fundholding also came under increasing scrutiny, critics claiming that it created a two-tier health service. Widespread reports of preference being given to fundholding GPs who were able to get quicker care for their clients, as opposed to those practices who were not fundholding, appeared regularly in the media. The

Labour Government claimed that this has resulted in the family doctor community being almost equally split in two, between GP fundholders and nonfundholders. On coming to power, the Labour Government seized on these issues and pledged that:

> In the 'new NHS' patients will be treated according to need and need alone. Cooperation will replace competition. GPs and community nurses will work together in Primary Care Groups. Hospital clinicians will have a say in developing local Health Improvement Programmes. (Department of Health 1997)

Implications for Nursing

Despite the furore, all was not doom and gloom over these years. For practice nurses and others concerned with the promotion of positive health, the strategy outlined in the Health of the Nation document promised new opportunities to raise their sights beyond the provision of health care to health itself. In the event, many practice nurses seized the opportunity offered by the publication of this strategy and, building on the previous opportunities offered by the implementation of the GP contract (Department of Health 1990a), began to work in new and innovative ways. It was around this time that practice nurses began formally to develop skills in health promotion and the management of patients with a chronic disease. Certainly as a result of Government policy on the organization and workload of general practice, practice nurses and primary health care teams have experienced and continue to experience a period of major and rapid change. Sines (1997) argues that this radical and sometimes traumatic rate of change in primary health care is influencing the very nature of community nursing practice. This issue will be returned to later in this chapter.

The New NHS – What Does the Future Hold?

The white paper *The New NHS. Modern. Dependable* (Department of Health 1997) sets out the Labour Government's proposals for action and change. Early on in this document the case for a primary care-led NHS is restated as follows:

> 'Most of the contact that patients have with the NHS is through a primary care professional such as a community nurse or family doctor. They are best placed to understand their patients' needs as a whole and to identify ways of making local services more responsive. Family doctors who have been involved in commissioning services (either as fundholders, or through

multifunds, locality commissioning or the total purchasing model) have welcomed the chance to influence the use of resources to improve patient care. The government wishes to build on these approaches, ensuring that all patients, rather than just some, are able to benefit.'

In relation to primary care the Government intends to:

'Establish primary care groups across the country, bringing together GPs and community nurses in each area to work together to improve the health of local people. Primary care groups will grow out of the range of commissioning models that have developed in recent years, but will give sharper focus to their work. They will have the benefit of strong support from their health authority and the freedom to use NHS resources wisely, including savings. With these new opportunities will go the need to account for their actions. They will be subject to clear accountability and performance standards' (Department of Health 1997).

These new bodies replaced GP fundholding in 1999. They were to build on the best of existing practice by offering an opportunity for innovative community nurses and GPs to spread the benefits of their experience. This should enable those who are willing to take the lead in shaping and influencing the early primary care groups. For those of us working in primary care this transitional stage is both exciting and challenging. It is vital that we get it right. Failure in the early stages could mean retrenchment. General practitioners already have a foot in the commissioning door and have powerful local medical committees to represent their interests – for most practice and community nurses this is new.

Functions of Primary Care Groups
The white paper states that the main functions of the primary care groups will reflect approaches already in existence in many parts of the country (Box 4.3).

The precise form of primary care groups will vary, depending upon what exists at present. The white paper acknowledges that in some areas there are already well-established GP-led groups of commissioners or fundholders, whereas in other parts of the country community trusts have taken the lead role. Whatever the situation it is expected that successful local arrangements will be built upon, not discarded. The document stresses that the approach will be bottom-up and developmental. Hence, practice and community nurses need to be articulate, skilled at their job and competent negotiators if they

> **Box 4.3**
>
> **Main functions of Primary Care Groups**
>
> ■ To contribute to the health authority Health Improvement Programme on health care, helping to ensure that this reflects the perspective of the local community and the experience of patients
> ■ To promote the health of the local population working in partnership with other agencies
> ■ To commission health services for their local population from the relevant NHS trusts, within the framework of the Health Improvement Programme, ensuring quality and efficiency
> ■ To monitor performance against service agreements they (or initially the health authority) have with the NHS Trusts
> ■ To develop primary care by joint working across practices, sharing skills, providing a forum for professional development, audit and peer review, assuring quality and developing the new approach to clinical governance, and influencing the deployment of resources for general practice locally (local medical committees will have a key role in supporting this process)
> ■ To integrate primary and community health services and work more closely with social services on both planning and delivery – services such as child health or rehabilitation, where responsibilities have been split within the health service, and where liaison with local authorities is often poor, will particularly benefit

are to help shape the organization and delivery of primary care as a member of a primary care group

Although not prescribing the function of primary care groups, the white paper suggests that the groups could adopt one of the following options:

■ have a minimum role advising health authorities on commissioning services
■ take responsibility for a devolved health care budget but within the health authority
■ become established as free-standing commissioning bodies accountable to the health authority
■ become established as free-standing commissioning and community health-providing bodies accountable to the health authority
■ eventually the groups, which it is anticipated could serve a population of 100 000 patients, would have the chance to become primary care trusts in their own right.

Each group has a governing body, which includes community nurses, GPs and social services. They have clear arrangements for public involvement, including the holding of open meetings. They are also expected to meet financial targets agreed with the health authority. They have a share of funds for hospital and community health services, prescribing and GP infrastructure to use for the provision of health care services and commissioning.

In relation to needs assessment the white paper states that health authorities will have a stronger strategic role in the assessment of health need in the local population. They will be required to use this information to plan health improvement programmes.

As has been suggested earlier in this chapter the previous Conservative Government's health policies were limited and failed to acknowledge the contribution of government departments other than that of the Department of Health. As a consequence, the concept of health and health promotion were redefined as the Government set targets for health that were illness focused. The *Health of the Nation* strategy could not hope to bring about the improvement in health it set out to achieve without a commitment to tackle inequalities in health in active partnership and collaboration with others.

The 'Third Way'

According to a Labour Government spokesman this is about to change – a new approach to health, a 'third way', was proposed in the white paper. The Minister for Public Health announced that the Government wished to pursue a 'third way' between the old extremes of 'victim blaming' on the one hand and control by the 'nanny state' on the other. This 'third way' involves the creation of a national contract for better health. This proposed programme for public health is to be welcomed as the first attempt by a British government to formally acknowledge in a strategy document a link between poverty and ill-health. Public health is at the heart of the new NHS. According to a government spokesman the aim is to improve the health of the most deprived at a faster rate than the overall national rate of improvement in health. For this goal to became a reality, however, there will be a need for collaborative, cooperative working between individuals, the Government, and local communities.

In this respect the white paper makes it clear that:

- the Government will help to assess the risk to health and will provide accurate, credible and understandable information
- health authorities will lead local alliances in developing health improvement programmes
- local authorities will have a duty to promote the economic, social and environmental wellbeing of an area
- individuals will be encouraged to take responsibility for their own health
- voluntary bodies will act as advocates for local people
- businesses will be responsible for improving the health and safety of their own employees

Therefore, health authorities will be expected to work in partnership with local authorities 'to identify how local action on social, environmental and economic issues will make most impact on the health of the local people'.

The importance of collaboration with other agencies is also stressed in rather strong language in the green paper on health (Department of Health 1998) which says:

> 'The Government will ensure the NHS works locally with those who provide social care, housing, education and employment, just as the Government itself will work nationally across Whitehall to bring about lasting improvements in the public's health.'

Throughout the legislation the subject of collaborative working is emphasized, the Government making the point that as a result of the impact of the internal market there had been little real attempt, or indeed incentive, over the past few years to provide collaborative care. This is to change – in the new NHS all those charged with the task of providing and planning health and social care services for patients will be required to work to jointly agreed local health improvement programmes. This will govern the actions of all parts of the local NHS to ensure consistency and coordination.

In summary, the Government set itself a formidable challenge in aiming:

- to replace competition with cooperation
- to explore new flexible local ways of delivering health and health care
- to develop a new approach to partnership for the 1998–1999 commissioning round
- to improve efficiency by reducing management costs
- to tackle waiting lists and times
- to rebuild public confidence

The Government itself recognizes the enormity of this task and to help to focus and develop health contracts in an organized structured way across the age range, the following are specified:

- focus on children – healthy schools
- focus on adults – healthy workplaces
- focus on older people – healthy neighbourhoods

In addition to the long overdue focus on wellness and public health, four priority illness areas have been identified for action. Government targets have been set for improvement in each of the following areas by the year 2010:

- heart disease and stroke
- accidents
- cancer
- mental health

This list is considerably shorter than the list of targets related to ill-health outlined in *The Health of the Nation* (Department of Health 1992) strategy. In this way it is expected that all local care agencies will set their own targets based on the assessed health need of their local population. As previously stated these goals can only be achieved in collaboration with a range of other agencies. This will involve the creation of a variety of local multidisciplinary initiatives; the white paper outlines the concept of healthy living centres, health improvement programmes and health action zones. Only time will tell how successful the Government has been in seeking to introduce health policy that is more broadly based, but there is no doubt that many will welcome the opportunity to deliver a 'health' rather than ill-health programme.

Nursing Input

So, what are the implications of this for practice and other community nurses? The white paper states that:

> 'for the first time in the history of the NHS all primary
> care professionals, who do the majority of prescribing,
> treating and referring, will have control over how
> resources are best used to benefit patients'.

The document goes on to say, 'there will be a spectrum of opportunities available for local GPs and community nurses'. Indeed, if the goals set out in the policy document are to become a reality, nursing input on primary care groups will be essential, a view shared by Yvonne Moores, Chief Nursing Officer, who in an interview for the journal *Health Visitor*: stressed that 'the quality of nursing input will need to be of a very high quality'. Bearing in mind that GPs already have a foot in the commissioning door and have powerful local medical committees to represent their views, nurses will need to get their act together quickly.

The white paper acknowledges the contribution that nurses have to make and specifically states that NHS trusts will be expected to strengthen the nursing contribution. The Government recognizes that nurses will need help and guidance as they move into new roles, for nursing, midwifery and health visiting. Against this backdrop of opportunity it is vital that as a profession we rise to this challenge. We cannot afford to get it wrong or we may lose the opportunity to influence and shape the service. As a profession we need to actively prepare individuals to accept the challenge these opportunities bring. In general practice settings this may not be easy because questions of funding, cover for time off and accountability are certain to raise their head. Yet, the current policy direction offers a window of opportunity few nurses even dreamt of a few years ago. We need 'to go for it'. Now is not the time for interprofessional nursing squabbles over who does what.

Implications of Policy Changes for Nursing

As a result of policy changes many activities over the past decade have been transferred from secondary to primary care; for example, most people who have a chronic disease such as asthma, diabetes mellitus or hypertension are almost exclusively cared for by their GP and other members of the primary health care team. The introduction of the GP contract in 1990 also brought about an increased workload as child health surveillance, immunization programmes and family planning services were gradually absorbed into general practice. These changes are vast and as Rashid et al (1996) suggest, if GPs are to cope with the continued changes there is an urgent need to explore the changing relationships of those working in primary health care settings with a view to determining roles and responsibilities.

Collaboration in Action – the Development of Nurse Triage

Across Hampshire the impact of these changes in the organization and delivery of primary health care, including the need to provide an out-of-hours service in general practice and the increasing demands on primary health care staff, was explored and discussed with a range of key personnel including representatives from the health authorities, the local medical committees, members of the Practice Nurse Consultative Committee and primary health care nurses.

These discussions took place over the summer of 1996, with questions of autonomy and accountability, and issues relating to tightly defined territorial professional boundaries being raised in most sessions. In the early stages there was considerable confusion with terminology, particularly with the titles 'practice nurse' and 'nurse practitioner'. Some GP colleagues were certain that what they really required was a 'nurse practitioner', most not fully understanding the difference between extended and expanded nursing roles and how these fit in with the notion of specialist or advanced practice. Some GPs who did understand the concept of 'nurse practitioner' were somewhat threatened by the whole idea, but everyone wanted to explore issues of skill mix and reprofiling within the context of teamwork in general practice. A similar degree of anxiety and indeed confusion was apparent from the nurses themselves in so far as some of the practice nurses, health visitors and district nurses involved in the discussion did not see what the fuss was about; they claimed to have been working in a triage role for some time! Despite the tensions, there was a real sense of excitement and anticipation as new ways of working were explored and important community and primary health care issues were discussed across professional boundaries.

At the beginning of the discussions there was no real unanimity as to the way forward in so far as the three health authorities and various professional representatives all had slightly different agendas. But, very early in the discussions one of the primary health care managers approached the University of Southampton and asked if we would mount a triage course. This proposal was formally presented and discussed with all the main stakeholders and resulted in the decision to mount an English National Board (ENB) triage course for nurses working in primary health care settings. It was agreed that this course would be primarily skill based and should carry an academic credit rating at level two. From the outset, and as a result of detailed discussion, it was acknowledged that the triage course would not prepare a nurse to practise as a nurse practitioner or at the specialist level required of the community health care nurse.

Triage was considered the most appropriate way forward because practice nurses and other community nurses are increasingly required to make an immediate assessment of health need and to intervene as appropriate. From this premise, it is believed that these nurses, with adequate preparation and working towards carefully defined protocols, are well placed to expand their role within the context of primary health care settings. The emphasis throughout the project was to produce a practitioner who is able to communicate in an effective and appropriate manner, competent and confident to work alongside GPs in a triaging capacity, professionally aware of their own accountability and levels of responsibility and proactive in encouraging the appropriate use of services available to the client group.

In an attempt to ensure that the education appropriately met the needs of the main stakeholders it was agreed that the course would only be available to nurses who were working in primary health care settings and were willing to participate in a triage programme. Hence, it was required that the infrastructure of the setting in which the nurses were working had to be willing and able to accommodate the available service. This included an ability to develop clinical protocols and the provision of a mechanism through which nurses could access immediate advice and guidance from a medical practitioner. This decision came to be challenged many times, but on evaluation of the first course members, it was an important prerequisite. It certainly lent weight and credence to the nurse's request for teaching and guidance in the practice situation.

Early Evaluation

The range of interprofessional involvement evident throughout the project was higher than at first anticipated, and the degree of collaboration and team working between all parties was commendable. This supports one of the basic premises underpinning the course, that triage, although shifting the context of delegation and consultation across professional boundaries, can also impact on collaboration and teamwork. Early evaluation showed that most students had a flawed understanding of the concept of triage on entry to the course. Most thought that as nurses working in a triage setting they would undertake tasks previously carried out by GPs without fully considering notions of autonomy and accountability. This perception of role fits with the view of extension, as opposed to expansion, of the nurse's role as expressed by the UKCC (1994). By the end of the course however, most practitioners had modified their views and were able to critically examine the issues surrounding nursing triage in primary care settings. Most had developed a range of skills enabling them to intervene safely and effectively in a variety of settings.

Overall, most nurses felt supported in practice, but for some life was not easy. Despite the fact that every effort was made to ensure that the course would be available only to nurses working in primary health care settings who were willing to participate in a triage programme, the failure – for whatever reason – of other staff to acknowledge this new way of working and reservations about delegation and teamwork occasionally surfaced. This finding is hardly surprising; the notion of delegation in general practice has been around for some time. Indeed, in the early 1990s Robinson (1990) suggested that delegation to nurses could be used as a solution for GPs struggling to cope with their increased workload – a view that was supported some years later by the findings of the 'York' study, which explored issues of skill mix in primary care (Jenkins-Clarke & Carr-Hill 1996).

While acknowledging that disputes about delegation, roles and boundaries still exist, the experiences of nurses who have completed the triage course have been positive. Ongoing evaluation will seek to explore whether or not this programme of care reflects patient need, recognizes the distinctive contribution of professionals and, where appropriate, helps to integrate primary and secondary care services.

The triage course is only one example of recent developments in practice nursing that have been driven by government policy and changes in the organization and delivery of health care. Another example is NHS Direct, the 24-hour nurse-led telephone advice line that offers callers a 24-hour service.

NHS Direct

According to the Minister of Health, NHS Direct, the 24-hour nurse-led telephone advice line that offers callers an around-the-clock service is a key component of the Government's 10-year plan to modernize the NHS. Initially three pilot sites envisaged in the white paper were established, based at NHS Ambulance Services Trusts. According to a government spokesperson, a Department of Health analysis of these three pilot schemes after the first 5 weeks has proved very positive.

The Findings

On analysis, the Department of Health evaluation showed that in the first 5 weeks of operation, approximately 70% of callers were redirected to the services they required or were helped to care for themselves at home. Approximately 700 people (25% of callers) were given advice on how to help themselves at home. Around 130 people were reassured that their needs could be met by a routine visit to their doctor. However, 40 callers were unaware that they needed urgent help from the emergency services and were diverted to 999.

Commenting on the success of the pilot schemes, Alan Milburn, Minister of Health said 'NHS Direct is already proving its worth for patients. It has put patients in touch, quickly and easily, with expert advice and help, 24 hours a day, 365 days a year'.

As a result the service expanded to cover up to 15 million people through a second wave of pilot sites.

Conclusion

Other examples of nurse-led initiatives could be cited, but in this brief discussion it is necessary to be selective. What is certain is that for practice nurses and other nurse members of the primary care team, the future looks good. General practice is at the centre of change and as such needs nurses who are able to communicate effectively, are competent negotiators, professionally aware of their own accountability and proactive in encouraging appropriate use of services to their client groups. Against this backdrop of opportunity it is vital that as a profession we rise to this challenge. We cannot afford to get it wrong or we may lose the opportunity to influence and shape the service.

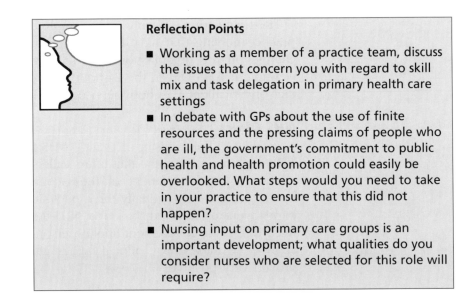

Reflection Points

- Working as a member of a practice team, discuss the issues that concern you with regard to skill mix and task delegation in primary health care settings
- In debate with GPs about the use of finite resources and the pressing claims of people who are ill, the government's commitment to public health and health promotion could easily be overlooked. What steps would you need to take in your practice to ensure that this did not happen?
- Nursing input on primary care groups is an important development; what qualities do you consider nurses who are selected for this role will require?

In summary:

- the white paper *The New NHS* (Command 3807, 1997) sets out the government's proposals for action and change. The case for a primary care-led NHS is restated in this document
- according to government policy the overall objective of a primary care-led NHS is to improve the health of the nation and the efficiency and effectiveness of NHS care
- the New NHS will pursue a new approach to health, a 'third way', which involves the creation of a national contract for health that formally acknowledges a link between poverty and ill-health
- the establishment of primary care groups and Trusts is at the centre of the new health service
- as a result of government policy, the organization and workload of general practice and nurses working in primary health care settings have experienced and are experiencing a period of rapid and major change.

Annotated Further Reading

- Jenkins-Clarke S, Carr-Hill R 1996 Measuring skill mix in primary care: dilemmas of delegation and diversification. Discussion paper 144. Centre for Health Economics, University of York, York *This paper outlines some of the issues surrounding skill mix in primary care settings. It also discusses issues related to the delegation of tasks.*

- Gordon P, Hadley J (eds) 1996 Extending primary care. Radcliffe Medical Press, Oxford. *This book explores some of the current developments in primary care. It also examines what is meant by primary care.*

- Fatchet A 1994 Politics, policy and nursing. Ballière Tindall, London. *This book addresses some of the main reforms in the provision of health care. It also challenges the reader to consider their response to some of these issues.*

References

Baggott R 1994 Health care in Britain. St Martin's Press, London

Department of Health 1986 Neighbourhood nursing: a focus for care. The Cumberlege report. HMSO, London

Department of Health 1989a Working for patients. Command 555. HMSO, London

Department of Health 1989b Caring for people. HMSO, London

Department of Health 1990a General Medical Service Council – new GP contract. HMSO, London

Department of Health 1990b NHS and community care act. HMSO, London

Department of Health 1992 The health of the nation. HMSO, London

Department of Health 1997 The new NHS. Modern. Dependable. HMSO, London

Department of Health 1998 Our healthier nation. HMSO, London

Dooris M 1998 Working with unemployment and poverty: a training manual for health promotion. South Bank Polytechnic, London

Disken S 1990 Models of clinical management. Institute of Health Services Management, London

Enthoven AC 1985 National Health Service: some reforms that might be politically feasible. Economist 295(7399):19–22

Fatchet A 1994 Politics, policy and nursing. Ballière Tindall, London

Glennerster H, Matsagnis M, Owens P, Hancocks S 1994 Implementing GP fundholding. Wild card or winning hand? Open University Press, Buckingham

Gordon P, Hadley J (eds) 1996 Extending primary care. Radcliffe Medical Press, Oxford

Gordon P, Plampling D 1996 Primary health care – its characteristics and potential. In: Gordon P, Hadley J (eds) Extending primary care. Radcliffe Medical Press, Oxford

Griffiths R 1983 Report of the NHS management inquiry. DHSS, London

Harrison S, Schulz RI 1989 Clinical autonomy in the UK and the US: contrasts and convergence. In:

Freddie G, Bjorkam JW (eds) Controlling medical professionals. Sage, London

Holliday I 1992 The NHS transformed. Baseline Books, Manchester

Jenkins-Clarke S, Carr-Hill R 1996 Measuring skill mix in primary care: dilemmas of delegation and diversification. Discussion paper 144. Centre for Health Economics, University of York, York

Mackenzie A, Ross F 1997 Shifting the balance in primary health care. British Journal of Community Nursing 23:139–142

NHS Management Executive 1992 The nursing skill mix in district nurse service. HMSO, London

NHS Management Executive 1993 New world, new opportunities: nursing in primary health care. HMSO, London

NHS Management Inquiry Team 1983 The Griffith report. HMSO, London

Peckham S 1996 NHS policy developments. In: Gastrell P, Edwards J (eds) Community health nursing frameworks for practice. Baillière Tindall, London

Ranade W 1994 A future for the nurse in the 1990s. Longman, London

Rashid A, Watts A, Lenehan C 1996 Skill mix in primary care: sharing clinical workload and understanding professional roles. British Journal of General Practice 46: 639–640

Robinson G 1990 The future for practice nurses. British Journal of General Practice April: 132–133

Royal College of GPs 1996 Skill-mix in primary care – sharing clinical workload and understanding professional roles. Report no: C82. Royal College of General Practitioners, London

Sines D 1997 The search for constancy in community health nursing. British Journal of Community Nursing 2(5)

Smail J 1996 Shifting the boundaries in practice nursing. In: Gastrell P, Edwards J (eds) Community health nursing frameworks for practice. Ballière Tindall, London

Taylor D 1991 Developing primary care: opportunities for the 1990s. King's Fund Institute, London

UKCC 1991 Report on proposals for the future of community education and practice, post registration and practice project. United Kingdom Central Council for Nursing, Midwifery and Health Visiting, London

UKCC 1994 The future of professional practice – the Council's standards for education and practice following registration. United Kingdom Central Council for Nursing, Midwifery and Health Visiting, London

World Health Organization 1978 Alma-Ata: primary health care. World Health Organization, Geneva

World Health Organization 1984 Regional targets in support of the Regional Strategy for Health for All. World Health Organization Regional Office for Europe, Geneva

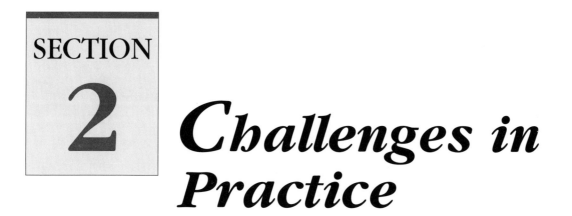

SECTION
2

Challenges in Practice

5 Conceptual Frameworks for Practice

Lynda Carey

Introduction

Practice nursing is undergoing a period of change influenced not only by the development and maturing of the role in general practice, but also by the changing structure and nature of health care delivery within the United Kingdom. As the organizational and structural changes impact upon practice nursing there is a grave danger that the very essence of nursing and its core philosophy may be overlooked in a drive for nurses to meet the short-term goals of a health service and their employers. The potential loss of the essence of nursing is undoubtedly pertinent to all nurses, but perhaps more so for practice nurses, given the isolation and domination of their workload by GPs (Jones 1997). If nurses working in general practice are to be recognized as complementary practitioners to the GP and move away from the perspective of the handmaiden or doctor's assistant (Greenfield et al 1987), they will need to identify and define their own unique contribution to primary care provision and gain professional recognition of their status (Graham 1996). In moving towards this goal the recognition of a unique and distinct body of knowledge is vital. Nursing theory's contribution to the development of practice nursing as a discipline cannot be underestimated, for as nursing theory has the potential to contribute to practice development, so will the development of nursing practice within general practice add to the growing body of nursing knowledge.

In examining the impact of nursing theory on practice nursing this chapter will explore the concept of nursing theory and its relationship to practice nursing. Recognizing the influence of a medical model of care on existing practice, it will argue that the development of nursing practice and its subsequent influence upon the primary health care agenda must value nursing knowledge and question why nursing knowledge and theory have failed to add to the development of practice nursing. The chapter will contest that in recognizing the value and development of nursing theory practice nurses will be able to identify the positive contribution nursing plays to the patient relationship.

Key Issues

- Nursing theory – what is it?
- Nursing philosophy – how is it impacting on current nursing practice?
- Using nursing models to identify the contribution of

nursing to the development of nursing practice
- Critical care pathways – what use for nursing in general practice?

Defining Nursing

To identify and distinguish the contribution of nursing theory to practice, it is perhaps important first to define the wider concept of nursing. This is not as easy as one might first expect. Nightingale in her *Notes on Nursing*, 1860 explicitly identifies the core problem of role definition stating 'I will use the word nursing for want of a better' (Nightingale 1978).

It is daunting to consider that Nightingale was unable to clearly define the emerging discipline, although perhaps not as disturbing as her belief that patients' need for nursing care, spiritual support and a healthy environment were secondary to the overriding needs of the medical profession to have an assistant (Salvage 1985).

Nevertheless, since Nightingale's first naive attempts at defining nursing many theorists have subsequently attempted to quantify nursing – each with only limited success. Peplau (1988) defined nursing as '... a healing art, assisting an individual who is sick or in need of health care'.

This emphasis on sickness is further developed by Salvage (1985) who defines nursing as 'looking after sick people'. This apparently clear definition is not without its initial problems, for as Salvage herself states, the concept of care is not the sole prerogative of the nurse, with the majority of care being provided outside the formal framework of nursing. Similarly, the concept of 'sickness' is in itself difficult to define; Naidoo & Wills (1994) state the issue of concept of health and sickness for the individual is not absolute, instead it is a social construct negotiated between individuals and dependent upon society's perceptions and expectations of health. This is clearly evident in individuals' presentation and definition of their own levels of ill health. Salvage's definition is also criticized for its failure to recognize the health promoting content of the nurse's role. Bryar (1994) and Kulbok & Baldwin (1992) identify this as a fundamental component of nursing, and particularly appropriate for practice nurses for whom the core of work does not centre on the management of sick people, but rather the promotion of health (UKCC 1996). In contrast to Peplau's and Salvage's core component of sickness, Virginia Henderson defined nursing as:

'... assisting the individual (sick or well) in the performance of those activities contributing to health, or its recovery (or peaceful death) that he would perform unaided if he had the necessary strength, will or knowledge' (Harmer & Henderson 1955).

Although dated, Henderson's definition has been a seminal piece of work from which a number of nursing models have subsequently developed. In contrast to Peplau's definition it focuses on the concept in health, although the concept of health is as problematic to define as that of sickness.

The debate and attempts in defining nursing continue, with a failure to offer any real clarity to the issue of what nursing itself is. A more recent definition is offered by the American Nurses Association (1980) who aim for precision in defining nursing as 'the diagnosis and treatment of human responses to actual or potential problems'.

This definition offers both simplicity in its role and importantly focuses on the human context of nursing care provision. Yet, Rogers (1990, cited in George 1995) argues that defining nursing is a complex issue, taking upon board both a theoretical and hands-on approach. The centrality of the human experience is expounded by Rogers (1990) in describing nursing science as 'a science of humanity – the study of irreducible human beings and their environments'.

In placing the human experience at the centre of nursing, Rogers' work clearly highlights the contribution of both the theoretical and practical component of nursing as a discipline. The value of a theoretical perspective to nursing care has long been established, as witnessed by Nightingale's vision for nursing, in recognizing the importance of a theoretical framework for practice (Nightingale 1978). Dale (1994) supports the contribution of the underlying theoretical framework, arguing that without such a framework, nursing will become a series of unplanned events. The theoretical framework allows nursing to describe, explain, predict and therefore control nursing events (Dale 1994). It is this contextual framework for nursing that is fundamental to the development of a clearer definition (Waterman, Webb & Williams 1995).

The lack of consensus of definition is a fundamental issue in the development of a professional base from which nursing can develop and achieve professional recognition for its contribution to care provision (Oldnall 1995). It is particularly consequential for practice nursing, for as Karen Gupta discusses in her chapter, there is even less clarity about the role and function of the practice nurse. The tradition of naming rather than defining of nursing has enabled the categorization of individual practitioners, and thereby failure to identify the unique nature of nursing. This is compounded by the fact that nursing is not one single discipline, but rather a series of disciplines that share one common basic training element, but thereon after very little. The subsequent labelling of different groups of nurses has the potential and reality of fragmenting nursing, and thereby undermining the core elements of nursing practice; the RCN (Salvage 1985) highlights the strength in nursing as lying in its 'adaptive and generalist nature'. Yet, the drive for recognition has led nurses to become divisive as each grouping competes for control and power over another group, subsequently with nursing perceived as the higher status technical tasks (Salvage 1985).

What Then is Nursing Knowledge?

The lack of consensus in defining nursing as a discipline results in the further difficulty in defining nursing knowledge, for if there is a lack of consensus in defining nursing then it is understandable that there is likely to be difficulty in defining what constitutes nursing knowledge. The importance of identifying the distinctness of nursing knowledge, and specifically that of practice nursing knowledge, cannot be overlooked in shaping the professional distinction of nursing and thereby identifying its contribution to care provision. Traynor (1996) reasons that the importance of identifying the underlying philosophical and moral base that defines nursing knowledge is particularly vital at a time when there is the dominance of the market rationalism. The necessity to identify unique knowledge, however, has only latterly been adopted within nursing. As late as 1974 Johnson maintained that nursing was 'a field of practice without a scientific heritage … a profession without the theoretical base it seems to require' (Johnson 1974). This is a pertinent comment given that Nightingale in her writing identified the importance of an underlying theoretical basis to practice (Trolley 1995). However, it can be argued that it was Nightingale's own emphasis on tasks and procedures that has contributed to the reluctance of nursing to adopt a theoretical base, and led to the subsequent emphasis of nursing as solely a practical discipline.

The difficulties in defining nursing have led nurses to be unsure of the relevance of a wider theoretical approach to the subject. The argument for a theoretical framework to practice is strong; however, in reality nursing is still perceived as a practical discipline. It is this more traditional perspective of nursing that identifies nurses as 'good nurses are born and not made' (Salvage 1985, p. 3). This is further developed in the context of practice nursing, and specifically the belief that the characteristics of the good practice nurse are close to the ideal of a 'good mother' than that of a professional (Greenfield et al 1987). The ensuing rejection of a theoretical base is a belief held by nurses who perceive nursing to be a hands-on approach and not a theoretical discipline. This perception is prevalent in practice nursing, with analysis of reasons for the move into this field of nursing being the proximity of patient contact. The reluctance to adopt a theoretical framework is evidenced in nursing's hesitance, until recently, to embrace higher education as a move towards professionalism (Dale 1994).

The value of knowledge is not purely concerned with the recognition of professional status and thereby the power acquisition that may accompany this. Instead Salvage (1985) stresses the value of knowledge specific to the preparation for caring. The core value of care in nursing has not at times been perceived as legitimate knowledge by nursing as a profession, given that nursing has traditionally looked to explicit or formal knowledge over intuitive knowledge, preferring to place a greater status on 'knowing that' rather than 'knowing how' (Rhead & Strange 1996). This raises the question of 'what then constitutes nursing knowledge'? This question is not without its complications; both Traynor (1996) and Rafferty, Allcock & Lathlean (1996) characterize nursing knowledge as a historically and socially constructed phenomenon. This is identified in the tradition of nursing using the male-constructed values of science in defining its knowledge needs to gain autonomy and social status (Traynor 1996). However, in attempting to gain social status the continued reliance on male-dominated scientific approaches devalues the very essence of nursing, namely the art of caring (Hagell 1989). Hagell (1989) argues that nursing knowledge is 'based in part on their situation as women in a patriarchal society and in part as women involved in a specific gender defined occupation – nursing which is given little value in society'. This raises a concern surrounding distinct practice nursing knowledge, given its relatively short historical development and the continued dominance by medicine and medical practitioners.

In contrast to the traditional development of knowledge, Carper (1978) argues that nursing knowledge cannot be limited to a purely positivistic approach, instead categorizing nursing knowledge into four distinct categories (Box 5.1).

The concept of the art of nursing equates to Benner's concept of expertise where the nurse is aware of the stimuli given to the patient and uses both experiential and positivistic knowledge in giving care (Benner 1984). Carper (1978) argues that comprehension is not reliant upon one form, but must include all four components for nursing knowledge to be achieved. Recognizing the different forms and patterns of knowledge is crucial to the development of nursing practice (Huntington, Gilmour & O'Connell 1996). Without such a comprehensive approach Chinn & Jacobs (1987) argue that nurses focus on only one particular aspect of a problem and not the problem as a whole.

Box 5.1

Categories of Nursing Knowledge (Carper 1978)

■ Empirics – the science of nursing – this traditional perspective of knowledge encompasses a positivistic scientific view of nursing, based upon testable assumptions

■ Ethics – this category classifies the moral knowledge that is held by nurses in the care decision process

■ Personal knowing – in recognizing the complexity of knowledge, Carper recognizes the contribution of experiential learning that develops as practitioners gain experience; it is the personal knowing or experiential learning that allows the nurse to gain an understanding of the events (Dale 1994)

■ Aesthetics – the art of nursing – this is a complex concept but primarily centres upon the knowledge that the nurse brings to the interaction with the client or patient.

Although Carper's work enables nursing to examine the concepts that jointly compose the totality of nursing knowledge, it does not explicitly define what constitutes the positivistic element of knowledge relevant to nursing. This lack of clarity concerning the positivistic constituent of nursing knowledge has led nursing, in its attempt to reject medical domination, to favour a social science approach (Oldnall 1995). This is evidenced by the inclusion of the 'ologies' within nursing curricula (Trnobranski 1997). This approach is unhesitating in its move away from a biomedical approach, but it is questionable whether it addresses the issue of providing knowledge that facilitates the development of care. The lack of research and investigation in this perspective (Oldnall 1995) has led nursing to continue to look to other disciplines to define its knowledge base.

What Knowledge do Practice Nurses Use?

The difficulty in defining nursing knowledge is equally valid within the discipline of practice nursing. Although a real issue for all nurses, practice nurses are further hindered by both their lack of heritage, and importantly by the uncertain nature of the presenting issue of many clients. These two factors further cloud the development of a core body of knowledge specific to practice nursing. Nevertheless, within the United Kingdom, the contextual knowledge for practice nursing is defined by UKCC, within the standards for specialist practitioner status as a higher level of knowledge surrounding the provision of practice nursing care. This includes assessment, diagnosis and treatment, health screening and health management programmes for chronic disease (UKCC 1996).

This short definition by the UKCC emphasizes the inherent difficulties in defining both roles and the underpinning knowledge

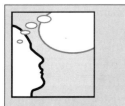

Reflection Points

■ Consider how practice nurses aim to define their professional standing

■ How do you use your own nursing knowledge base?

that is fundamentally a behavioural discipline based upon human interaction. However, the challenge for practice nursing is to gain recognition and parity in professional standing, because it is through this process that practice nurses will have the greatest opportunity to recognize and articulate their contribution to care. The difficulties for practice nursing therefore lie not only in the lack of clarity surrounding the role, but also the lack of a unique body of knowledge to underpin practice. Development of nursing theory is a means of professionalizing nursing, with the greater the degree of abstract knowledge the greater social status afforded to a profession (Rafferty et al 1996).

Nursing Theory in Practice

The difficulties in defining nursing and identifying the specifics of nursing knowledge have implications for the development of theoretical perspectives from which nurses practice. Specifically, the fundamental problem in defining nursing is that the definitions mean little or anything to nurses in their actual practice setting. Indeed the difficulty in defining practice in a meaningful context has led to a number of theorists instead to define nursing in terms of its theoretical concepts. Fraser (1996) defines nursing as a 'series of concepts', with nursing models characterized as the different ways in which nurses can frame a situation. This proposition identifies little difference between a nursing theory and a conceptual model for practice (Barnum 1996); instead they can be classified as a means of understanding and developing practice.

This perspective may be disputed for its naivety because nursing theory is more than a simple set of concepts and must also incorporate the relationship with the client or patient. This is what Dickoff & James (1968) argue is a 'situation-producing theory' and as such will increase relevance to practice – a fundamental issue as nursing is concerned with gaining knowledge for the purpose of assuring sound practice (Cook 1991). The move towards a situational base theory, Trnobranski (1997) argues, is consistent with nursing's present drive to refocus itself away from a biomedical model towards a holistic model. This move away from the medical model of care is prevalent in many nursing disciplines (Barker, Reynolds & Stevenson 1997) and can be argued as the most influential factor presently shaping nursing's theoretical development.

Given that nursing incorporates the human relationship based on the need for care it is wrong to suppose that nursing theory will be identified in a simplistic approach. Barnum (1996) highlights the value of the complexity nursing theory as offering a contextual human-based approach, which facilitates the nurse to make sense of the situation. He argues that without such a complex approach nursing cannot be placed within the reality of the care situation and will therefore be rejected by practitioners. In this approach, the impact of nursing theory, research and practice are recognized as codependent variables that impact upon the practice of nursing.

However, for nursing, the issue is often the division between the theory and practice gap. Rafferty et al (1996) argue that this divide between practice and theory is perceived as a key problem for the development of nursing. The underlying assumption is that the division of practice is separate to theory, yet they are intrinsically linked – a circular link between theory and practice.

Barnum (1996) argues for the interdependence of theory, research and practice; in reality there has been a reluctance by nurses to use nursing theory in practice. The reasons for the rejection of nursing theory are highlighted by Basford & Slevin (1995) as a lack of time, support for change and preparation and the individual's perception that what they are doing is right. However, the perceived lack of impact on practice is the strongest argument for the rejection of all theoretical concepts within the practice setting (Francke, Garssen & Huijer Abu-Saad 1995).

The apparent reluctance to use theoretical models for practice has led to a long debate in nursing about the apparent theory–practice gap, and the implications of this on nursing care provision. Trolley (1995) contests that the theory–practice gap is a manifestation of the underlying power struggle for moral supremacy that exists between nursing theorists and practitioners. The underlying assumption that there is a direct correlation between theory and practice can lead to a situation where either the practitioner or theorist is perceived as failing in the implementation of a theoretical perspective. Rafferty et al (1996) argue that this approach is fundamentally detrimental and hinders practitioners in taking responsibility for their own work.

The difficulty has in part arisen from the perception that there is one nursing framework or model that will offer nurses insight into all care activities. This perception is undoubtedly false and no single model is appropriate given the complexity of the situations in the delivery of nursing care (Waterman et al 1995). Furthermore, Fraser (1996) argues that no model will provide all the answers – therefore the adoption of multimodel analysis is recommended, although the choice of model is linked to the reflective decision making.

In response to the apparent stark division between theory and practice, a new concept for analysis has developed from the belief that the two are intrinsically linked and should not be separated (Rolfe 1993). This new concept, defined as praxis theory, fails to accept formal theory as valuable to nursing practice. In contrast to the belief that nursing theory and practice are separate codependent concepts, the premise builds directly on Kolb's (1984) contention that 'knowledge is created and recreated through experience in context'. Nursing praxis is defined as the bridging of theory and practice, involving a continual process of hypothesizing and testing out new ideas (Rolfe 1993). The development of theory from practice is central to realizing the potential and influence of nursing actions, thereby articulating the contribution of nursing to care provision.

The recognition of the complementary nature of nursing theory to practice in practice nursing will be crucial for future development given that at present there is little development of new nursing theory within this approach. In response to this, praxis theory has identified the value of informal theory generated from practical situations by reflection in action. This approach facilitates development and change in practice through the development of a reflective approach, which facilitates the application of theory back to practice. Such an approach is based upon a core philosophy of nursing that believes that 'becoming a nurse is more than learning from practice, it is learning through it' (Keen & Shannon 1991). The importance of learning from practice is articulated by Benner (1984), who argues that through an experiential approach nurses are able to develop their skills and perceptions. The resultant awareness of patient needs, Benner maintains, enables nurses to develop an intuitive perception, and thereby pre-empt patients' needs. This approach she identifies as 'expert' practice. Although not achieved by all nurses, this level of practice is evolved through a reflective basis of examining one's own practice and individual interaction with clients.

For this approach to be widely adopted there is a need for nurses to be able to reflect upon their own practice; without such an approach, learning, and therefore the development of practice, will not be achievable. Yet in reality, nurses in practice have been slow to adopt a reflective approach to their own practice, highlighting difficulties in implementation, such as a lack of time and knowledge of the process of reflection. Although an admirable concept it is still relatively new for many nurses and has only been widely adopted into nurse education over the past decade. Disconcertingly, the adoption of such an approach is often perceived with negativity, given that it encourages nurses to examine their own practice. The issue of a change in the control and perspective of nursing is most dramatic because as nurses we have traditionally been socialized into accepting and not encouraged to question practice for ourselves. Indeed, the strong socializing element of nurse education up to the mid to late 1980s can be seen to make an appreciable contribution to the development of practice nursing and the incorporation of nursing theory into practice. As Atkin et al (1993) identified, most practice nurses undertook nurse training before this period and were therefore not exposed to the concepts of nursing theory and reflection as younger nurses have been. Similarly, until relatively recently nurses were conditioned to be nonchallenging in the application of practice (Wiles 1997). It is, therefore, even more important that practice nurses consider the issue of reflective practice and its potential impact upon practice development.

However, even in acknowledging the present reluctance to adopt a reflective approach to practice, the development of praxis theory has been criticized. In particular, criticism has been levelled because it places greater responsibility at the hands of the practitioner, and builds upon the values of self-reliance and self-improvement (Powell 1989). The approach is also criticized for encouraging introspection at the expense of looking outward at the wider political context. Powell (1989) argues that it fails to recognize the impact of the political environment, and therefore the complexity of the implementation process. Indeed, Rolfe (1993) highlights that instead of hindering practice development the gap between theory and practice is positive in encouraging change and development that impact upon practice.

What Value Then of Nursing Theory to Practice Nurses?

The debate over the value of nursing theory to practice is crucial to practice nurses given the challenges faced by a changing structure of a health services and the subsequent growing emphasis on demonstrating clinical effectiveness. However, the continued definition of clinical effectiveness as measurable outcomes is particularly difficult for nursing because the contribution of nursing to care has been seen to be immeasurable (Rafferty et al 1993). Kitson (1993) identifies the value of a nursing theory as a means of 'explaining what nurses do'; nursing theories are a means of quantifying nursing action and therefore can have an impact upon both care outcomes and nursing status. This is particularly fundamental for practice nursing, for without the adoption of a nursing framework for practice, practice nurses will only be perceived as nurses undertaking a series of delegated tasks (Damant, Martin & Openshaw 1994).

Identifying nursing as simply a series of tasks is potentially dangerous for practice nursing on two levels. First, it fails to recognize the human context of nursing and the impact of this on patient and client welfare. This is evident in the value placed by patients on having someone to talk to, a quality that is difficult to measure or quantify. Similarly, this approach raises the problem of how nursing is perceived and the inherent variation between nurses' definition of the discipline and the public's perception. Nurses are still appreciated by the general public for their caring, warm approach, with little consideration given to their professional training and underlying theoretical knowledge.

Second, the focus on tasks alone leads to an issue of skill mix for practice nursing and the potential for tasks to be undertaken by either support workers or other groups of nurses. The value of nursing theory is important on a third level in recognizing the inherent value of nursing theory to care provision (Traynor 1996). Traynor stresses that as nursing has sought to become professionalized, there is a drive to define the underlying power base of the profession, and this is an important issue for practice nurses if they are to move away from the dominant medical model. For professional development to become reality, both practice nursing and individual nurses must articulate their objectives and demonstrate and measure their impact using identified criteria (Bloomfield et al 1982, cited in Traynor 1996).

Applying Nursing Theory and Models to Practice Nursing

Practice nursing has traditionally been dominated by the overriding beliefs and dominance of the medical model of practice. In contrast to the medical model, nursing models offer a means of understanding the situation and of achieving results based on the underlying philosophy of the nurse, namely caring. However, an analysis within the general practice setting, suggests little evidence of their widespread use by nurses (Carey 1994). If models of care are identified there is a concentration around Roper, Logan & Tierney's *Activities of Daily Living* model of care. Although this is a useful model in advocating the move towards independence of patients, it is questionable whether it is wholly applicable within the general practice setting. Indeed, for models of nursing care to be used it is vital that they are relevant to the individual situation faced by the nurse (Walsh 1998).

McMurray (1993) in examining the application of nursing models to community nursing, argues that it is critical that models identify individuals in terms of their wider social structure and environment. This may be particularly relevant in terms of considering the interaction of patients with practice nurses because the interaction is often only limited in time span. The practice nurse has the potential to understand and actively consider the environment within which the client lives, given the relatively static nature of populations and knowledge of the local environment. The emphasis on the contextual nature of the individual nursing situation focuses nurses away from the use of single models of care for all patients and clients towards choosing the most appropriate model for each situation.

The following section offers the opportunity to examine models of care that have the potential to facilitate the development of nursing care for the individual client. In exploring these issues it is necessary to recognize that models of care are not prescribed methods of care, but seek to offer a blueprint for practice; as Walsh (1998) highlights, it is vital to acknowledge that there is a need to modify the model according to the client needs. The model should aid the nurse in identifying client needs and not, as is often perceived, identify client needs within an inappropriate model.

Orem's Self Care Nursing Model

Developed in the United States, this model of care has been widely used within the United Kingdom, although predominantly within the field of mental health nursing. The emphasis of the model identifies nursing intervention in the maintenance of self care activities in the acute illness episode and normalization and integration of the individual within society. The model is based upon the fundamental principle that when individuals are able to care for themselves, they do. When they are not in a position to do this the nurse interacts to care for the individual (Orem 1995).

Orem's model of nursing care is built around the two categories of self care demands (Box 5.2). Self care demands are the needs of the individual in relation to their ability to self care.

Box 5.2

Orem's Model of Self Care – Self Care Demands

1. Universal self care – this category incorporates the actions the individual will undertake to maintain basic human needs. These incorporate:
   — air, food and water
   — excretion
   — activity and rest
   — solitude and socialization
   — hazards to life and wellbeing
   — normalization – the effort the individual places on being identified as normal
2. Health deviation category – this occurs when the individual is not able to sufficiently meet their own self care needs as a result of changes in their body structure, physical environment, behaviour or activities of daily living (Fraser 1996) – if the individual is unable to make up for this deviation themselves they may need assistance from a nurse – Orem defines this intervention as a nursing agency (Orem 1995)

Box 5.3

Self Care Requisites identified by Orem (1995)

■ Acting for
■ Teaching
■ Guiding
■ Supporting
■ Encouraging development

Nursing Intervention

The nursing intervention is structured on determining why the individual needs nursing intervention. This involves the ability of the individual to self care now and in the future, and identification of any deficits they may have in self caring. The role of the nurse is to wholly compensate for the present self care deficits (this may be more appropriate in an acute episode of care), partly compensate (e.g. in a rehabilitative situation) or provide an educational approach. It is this educational approach that it can be argued is most appropriate for the community and general practice setting. The nursing plan is then implemented using the five categories of self care requisites (Box 5.3).

Using Orem's Model in General Practice

Orem's model within a general practice setting is best considered in the management of individual clients who have long-term chronic illness. The role of the practice nurse within this situation is often not the management of the disease, but to work with the individual to enable them to self care. Through such an approach individuals are able to examine the impact of their physical condition upon their lifestyle and behaviour. As the model is not based upon direct caring for clients within the community setting, it facilitates the nurse to plan her intervention in a structure that identifies her role as advocate, educator and supporter in achieving individual development.

Neuman's Model of Care

Like Orem's model, Neuman's model of care (Box 5.4) was developed in the United States (Neuman 1989). This model promotes a philosophy of holistic care provision. In adopting such an approach to nursing care Neuman argues that it is important for nurses to consider the impacts of life upon the individual, and these are identified as both external and internal stressors. In promoting her model of nursing care Neuman defines health as a degree of stability maintained by the body and identifies this stability as existing along a continuum between wellness and illness (George 1995). The concept of health occurring on a continuum offers the opportunity for the individual to define themselves as healthy even though they are nearer

Box 5.4

Newman's Model – components that impact upon the individual's health and identified by Neuman in structuring her model of nursing care

1. Basic structure and energy resources
   — the basic structure for the individual consists of the genetic structure of the individual, and the functioning of the body systems
   — for the individual to achieve system stability or homeostasis, there must be more energy input than is used by the body systems
2. Client variables – these are the factors that influence the individual's ability to achieve optimum stability and are identified by Neuman as:
   — physiological variable
   — psychological variable (based upon the individual's relationships and mental health status)
   — sociocultural variables (those related to the social, cultural expectations and activities undertaken by the individual)
   — development variable (this relates to the individual's development in relation to their expectations in terms of lifespan)
   — spiritual variable (Neuman argues that this is the least understood variable within nursing and highlights the importance of the individual's spiritual beliefs in achieving holistic care provision for individuals)
3. Lines of defence – these are defined as the processes that protect the body when activated by environmental stressors (e.g. the body's immune system)
   — normal line of defence (this is defined by Neuman as the usual level of stability that may change over time as a result of reaction to external factors)
   — flexible line of defence (similar to the normal line of defence, but acts as a flexible line and a buffer to attacks to the line of defence)
4. Environment – these are all the internal and external factors or influences on the individual and are further subcategorized into:
   — internal environment (defined as factors within the individual's body system)
   — external environment
   — created environment (defined by Neuman as the individual's response to stressors from the individual's perception)
   — neuman argues that it is crucial in the delivery of nursing care to examine all aspects of the environment in relation to the client

> **Box 5.4** Cont'd
>
> 5. Stressors – these are the stimuli that have an influence upon individuals and their body system and may be
>   — intrapersonal in nature, namely, from within the body (e.g. the immune system)
>   — interpersonal, that is outside the body but related to the individual (e.g. role expectations)
>   — extrapersonal (i.e. affect the individual but are not related to the individual)

the illness end of the continuum than wellness. This may be particularly important in the management and support of those individuals who have a chronic disease and who themselves feel healthy.

Having defined the concept of health, Neuman describes the key issues for the model as stress and reactions to stress – these may have both a positive and a negative effect upon the individual. As Neuman's model is based upon adaptation, the individual is constantly adapting to the environment, with the environment being influenced by the individual. When the optimum stability is achieved, Neuman identifies this as a revitalizing process.

Nursing Intervention

Given that Neuman's model is perceived primarily as an assessment tool, Neuman defines the role of the nurse as involvement in terms of prevention at a primary, secondary and tertiary level. Primary prevention is in the format of preventing a stressor occurring (e.g. health promotion). Secondary prevention focuses on strengthening the lines of resistance (e.g. treatment). Tertiary prevention is the process to protect the individual's system through supporting existing strengths and maintaining energy.

In using the model in the organization of nursing care, Neuman identifies three key stages. The first stage is that of nursing diagnosis – at this point the nurse identifies the move from health based upon the impact of the variables. These are then negotiated with the individual (the nursing goals phase). The final stage is the setting of nursing outcomes, which are identified using the prevention modes.

Using Neuman's Model in General Practice

Neuman's model has as its core philosophy the belief that the individual is a partner in care provision and therefore offers the mechanism for the practice nurse to work with the individuals in identifying those stressors that have altered their 'stability'. The recognition of stressors and their impact upon health is particularly relevant to practice nurses working with clients who are experiencing either nonacute episodes of illness or are chronically ill because this model facilitates the nurse to examine the wider environment upon health. Walsh (1998) highlights the value of the model in enabling the nurse to gain an understanding of both the stressors and also the patient's own perceptions of them. The model's key strength is in offering a structure that facilitates an assessment of the individual's needs at primary, secondary and tertiary levels.

The Roy Adaptation Model

Like Neuman's model the Roy adaptation model is built on the premise of holistic care provision by the nurse. However, this model recognizes that the individual parts of what constitutes a human being work together to form the whole being, and that there is a constant interaction between the individual and the environment (George 1995).

This model of care recognizes the importance of the individual to adapt to stimuli, which are categorized by Roy as focal, contextual and residual. The focal stimuli are those that directly impact on the individual, the contextual stimuli are those stimuli that can have a positive or negative effect on the individual, and finally, the residual stimuli are those factors for which the impact is not yet known. Roy assumes that as the individual adapts a series of output responses may occur, which can be negative or positive. If the individual is able to meet the output then they are exhibiting adaptive responses. Adaptive responses enable the individual to meet the goals of survival, growth, reproduction and mastery. If the outcomes do not meet these goals then they are identified as ineffective responses (George 1995). These adaptive responses are controlled by what Roy defines as coping mechanisms (Box 5.5).

Nursing Intervention

Within Roy's model the focus of the nursing interaction is to promote adaptive responses in the individual because these adaptive responses promote positive health. As the individual's ability to adapt will vary from time to time, the role of the nurse is to manage the stimuli, thereby enabling the individual to adapt as necessary.

In using this model the nurse must first assess the individual's behaviour in relation to the four adaptive modes; this ensures that the assessment is both holistic and systematic in its approach. Following the behavioural led assessment the nurse identifies the patterns of behaviour that are ineffective or adaptive responses requiring support. From this the nurse aims to identify the internal or external stimuli affecting behaviour. This leads to the identification of assessment goals being set in negotiation with the individual.

Using Roy's Model in General Practice

The potential benefit of Roy's adaptation model to nursing care within general practice is primarily in facilitating the nurse to assess

Box 5.5

Categories of Assessment within Roy's Adaptation Model

In using this model for nursing practice Roy identified four categories for assessment of behaviour that occur as a result of the individual's coping mechanisms. These categories (see below) allow the nurse to assess the individual.

- Physiological mode
    - this is the physical response to external stimuli – the basic needs of the body of oxygenation, nutrition, elimination, activity, rest and protection must be maintained
- Self concept mode
    - this relates to the individual's psychological and spiritual needs and incorporates the issues of body image and self ideal
- Role function mode
    - Roy identifies this as the patterns of social interaction exhibited by the individual in relation to others in society – it is reflected at three different levels
        - at a primary level it is determined by an individual's sex, age and development stage
        - at a secondary level, it is the associated roles and expectations in society dependent upon the primary level (e.g. the expectations of women's behaviour within society)
        - the tertiary roles are those that are chosen freely by the individual
- Interdependence mode
    - as Roy's model is built upon humanistic beliefs, this mode centres on the patterns of human value, affection, love and affirmation, which occur through the process of human relationships

the individual's key needs. The move away from an emphasis on physiological processes encourages the practice nurse to examine the impact of the disease process on the individual – this is central in planning nursing. The examination of both self image and the social interaction are particularly important to consider in assessing the needs of individuals who have chronic disease.

The models identified within this chapter are obviously not exhaustive, but have been chosen as potential frameworks for nursing care in general practice. All demonstrate an approach that incorporates wider environmental issues that impact upon health and also offers a holistic perspective to health. Indeed, in identifying potential models for nursing care practice within the general practice setting, this chapter has deliberately excluded the model devised by Roper, Logan & Tierney (1985). This model draws heavily on the identified activities of daily living as a means of planning care, with a core philosophy that identifies the nurse's role as assisting the individual towards a state of independence, the role of the nurse being to assist the individuals if they have any dependent needs. Although a useful model, it does not address the wider issues of environmental factors, instead favouring an examination of the influences on the individual.

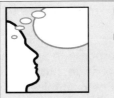

Reflection Point

■ Consider using the models of care within your practice. How does your identification of patient needs differ from not adopting a nursing framework? If so in what manner?

Using a Nursing Model for Practice – the Practical Issues

Given that nursing models offer the practice nurse the opportunity to assess individual needs holistically, it is surprising to encounter a reluctance to use models in the general practice setting. Yet, practice nurses do not use nursing frameworks, often citing practical difficulties in their implementation. To use a nursing model, it is therefore important to consider the issues of time and documentation. This will be fundamental in facilitating the move towards a systematic approach to nursing care delivery within general practice away from the medically dominated task-orientated approach to care delivery.

Time

Faced with many patients to see, nurses often complain that they do not have time to undertake such a detailed assessment. The time allotted to nursing activities has been traditionally set by the traditions of medical practice. Paxton et al (1996) argue that such an approach undermines the contribution of nursing to care provision within general practice. The first meeting with a patient is important for the nurse to build and develop a trusting and supporting relationship (Burnard & Morrison 1991). Such an approach is central to nursing activity and therefore requires the appropriate time to allow the relationship to develop to meet the needs of the individual. The use of a nursing model can facilitate this approach, but requires time. The challenge for practice nurses is to identify and claim the right for appointment times that allow a holistic assessment. This has been achieved by other nurses in general practice, namely, nurse practitioners, whose appointment times are appreciably longer than those of the GP.

Documentation

Recording of information and application of a nursing model are fundamental to the recognition and legitimization of the nursing model, yet within the general practice setting there is reluctance to write detailed notes within the compact Lloyd George notes (Carey 1994).

The justification for this failure to adopt nursing theory was identified as a lack of effective documentation. Although encouraged to write in patients' notes, nurses were positively encouraged to keep notes to a minimum because the doctors were not interested in reading nursing notes, but only in ensuring that the completed task was appropriately recorded. Nevertheless, the recording of the information collected is important both in recognizing the thought process undertaken by the nurse and evidencing the effectiveness of nursing intervention (Girvin 1998). This issue may become less of an obstacle as nurses increasingly use A4 notes within the general practice setting.

Recording of information is now no longer confined to written information, but can be as easily recorded using information technology. Recording detailed information of an individual patient's circumstances can provide an invaluable source of data for identifying practice-based population needs and evaluating the effectiveness of nursing practice.

Limitations to Nursing Theory and Models

The use of nursing theory and models is not without criticism from nurse academics. Most notably, Patricia Benner (1984) has been critical of the reluctance of nurse theorists to recognize and value the contribution of intuitive knowledge. Benner (1984) argues that as nurses move towards expert practitioners, the contribution of nursing models is less explicitly used as information becomes internalized by the nurse. Benner, however, does recognize the contribution of nursing models for nurses not working at this level of practice.

In a more disparaging manner Barker et al (1997) are concerned about the extent to which the scope of the theory is clearly delineated. They highlight that without an explicit definition of the boundaries of the model the nurse may not be aware of its inherent limitations. Similarly, they argue that models must only be used if they are relevant to the patient's problem. In recognizing this they believe that it is important for nurses using models to consider the questions in Box 5.6 to identify the most appropriate model of care.

Box 5.6

Questions to Consider to Identify the Most Appropriate Model of Care

- Does this theory assist me in identifying and understanding my patient's responses to health problems and their consequences?
- Does this theory enable me to identify interventions that will help my patients move toward optimum health?

The issue of aiding patients to achieve their optimum level of health is contestable given that the factors impacting upon health are so great (Naidoo & Wills 1994) and not always in the control of either the patient or the nurse. It is perhaps naive to expect the patient to achieve optimum health, although the move towards this status may in itself be valuable. Given the limitations of nursing models within their purest sense it is necessary to examine how models of care can be used within a wider framework of multidisciplinary care, namely through the use of care pathways.

Care Pathways – Incorporating a Nursing Model into Multidisciplinary Care Provision

Walsh (1998) states that the use of a care pathway in planning care delivery will afford nurses the opportunity to effectively incorporate holistic models of care into practice. Care pathways offer an effective means of reducing the time spent in planning care and the need for detailed written notes, while maintaining a holistic approach (Walsh 1998). Walsh (1998) argues that they are valuable in identifying the effectiveness of nursing care, unlike the nursing process. The fundamental weakness of the nursing process has been that it fails to facilitate the nurse to process information. Nurses need to inform the process around the issues of task, environment and problem – and thereby adopt a problem solving strategy – this can be achieved within the care pathway framework (Walsh 1998). Information processing theory can offer practice nurses the greatest opportunity to use nursing theory in an approach that facilitates the development of a multidisciplinary approach to care delivery in general practice. Indeed, care pathways afford practice nurses the opportunity to articulate nursing intervention in care delivery.

Care pathways offer a different approach to the planning of care delivery in enabling a multidisciplinary approach to care planning. The care pathway facilitates individuals to come together to work together to agree standards of care and expected outcomes for a specific group of patients (Walsh 1998). Tallon (1995) identifies care pathways as 'defacto standards of care', a familiar concept for general practice, where the use of protocols has long been advocated, if not always adopted. Care pathways are not, however, simply protocols; instead they offer a more structured approach to care delivery that takes as their baseline the concept of time, with activities and interventions planned around a specific time scale. In identifying care around the baseline of time the evaluation of both the process and outcomes of care is determined in advance. The development of a framework of care for a specific group of patients allows the care team to evaluate the care delivery at a number of points, both in its effectiveness, and also in the individual's needs in relation to the care pathway.

The use of a general framework enables the practitioner to record only the patient's variance from the pathway. This can only be achieved if the care pathway sets out clear measurable outcomes at various stages of the process. Any variance is problem-solved by the care team in relation to both the care pathway and the patient needs – this approach ensures that individualized patient-centred care is maintained. Indeed, the care pathway is not written to meet the needs of all patients – this is not possible – instead it will only be suitable for the majority of patients. To determine its continued suitability for the target group it is necessary to review the care pathway at regular intervals. At this stage it is important to re-examine the number of patients who vary from the pathway – this analysis may lead to a need to modify the pathway or may raise possible future research issues.

Writing a Care Pathway in General Practice

The fundamental issue for care pathway development is the need to incorporate all those who will deliver or impact upon the care delivery within the writing process. This may sound daunting, but the investment at this initial stage is crucial for a successful implementation. The process of the team writing and agreeing a care pathway requires all participants to compromise to reach a consensus. The byproduct of such an approach can be greater understanding of roles within the team, and the potential for improved team working.

In the process of writing the pathway it is important to avoid a task-orientated approach, which is often a criticism levelled at protocols. In addressing this issue Woodyard & Sheetz (1993) suggest that the outcomes of care should incorporate outcomes from the following categories:

- physiological parameters
- activity and behaviour
- knowledge and discharge planning

It is crucial to clearly define the population or group for which it will be used, for example, patients who have ischaemic heart disease. This appears relatively straightforward; however, given that a marked number of patients within general practice experience comorbidity, it is inappropriate to identify their care within one disease-specific care pathway.

Role of the Nurse

The role of the nurse in the management of care within a pathway approach can include the initial assessment of patients to determine their suitability for the care pathway. It is at this stage of the process that the nurse uses a nursing model to assess patient needs and this is best approached using an interactionalist nursing model, as identified earlier.

Benefits of Care Pathways for Practice Nursing

As identified earlier, the benefits of care pathways are undoubtedly the reduced time needs after initial assessment and increased communication within the team. Walsh (1998) states that care pathways offer the capacity to increase patient involvement in care delivery, and thereby aid in the empowerment process. This can only be achieved if the patient is able to have access to the pathway. The increase in both patient involvement and a team approach to care delivery requires all practitioners to be accountable and responsible for their aspect of care delivery and requires the individuals to keep their knowledge base up to date.

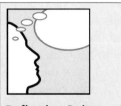

Reflection Point

What benefits can you see in a care pathway approach to care delivery?

Conclusion

Nursing theory is vital for nursing practice – it enables nurses to define their practice and articulate the nursing intervention and its impact upon care delivery. As practice nursing moves towards its next evolutionary phase it is important for nurses to define their contribution to care and not be defined by the needs of the medical profession and government. Nursing theory facilitates this process. The challenge for practice nursing is to use explicit nursing frameworks within the medically dominated environment of general practice. If practice nurses continue to fail to acknowledge and use nursing theory, the continued dominance of the medical model will only further hinder the development of practice nursing, both in its drive towards professional recognition and ability to deliver effective measurable nursing care.

Further Reading

- Walsh M 1998 Models and critical pathways in clinical nursing, 2nd edn. Baillière Tindall, London

References

American Nurses Association 1980 Nursing: a social policy statement. ANA, Kansas City

Atkin K, Lunt N, Parker G, Hirst M 1993 Nurses count: a national census of practice nurses. Social Policy Research Unit, The University of York

Barker PJ, Reynolds W, Stevenson C 1997 The human science basis of psychiatric nursing: theory and practice. Journal of Advanced Nursing. 25:660–667

Barnum BS 1996 Spirituality in nursing: from traditional to new age. Springer Publishing Company, New York

Basford L, Slevin O (eds) 1995 Theory and practice of nursing. Campian, Edinburgh

Benner P 1984 From novice to expert: excellence and power in clinical nursing practice Addison Wesley, California

Bloomfield B, Coombs R, Cooper D, Rea D 1992 Machines and manoeuvres: responsibility accounting and construction of hospital information. Accounting Management and Information Technologies 2(4):199

Bryar R 1994 An examination of the need for new nursing roles in the primary health care team. Journal of Interprofessional Care 8(1):73–75

Burnard P, Morrison P 1991 Client centred counselling: a study of nurses attitudes. Nurse Education Today 11:104–109

Carey L 1994 The role of the nurse in general practice: a comparative study of the role of the practice nurse and nurse practitioner. Unpublished MSc dissertation. University of Liverpool, Liverpool

Carper B 1978 Fundamental patterns of knowing in nursing. Advances in Nursing Science 1:13–23

Chinn P, Jacobs M 1987 Theory and nursing: a systematic approach. Mosby, St Louis

Cook SH 1991 Mind the theory/practice gap in nursing. Journal of Advanced Nursing 16:1462–1469

Dale AE 1994 The theory–theory gap: the challenge for nurse teachers. Journal of Advanced Nursing 20:521–524

Damant M, Martin C, Openshaw S 1994 Practice nursing: stability and change. Mosby, London

Dickoff J, James P 1968 A theory of theories: a position paper. Nursing Research 17:197–203

Francke AL, Garssen B, Huijer Abu-Saad H 1995 Determinants of changes in nurses' behaviour after continuing education: a literature review. Journal of Advanced Nursing 21:371–377

Fraser M 1996 Conceptual nursing in practice, a research based approach, 2nd edn. Chapman & Hall, London

George JB 1985 Nursing theories, the base for professional nursing practice, 4th edn. Prentice Hall International, London

Girvin J 1998 What makes a good nurse leader? Elderly Care 10(4):34–35

Graham I 1996 A presentation of a conceptual framework and its use in the definition of nursing development within a number of nursing development units. Journal of Advanced Nursing 23:260–266

Greenfield S, Stilwell B, Drury M 1987 Practice nurses: social and occupational characteristics. Journal of the Royal College of General Practitioners 37:341–345

Hagell E 1989 Nursing knowledge: women's knowledge. A sociological perspective. Journal of Advanced Nursing 9:77–82

Harmer B, Henderson V 1995 Textbook of the principles and practice of nursing, 5th edn. Macmillan, New York

Huntington A, Gilmour J, O'Connell A 1996 Reforming the practice of nurses: decolonization or getting out from under. Journal of Advanced Nursing 24:364–367

Johnson D 1974 Development of theory: a requisite for nursing as a primary health profession. Nursing Research 23(5):372–377

Jones D 1997 The changing role of the practice nurse. Health and Social Care in the Community 5(2):77–83

Keen T, Shannon A 1991 Fish are the last to discover water. Senior Nurse 11(1):36–38

Kitson A 1993 Nursing: art and science. Chapman & Hall, London

Kolb D 1984 Experiential learning. Prentice Hall, London

Kulbok PA, JH Baldwin 1992 From preventive health behaviour to health promotion: advancing a positive construct of health. Advanced Nursing Science 14(4):50–64

McMurray A 1993 Community health nursing, primary health care in practice, 2nd edn. Churchill Livingstone, Melbourne

Naidoo J, Wills J 1994 Health promotion: foundations for practice. Ballière Tindall, London

Neuman B 1989 The Neuman systems model, 2nd edn. Appleton & Lange, Norwalk

Nightingale F 1978 Notes on nursing: what it is & what it is not. Gerald Duckworth & Co., London

Oldnall AS 1995 Nursing as an emerging academic discipline. Journal of Advanced Nursing 21:605–612

Orem DE 1995 Nursing concepts of practice, 5th edn. Mosby, London

Paxton F, Heaney DJ, Howe JC, Porter AM 1996 A study of interruption rates for practice nurses and general practitioners. Nursing Standard 10(43):33–36

Peplau HE 1988 The art and science of nursing: similarities, differences and relations. Nursing Science Quarterly 1:8–15

Powell JH 1989 The reflective practitioner in nursing. Journal of Advanced Nursing 14:824–832

Rafferty AM, Allcock N, Lathlean J 1996 The theory/practice 'gap': taking issue with the issue. Journal of Advanced Nursing 23:685–691

Rhead M, Strange F 1996 Nursing lecturer/practitioners: can lecturer/practitioners be music to our ears? Journal of Advanced Nursing 24:1265–1272

Rogers ME 1990 The space-age paradigm for new frontiers in nursing. In: Parker ME (ed) Nursing theories in practice. National League for Nursing, New York

Rolfe G 1993 Closing the theory–practice gap: a model of nursing praxis. Journal of Clinical Nursing 2:173–177

Roper N, Logan W, Tierney A 1985 The elements of nursing: a model for nursing based on a model of living. Churchill Livingstone, London

Salvage J 1985 The politics of nursing. Heinemann Nursing, London

Tallon R 1995 Critical paths for wound care. Advances in Wound Care 8(1):26–34

Traynor M 1996 Looking at discourse in a literature review of nursing texts. Journal of Advanced Nursing 23:1155–1161

Trolley KA 1995 Theory from practice for practice: is this a reality? Journal of Advanced Nursing 21:184–190

Trnobranski P 1997 Power and vested interests – tacit influences on the construction of nursing curricula? Journal of Advanced Nursing 25:1084–1088

UKCC 1996 Standards for education and practice following registration: specialist practice transitional arrangements. Registrar's letter 14/199b. United Kingdom Central Council for Nursing, Midwifery and Health Visiting, London

Walsh M 1998 Models and critical pathways in clinical nursing, 2nd edn. Ballière Tindall, London

Waterman H, Webb C, Williams A 1995 Parallels and contradictions in the theory and practice of action research and nursing. Journal of Advanced Nursing 22:779–784

Wiles 1997 Empowering practice nurses in the follow up of patients with established heart disease: lessons from patients' experiences. Journal of Advanced Nursing 26:729–735

Woodyard L, Sheetz J 1993 Critical pathway patient outcomes: the missing standard. Journal of Nursing Care Quality 8(1):51–57

6 *From Health Education to Community Development: Defining the Practice Nurse's Role*

Michelle Creed   Daria McCusker
Roslyn Hope   Maureen Morgan

INTRODUCTION

The move towards primary care-led health services has raised the value of health education and promotion in primary care, most notably in the shaping of the practice nurse's role. In examining this move this chapter will explore different approaches to the promotion of health.

The first section will review the different approaches to health education adopted within general practice, whereas the second component will explore the concept of user involvement and how practice nurses can encourage greater participation in the shaping of the service they deliver. The final portion of the chapter explores the concept of public health, with specific reference to the potential for practice nurse role development.

Key Issues

- Health education approaches
- Implementing effective health education within general practice
- Involving users in care provision-policy and reality
- Public health – applying the principles to general practice nursing

---

PART 1

Using Health Education in the Management of Chronic Disease

Michelle Creed   Daria McCusker

INTRODUCTION

The value of educating patients about their health has been central to nursing practice since Florence Nightingale (Clarke 1991). This is particularly crucial for practice nurses, given the anticipated rise in the demand for health care provision, an ageing population and an increasing incidence of chronic disease. This scenario ensures that health education in itself is no longer a luxury, but now a necessity for all care providers (Noble 1991). Individuals listen to health professionals for advice on topics such as diet, exercise, and smoking habits (lifestyle advice). The advice may not always be responded to; however, the individuals are armed with the information to make informed choices in their own health, work and social environments. For individuals to be in control of their own health requires a change from being dependent or reliant on health care professionals, as has been the case, to empowerment, independence and self reliance. Traditionally health professionals have tended to follow national guidelines and strategies and attempted to implement them at local level. Yet, the problems in dealing with health-related behaviour and specifically chronic disease, must be examined at a local level and fed back to the national agenda. If as practice nurses we are to provide a needs-led service and enable nursing to evolve, then we should be targeting local health policy with a view to influencing national policy.

Key Issues

- Influences upon health behaviour
- Definitions of health education
- Role of the practice nurse in delivering health education

The chapter will draw on critical incidents from practice as a means of exploring the issues. The incidents are centred around chronic disease management because this is the area in which practice nurses describe the most health education activity occurring.

Influences Upon Health Behaviour

Before the analysis of health education strategies within the general practice setting it is critical to examine the factors that influence the individual's health behaviour. An analysis of these factors will enable the nurse to determine the most effective health education strategy to ensure health gain. The key influences upon health education uptake are identified as poverty, social expectations, access to health care services and cultural and individual perspectives of health (Ewles & Simnett 1992). These will each be addressed in turn.

Poverty

Poverty has the biggest impact upon an individual's health status and the burden of disease is much higher among the poor (Townsend 1980). This is perhaps best evidenced by an examination of the incidence of asthma. The standardized mortality ratio (SMR) for asthma shows sharp increases between social class one and social class five, with children in lower socioeconomic groups being more likely to sleep on older mattresses and bedding, have older carpet in their rooms and live in older houses or apartments (Department of Health Centre Monitoring Unit 1995). These factors increase the exposure to ill health. The influence of social and economic deprivation on health is further exaggerated when considering dietary needs for individuals who have diseases such as diabetes mellitus and access to rehabilitation services for individuals who have mental health problems, and ensuring adequate housing for those who have chronic heart disease or stroke. (Benzeval, Whitehead & Judge 1995, Black 1980, Leather 1992, Whitehead 1987).

Those people who require the most help to improve their health are usually the least likely to attend clinics, so unless an appropriate and sensitive approach is taken the health divide between the 'haves' and 'have nots' may actually increase. Similarly, people may not have the freedom to choose a healthier lifestyle because of their economic or social conditions. Therefore, health education is more difficult and time consuming in an area of high deprivation, given that the causes of ill health are outside the ability of the individual to change. This in itself poses one of the greatest challenges to practice nurses in their work.

Social Expectations and Health

The burden of disease is laid at the door of the poor and is exacerbated by societal exclusion of those with ill health. During the past century, the medical model of health has focused on disease (Bunton, Nettleton & Burrows 1995). The disease model examines only the disease process, yet chronic illness and disease have a social component.

Illness prevents the individual from working and maintaining social contact, affects economic status and in turn affects lifestyle (Bunton et al 1995). This perspective is represented in definitions of health, which now recognize that employment, economic status and social situation influence lifestyle, and can influence health (Bunton et al 1995).

Access to Services

Key factors in the success of health education are structural variables, namely access and equity of facilities. Funding from local or central government is required in areas of access and availability to increase resources available. If the population is close to a health centre that provides a variety of health promotion activities, is open all day, and offers a crèche facility for the children, then there is likely to be a higher use of the services than if the local surgery is open for set hours only and is staffed by just one doctor. The importance of this becomes apparent when we look at an area such as Liverpool, where 95% of all medical contacts are at a general practice level (Liverpool Health Authority 1997).

It is not only access to the building that may have its problems; other issues such as communication, gender, attitude, inflexible procedures and cultural barriers need to be addressed. Health needs assessments may vary in different cultures; however, the provision of services and access to these services need to be facilitated for all the population (Liverpool Health Authority 1997).

Individual Perspectives

It is a person's appraisal of their situation that affects their actions; it is beliefs and not necessarily factual-based information that will influence any decision making. Whether the individual has the power, the resources or the ability to take control of their own health, can be debated. The concept of internal or external locus of control discussed by Rotter in (1966), concludes that people who have an internal locus of control are largely responsible for their own destiny, whereas those with more external dimensions tend to feel life events are determined by luck, fate or chance; this is further expanded by Burgess & Hamblett (1994) to include not only control, but also an individual's personality and how he or she learns social behaviour throughout life.

Stainton-Rogers (1991) further questioned the possibility of other influences, referred to as 'powerful others', to include doctors, nurses, family and friends and the workplace. These 'others' may influence 'the health locus of control' and support the possibility that when looking at an individual we need to look at a more holistic picture and include the individual's environment, culture, workplace, and social background. This is defined as a multidimensional health locus of control (MHLC) (Stainton-Rogers 1991). Although critiqued by Olbrisch (1975), Stainton-Rogers (1991) and Wallston et al (1978) as there being no significant links between the MHLC scale and a wide variety of health-related behaviour, there is agreement that it is important to encourage individuals to play an active role in decisions affecting the management of certain conditions, such as diabetes mellitus and asthma.

The individual's perception of health is similarly influenced by culture; indeed Kenney (1991) reminds us that clients view health in broader terms than purely clinical measurements. Throughout history folk law has played a role in lay beliefs of health. In particular it concentrates on traditional and cultural story telling that believes strongly in common sense and wisdom. It is argued that this culture is only relevant to the era it was constructed in and then in later years, they become 'old wives tales' (Frost 1994). Blaxter (1983), in researching the 'lay theory' in relationship to women, concludes that older women influenced the views of their daughters during childhood and these influences had an effect on health, illness and lifestyle. It is therefore necessary to consider not only the individual's own perceptions but also the prevailing cultural experiences in delivering health education.

What do We Understand by the Term Health Education?

Ewles & Simnett (1992) define the goal of health education as raising health consciousness or awareness of health issues. It can be classed as primary, secondary or tertiary (Box 6.1). A central tenet of health education is the notion that appropriate encouragement and support by health care professionals assists individuals in behaviour changes which are thought to benefit them. Tettersall, Sawyer & Salisbury (1993) suggest that it also involves listening, counselling and helping people make decisions for themselves. It is therefore important that health education programmes are targeted at the appropriate group

---

Box 6.1

Defining Levels of Health Education Intervention

■ Primary (e.g. education about a healthy lifestyle – no smoking, diet, exercise)
  — target: general population
■ Secondary (e.g. stop smoking, reduce weight, increase activity)
  — target: at-risk individuals
■ Tertiary (e.g. education aimed at ensuring compliance with treatment) programmes. Aims to minimize complications and reduce the impact on an established disease
  — target: affected individuals (e.g. people who have asthma or diabetes)

and crucial to determine the level of health education necessary to improve health status. The different levels all require intensive health education, though all are distinct and as such it is not appropriate to identify only one strategy to meet the primary, secondary and tertiary health education needs for groups of individuals.

Having identified the levels of intervention Ewles & Simnett (1992) categorize five approaches to health promotion.

1. Medical Model

This approach involves medical intervention to prevent or ameliorate ill health – the classic example is a mass immunization programme. The key limitation of such an approach is that the dominant medical model, and therefore middle class values may be imposed on clients (Ewles & Simnett 1992). Such an approach is not always effective given that patients may not share the same value system as the health care professional.

2. Behavioural Change

The behavioural change model attempts to change an individual's behaviour and attitudes, encouraging them to adopt a healthy lifestyle. Many of the major causes of death today are from chronic diseases that are strongly affected by behavioural factors, such as smoking, high alcohol consumption and inadequate diet.

The limitations of this approach lie in the assumption that the individual's behaviour is the primary cause of ill health, whereas many people are 'trapped' in their social conditions and do not have the genuine freedom to choose. This has been referred to as the 'victim blaming' approach. Whitehead (1991) suggests that this method can be counterproductive by stimulating defensive reactions in certain social groups. This can lead the individual to reject advice offered and refuse to take part in any further health education strategies. Changes in behaviour in this area have long-term rewards and result in healthier lifestyle; however, there are no immediate benefits and therefore this creates barriers in changing health-related behaviours (Gatchel, Baum & Krantz 1989).

Cultural, social and economic factors are also important in influencing health behaviour; for example, is there any realistic health gain from increasing the dosage of inhaler devices for a patient who has asthma, who lives on the third floor of a tower block of flats, with no lift, in damp housing?

It has been suggested that 'a behaviour that is highly reinforced and motivated will not succeed unless enabling factors are also present. Similarly, an enabled and motivated behaviour that is socially punished or ridiculed will also not endure' (Gatchel et al 1989). This reinforces the notion that a holistic view of the social influences of health need to be remembered in consultations.

3. Educational Approach

This model has an underlying philosophy that centres upon information and knowledge giving. It assumes that as individuals have knowledge they will then be able to make rational informed decisions concerning their health and lifestyle choices (Ewles & Simnett 1992).

This model is criticized for its overt rational perspective. It therefore fails to recognize that health educators bring their own values to the learning situation and these will determine the subject matter to be studied. Hence, it is questionable if this approach can really be value free.

4. Client-centered Approach

This empowering model of health education places the role of the health educator as a facilitator. The facilitator works with the client to enable them to identify their own needs and make health choices. It is often criticized because it is difficult for clients to articulate their health needs. Similarly, clients are not always self directed and may become frustrated or disinterested if their expectations for direction are not met.

5. Societal Change Approach

The societal change model of health education rejects the individualistic approach advocated by the above methods in favour of promoting changes to physical, social and economic environments that enable the individual to adopt health damaging behaviour. An example of the societal change approach to health behaviour has been the seatbelt legislation within the United Kingdom. This approach is undoubtedly potentially effective, yet within the British culture there is rejection of an intrusive approach to individual behaviour, so this approach can be viewed as highly contentious and politically sensitive.

Applying Interventions

The five approaches categorized by Ewles and Simnett are not mutually exclusive and each should be considered for its appropriateness in different situations at different times. For example, as a practice nurse you may decide that you will advise all patients who have diabetes or asthma who smoke to give up (medical model/behaviour change), while only giving advice on smoking to other patients if requested (client-centred). You may wish to set up a support group for smokers to look at the issue (educational approach) as well as establish a policy on smoking in the surgery (societal change). However, it must be remembered that individuals will only change their behaviour if they have a personal desire for change (Noble 1991). Indeed, Noble (1991) suggests that as health status improves the need to know may not be as acute and the behaviour change will not be as longlasting. That is why it is imperative that any education programme is reinforced at each opportunity that arises.

Supporting the Individual to Change – The Role of the Practice Nurse

Clarke (1991) suggests that the role of the nurse as a health educator and role model has gained prominence in the current political and social climate where people are encouraged to take responsibility for their own health. This notion has also come to the fore in nurse education in the diplomate programmes where educating patients for health and self care is a priority (UKCC 1986). Nurses are close to patients at the point of care delivery and are therefore in an ideal position to assess each individual about their particular needs. The potential benefits of health education to patients include an increase in health knowledge, involvement in decision making and self empowerment (Latter et al 1992).

Close (1988) identifies health education as a two-way process for the nurse, with both a teaching and a learning experience, in an effort to facilitate optimum health for the patient. In this context it is therefore crucial to consider how to help patients deal with their social problems before they can even begin to improve their physical wellbeing. Clarke (1991) states that making relationships with patients that are based on warmth, respect, genuineness and empathy seems to be a more effective method of helping people make health choices that are pertinent to their lives. Therefore we must be flexible and realistic. Even the smallest lifestyle change can be extremely difficult for patients who live in areas of high deprivation, and must be regarded as an achievement that elicits positive reinforcement. In support of this, Bayliss (1993), using the example of coronary heart disease, highlights the importance of motivating and empowering individuals to make healthy choices. However, we have come to realize that working with individuals can only have a limited effect on the broader factors influencing health.

In promoting positive health with patients who have a chronic illness, individuals and families need knowledge to react appropriately to changing situations – this can be achieved through actively promoting a philosophy of self care. Coates & Boore (1995), however, acknowledge that 'whether patients put health care knowledge and skills into the practice of self management of chronic illness is known to depend on many variables including health beliefs, decision making ability, quality of physician communication and sense of power and control'. They suggests that for individuals to be autonomous in control of a chronic illness, health professionals need to:

■ impart knowledge that will enable integration into the individual's chosen lifestyle

- ensure that educational material is multicultural in origin and allows for various cultural beliefs and customs
- listen and learn from each individual and share that knowledge among others who have similar lifestyles
- allow for flexibility, compromise, tolerance and failure – the decision we may wish to take may not be the decision of the individual or family in the management of any chronic illness
- become a partner in the care offered, not the controller

Research into patient participation in chronic disease management is inconclusive in its findings (Biley 1992, Coates & Boore 1995, Rourke 1991, Steele et al 1987, Waterworth & Luker 1990). However, it is agreed that it requires more than compliance with a medical regime. It requires the individual to have active involvement in decisions and to be consulted (see Case Study 6.1). Furthermore it allows

---

Case Study 6.1

Questioning the effectiveness of health education approaches

Oliver is a 5-year-old boy who over the past 3 months has developed a cough, which is worse at night and consequently he has had a disturbed sleep pattern and has missed several days of school. His mother has noticed that when playing football with his older brother, he 'has to stop frequently' due to the cough and shortness of breath. He has an evident audible wheeze during the consultation.

Oliver has a history of atopic eczema and a family history of asthma via his paternal grandmother and brother (whose compliance with clinic attendance and medication is questionable). Both parents smoke cigarettes and the family are on the rehousing list because they live in a one-bedroom flat; both boys share one bedroom and the parents sleep in the lounge area. Oliver's mother is at present pregnant with the third child.

Oliver is started on beclomethasone 100 micrograms two puffs twice a day and salbutamol 100 micrograms two puffs as needed both via a Volumatic spacer device. He is given a peak flow meter and diary and his mother is asked to monitor his symptoms, peak flow rate and use of his salbutamol inhaler over the next 2 weeks and return to surgery with his diary for review. The inhaler devices and the peak flow meter are demonstrated to his mother in surgery and any questions answered.

- Ask yourself some questions about the family dynamics here.
- Oliver is reliant on his mother's support in getting his symptoms under control. Can you think of any support in helping her achieve this?
- There are educational issues that need to be ongoing with both parents about smoking; what ways do you envisage helping the children in the interim period to keep them in a smoke-free environment?

for questions to be asked and answered, preferences to be considered and opinions respected, but more importantly it allows the individual to be heard.

Collaborative Approaches to Health Education

It is assumed that the primary care setting is an appropriate setting for health promotion advice and attitude change, given that patients are relatively 'well'. We would suggest that no setting is wrong or right – if the 'cue for action' is there it should be used – whether in nursery school or the workplace the messages are still the same and the long-term goals do not change. We are aiming for an improved standard of life. To achieve this all health care providers must work collaboratively within a multidisciplinary framework. It is through collaborative working and respect for each other's ideas that new preventative health education strategies will be formulated.

Although health promotion and education may influence behavioural changes in some individuals, the aim needs to be focused on community development strategies. Participation in decision making related to health issues encourages self esteem in the individual and creates a sense of community spirit. This approach is more likely to result in a change of lifestyle activities and deal with unhealthy habits (Benzeval et al 1995)

Health Education – Opportunistic or Structured?

In delivering health education it is worth considering whether within the general practice setting it is more appropriate to convey health messages opportunistically or through a structured approach. Opportunistic methods essentially rely on 'tacking on' health education when patients present at a general practice surgery. Their advantages lie in their simplicity, low cost and high uptake. Additionally Jolleys (1992) argues that opportunistic population screening on a nonselective basis is the only way to uncover otherwise unsuspected problems. Since 70–80% of patients consult with a GP at least once every 3 years (O'Brien, Beevers & Marshall 1995), it is possible to identify a large population of patients, for example, at risk from coronary heart disease. However, it fails to address the problem of nonattendees and may involve people who are not receptive, as well as being perhaps unrealistically time consuming in the normal consulting time.

On the other hand a more structured (i.e. clinical based) approach can attempt to reach a more specific group. This helps the nurse by increasing her knowledge in the area; however, it can also create an environment where the individual is labeled by the disease process, for example, 'diabetic' or 'asthmatic'. This in itself can alienate those who most need to attend. Similarly, the clinic times may not be convenient, particularly for patients who work. An inappropriate timing of clinics can be costly, resulting in a small number of patients attending, even though 2 or 3 hours of nursing time have been allocated.

Individuals, families or communities should be able to seek advice or guidance as they feel necessary or when they have the resources or access to do so. There should be no greater or lesser access with regard to social class or income, and health promotion strategies must be guided by local needs to improve health. Our experience in Liverpool confirms the view that health education should be delivered within a 'mixed economy', therefore avoiding the serious pitfalls of using an opportunistic approach alone.

Conclusion

No one health promotion strategy would enable any society to drastically improve health standards; however, an understanding of various cultures may enable health strategies to be tailored to fit a variety of settings. Health professionals must consider remodeling health promotion activities and ideals. Nothing should be laid in stone. As human beings we are apt to change with the times – cultures evolve with the times, peer groups have new 'fads' to follow and there is always a new generation of ideas. However, it has become clear that behavioural change can occur and to promote a healthier lifestyle in individuals health promotion activities should be provided on an individual basis.

Health education programmes as we know them are planned opportunities for people to learn about and undertake voluntary changes in behaviour. It is evident that these programmes only work with motivated individuals and are restrictive. Therefore, they may be more appropriate on a one-to-one basis, in a group such as smoking cessation, slimming or exercise class, or through mass media campaigns, health fairs, exhibitions or by providing a stand at a supermarket to reach a larger audience. Flexibility is the key and listening to what individuals and communities want themselves is essential.

In the real world people at times lack knowledge and resources, and have diverse cultural beliefs. However, these factors should not starve them of a form of lifestyle that improves health opportunities, taking into account their personal and cultural beliefs. We should therefore all strive to improve the general quality of life, no matter how small the change is.

References

Bayliss SJ 1993 Coronary heart disease prevention: an inner city problem. Medical Action Communications, London

Benzeval M, Whitehead M, Judge K 1995 Tackling inequalities in health. King's Fund Institute, London

Biley F 1992 Some determinants that effect patient participation in decision making about nursing care. Journal of Advanced Nursing 17:414–421

Black D 1980 Report on the working party on inequalities in health. DHSS, London

Blaxter M 1983 The causes of disease: women talking. Social Science and Medicine 9(10):698–703

Bunton R, Nettleton S, Burrows R 1995 The sociology of health promotion: critical analyses of consumption, lifestyle and risk. Routledge, London

Burgess C, Hamblett M 1994 Application of Rotter scale of internal–external locus of control to determine differences between smokers, non-smokers and ex-smokers in their general locus of control. Journal of Advanced Nursing 19:699–704

Clarke AC 1991 Nurses as role models and health educators. Journal of Advanced Nursing 16:1178–1184

Close A 1988 Patient education, a literature review. Journal of Advanced Nursing 13:203–213

Coates VE, Boore JRP 1995 Self-management of chronic illness: implications for nursing. International Journal of Nursing Studies 32(6):628–640

Department of Health Centre Monitoring Unit 1995 Asthma: an epidemiological overview. HMSO, London

Ewles I, Simnett I 1992 Promoting health. A practical guide, 2nd edn. Scutari Press, London

Frost J 1994 A means of empowerment: a psychosocial perspective on active asthma management. Professional Nurse 9(10):698–703

Gatchel R, Baum A, Krantz D 1989 An introduction to health psychology, 2nd edn. Newbury Award Records, USA

Jolleys J 1992 Reducing coronary heart disease in general practice. Medical Action Communications, London

Kenney J 1991 The consumer's view of health. Journal of Advanced Nursing 17:829–834

Latter S, MacLeod Clark J, Wilson-Barnett J, Mabbern J 1992 Health education in nursing: perceptions of practice in acute settings. Journal of Advanced Nursing 17:164–172

Leather S 1992 Less money, less choice: poverty and diet in the UK today. In: Your food, whose choice? National Consumer Council, London

Liverpool Health Authority 1997 Liverpool Public Health Annual Report. Liverpool Health Authority, Liverpool

Noble C 1991 Are nurses good patient educators? Journal of Advanced Nursing 16:1185–1198

O'Brien EJ, Beevers DG, Marshall HJ 1985 ABC of hypertension, 3rd edn. BMJ Publishing, London

Olbrisch M 1975 Perceptions of responsibility for illness and health related locus of control in gonorrhea patients. Unpublished. Cited in Stainton-Rogers 1991

Rotter J 1966 Generalized expectancies for internal versus external control of reinforcement. Psychological Monographs 80(609)

Rourke AM 1991 Self-care: chore or challenge. Journal of Advanced Nursing 16:4233–4241

Stainton-Rogers W 1991 Explaining health and illness: an exploration of diversity. Harvester Wheatsheaf, Exeter

Steele DJ, Blakewell B, Gitman MC, Jackson JC 1987 The activated patient: dogma, dream or desideratum? Patient Education Counselling 10:3–23

Tettersell M, Sawyer J, Salisbury C 1993 Handbook of practice nursing. Churchill Livingstone Edinburgh

Townsend P 1980 Labour and equality: a Fabian study of Labour in power, 1974–79. Heinemann, London

UKCC 1986 Project 2000: a new preparation for practice. UKCC, London

Wallston K, Wallston B, Kaplan G, Maides S 1978 Development and validation of the health locus of control (HLC) scale. Health Education Monographs 6:107–116

Waterworth S, Luker KA 1990 Reluctant collaborators: do patients want to be involved in decisions concerning care? Journal of Advanced Nursing 15:971–976

Whitehead M 1987 The health divide. Health Education Council, London

Whitehead M 1991 The concepts and principles of equity and health. Promotion International 217–227 Oxford University Press, Oxford

PART **2**

Involving the Public in Health Care Decision Making: User Involvement in General Practice

Roslyn Hope

INTRODUCTION

It is frequently asserted that GPs are in an excellent position to act as proxies for patients' health needs (Jordan et al 1998). There is, however, considerable evidence to show that doctors and patients have different perspectives. Equally, there is disparity between demand and needs. Many health professionals, including the primary health care team, see the proactive seeking out of need as secondary to the primary care responsibility for individual demand, and therefore perceive the knowledge held by people living locally as 'inferior' to that generated by clinical observation and diagnosis. Most illness, however, does not lead to a medical consultation, so professional knowledge cannot be assumed to reflect the experience of individual patients because presentation at the surgery may best be understood as only one expression of demand. One way of filling the gaps in understanding is to consult the community.

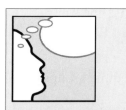

Reflection Point

It is worth reflecting for a moment on why it is important to enable the community and the individual health service user to participate in health care decisions

Key Issues	
■ Defining community	■ Involving users in health care decision making
■ Increasing participation in care	

Defining Community

Who or what is the practice nurse's community? Despite the influence of the World Health Organization in advocating for community participation in primary health care services, its influence on primary care is hard to detect.

For many health workers, community is equated with nonhospital based services. Such a definition is inadequate in clarifying how primary care should engage with the community. Brown (1994) in a study looking at the perception of community and participation of GPs and community nurses found three main interpretations of community (Box 6.2).

> **Box 6.2**
>
> **The Three Main Interpretations of Community (Brown 1994)**
>
> ■ Community as an area of locality: a geographical definition
>   — where there is a compact area around the surgery this is seen as a positive and appropriate description of their community; where, however, a practice serves a scattered area, there is no sense of a local community
> ■ Community as the practice population
>   — those in the study who do not value the concept of community for general practice view the practice population as an administrative detail; for those who see the community as important, there is strong support for the practice itself being a community of patients that relates to local populations from which the patients are drawn
> ■ Community as groups with shared interests
>   — groups with shared medical and social needs as part of the concept of communities of interest are another interpretation – this could be, for example, ethnic minority groups, people who have mental health needs, etc.

There is a tension between the individual focus of the practice population and the more collective focus on the community as a locality or groups with shared interests. Brown summarized these as follows:

■ individual focus
  — individual users
  — the Practice list
  — specific groups of users who have shared (medically delivered) needs
■ collective focus
  — a locality patch or area
  — groups who have shared interests (e.g. ethnic groups, social need)
  — shared institutions (e.g. schools)

The white paper *The New NHS: Modern, Dependable* (Department of Health 1997) will help to move the individual and collective divide through developing primary care groups, which are required to assess the needs of a locality population in partnership with other practices and other agencies. The Health Improvement Programme gives a structure through which this can be achieved.

Working as a practice nurse directly with individuals will inevitably lead you to take an individual perspective in the first instance. This can feed in to a broader collective process for health improvement.

Increasing Participation in Care

User involvement or empowerment has its roots in the dissatisfaction with services for specific devalued groups, such as people who have mental health needs or learning and physical disabilities. Barker & Peck (1996) comment that in the 1970s, the Civil Rights Movement in the United States, antipsychiatry, de-institutionalization, labelling theory and normalization led to the use of consciousness-raising methods established by women's groups for mental health users. Based on people's personal perspectives, a political movement was born to bring about change in services.

However, the 1980s saw the rise of the 'new conservatism' in the United Kingdom in which the consumer of services was to be given increased influence. Such approaches were intended to lead to greater choice, more responsiveness to complaints and service developments based on consumer wishes. At the same time, the government reflected a decreasing deference to doctors; Alan Langlands, Chief Executive of the NHS, told the Health Select Committee of Inquiry in Mental Health Services in 1992 'We are listening to carers and users, the people whom we think know best about services'. Simarly, the National Priorities Guidance *Modernising Health and Social Services 1999/2002* restates this in the context of multiagency working:

> 'There is now the opportunity to energise partnership
> working between organisations, with service users and
> their carers to reflect better their wishes, with locality
> communities and with the voluntary sector. This will not
> only improve the quality of treatment and care for the
> users, but also represent an efficient use of resources for
> the tax payer and be welcomed by staff' (Department of
> Health 1998b).

Engaging service users in health care decision making requires a fundamental shift in the historic health professional view of the patient as the passive recipient of services. Pritchard (1994) quoted William Pickle's GP father as saying 'If patients ask me what is wrong with them I tell them "that is my business – just take the medicine and you will get better"'. Although few health practitioners would espouse such views these days, the shift in the balance of power that is required for full participation to be meaningful is still an appreciable challenge in primary and secondary care.

Perkins (1996), considering the issue of user involvement, quoted Besio in saying that 'professionalism' is deep rooted:

> 'There is a pervasive societal belief that trained
> professionals are the only people who know how to

provide proper assistance. This attitude exists, whether our television needs to be fixed or we need help dealing with personal issues. We have grown accustomed to turning to professionals for help because we assume they have special expertise' (Perkins 1996).

Over the past decade, however, service users have increasingly been questioning whether doctor (or nurse) knows best. People have been seeking other sources for help and advice, for instance, homeopathy. They have also been making their own judgements about whether they will follow advice or take prescribed medication as instructed. In mental health, people who have been disillusioned with services at all levels have turned to each other for support and found that people who have suffered direct personal distress have been more able to understand their needs than professionals who have learned through education and training. This has led to a growth in self-help groups, user-led and user-provided services. Unfortunately, Gell (1996), a user consultant, comments that 'one area where there has been very little involvement is primary care (which) has always played an important role in the lives of most service users'.

Although much of the user involvement literature has come from the mental health field, the lessons learned are relevant to all aspects of health care. Brown (1994), in his study of GPs and community nurses, found two key dimensions for participation in primary care. These were described as: the 'individual–collective' and the 'professional control–lay control' dimensions.

The individual–collective concept at the individual pole of the continuum places emphasis on the rights of individuals as consumers and users of health care. Participation is about taking up mechanisms of information, choice and consultation. The collective pole includes 'health for all' policies and community-developed initiatives.

The professional control–lay control dimension highlights that user control is more acceptable at the soft end of involvement (e.g. information through newsletters), but much less acceptable, for example, in setting the agenda for the practice. A GP was quoted on the idea of a lay forum:

> 'I think there could be a problem if they tried to exert too much control over what we are doing. Obviously, we've got our own interests and they've got their own interests as well and there could be conflict between the two if they were participating in decisions about the practice management or something. I'd hate a patient group to exert their authority over what we are doing, although it would be nice to have some views about what we're doing and what they would like' (Brown 1994).

There is a real danger that in the light of the political imperative to develop and respond to the service user and carer agenda, work is carried out at a superficial or tokenistic level. If one were to consider how best to sabotage real user participation, it would be worth trying the following:

- expect the service user to represent the views of all users with the same diagnosis or need – as there is rarely a democratic constituency of service users to whom an individual can relate and therefore represent, this becomes impossible
- if the service user does not represent the views of others, treat his or her individual view with caution because it will probably reflect the idiosyncrasies of the person and can therefore be dismissed
- if more than one service user is involved, expect them to agree, otherwise you will not know whom to believe; equally, if you find the view of one more acceptable than another you can take that on board, ignore the others and still have responded to users' views!
- claim that there simply are not the resources available to deliver different services; this is probably true and means you can carry on using resources as they are currently invested
- if the user has a mental health problem, consider his or her opinion to be purely the result of their psychopathology; in this case, you will clearly know best; if, however, you are successful at talking them round to your point of view you can deem the person to be successful in gaining insight
- if you have no alternative to listening to the person, you can do so, but take no notice
- you can try to get the person to follow your suggestions by either limiting their information or giving it in an indigestible way, so that they cannot make an informed judgement themselves
- you can make services contingent on compliance with your proposed cause of action (e.g. the person will only be seen by the nurse if they take their medication)

All of these tactics are successfully deployed on a daily basis in the health service. Interestingly, Perkins (1996) believes that the shift from talking about the 'power' of users to the now popular user 'empowerment' is not purely a semantic change. Power is political and refers to structural conditions, to relationships between different groups:

> 'In empowerment, power is redefined as a state of mind in which users feel powerful, competent, worthy of esteem, able to influence events whilst leaving oppressive structures unchanged. This shift from a political to a psychological concept can enable a powerful group to

maintain conditions and power relationships whilst appearing not to do so' (Perkins 1996).

She concludes somewhat pessimistically:

> 'If real changes are to be effected and "user involvement" becomes more than empty rhetoric – a change in power relationships, rather than a feeling of power, is required. But it is rare for anyone to give up any power unless they are forced to do so' (Perkins 1996).

Nevertheless, Perkins offers an alternative model where health professionals place their expertise and services at the disposal of those who need them. As a practice nurse you may feel you are already only there to serve – this is where reflective practice can help you stand back and consider these issues.

What are the Important Issues for Users in Health Care Decision Making?

What people expect and what they desire from their GP are two different things. Valori et al (1996) described how research is increasingly showing:

> 'that patients' care often diverges from their expectation in important respects. Specifically, patients tend to receive more prescription than they expect and less information and explanation. Moreover, the fulfilment of certain expectations has been related to satisfaction with the consultation that would, in turn, improve compliance'.

Using a patient's requests form in two different practices, they identified the three key requirements and desires of people seeing their GP (Box 6.3).

Traditionally it is the third of these three elements that has been seen as the main purpose and value of a consultation. If there were

---

Box 6.3

Three Key Requirements and Desires of People Seeing Their GP (Valori et al 1996)

- Explanation and reassurance – given during the consultation
- Emotional support – a desire for empathy and counselling rather than information; this was equally relevant for people who had physical problems as for people who had emotional problems
- Technical services – drugs, investigation and referral

a better understanding of what is important to the user, it could alter the outcome of the consultation.

Misreading of patients' needs could explain why prescribing exceeds their expectations. It could also explain why requests by emotionally distrubed patients for support are misperceived as requests for intervention, which result in unnecessary prescribing or onward referral.

A study carried out by Britten (1994) of patients' ideas about medication aimed to examine whether their perceptions affected compliance. It was found that medicines were perceived as either positive or negative depending upon their generalized properties, for instance, antibiotics and penicillin were 'good'. Negative views clustered around medicines being unnatural, addictive, dangerous, etc. In looking at orientation towards medication, more was reported on negative views, including wanting to avoid strong drugs, taking drugs as a last resort, side effect aversion, it was an easy option instead of sorting things out personally. In examining appropriate and actual use of medicines, it was found that people who had a positive orientation took medicines according to instructions. People who did not comply did so because they forgot, they took them only as and when symptoms appeared and they stopped if they experienced side effects. It was concluded that:

> 'first it should not be assumed that medicines are an acceptable form of treatment in every situation. If appropriate, the patient could be asked what kind of treatment they would prefer. Secondly, it is worth establishing the patient's general orientation towards medication (i.e. whether they have fears about it). Finally, the doctor can enquire about the social context to establish if work or leisure commitments will affect adherence' (Britten 1994).

In short, asking user views can affect the outcome of the consultation and the treatment.

Similarly, in a recent study in South Staffordshire (personal communication) practice nurses and district nurses were trained in the use of a health risk assessment card (HRAC), published in the *Primary Mental Health Care Toolkit* (Department of Health 1997b). Patients who appeared to be distressed were screened using the HRAC. If they were found to be at risk of developing a mental health problem they were offered the following options:

- information on where to go for help (e.g. Citizen's Advice Bureau, Samaritans, Relate)
- a follow-up session around problem solving

The results showed that before the study the nurses had not known how to listen and respond to people when they presented with some distress. They had tended to ignore their emotional problems and dealt with something more practical or physical or they had referred them directly to the community psychiatric nurse. After their training, all considered that they were more skilled at dealing directly with problems presented, being empathic and giving appropriate information. Furthermore, there was a drop in the referral rate to the secondary mental health service. Although the intention of the study had not been to directly address user-defined priorities it clearly addressed the issues identified in the study by Valori et al (1996).

In further considering what aspects of care are important to the person using health services, Wensing, Grol & Smits (1994) carried out a literature analysis on how patient reports have been used as a method of quality assurance. They used aspects of care based on the perspective of the patient, which is generally adopted in the Netherlands, as a measure of analysis (Box 6.4).

They found that patients in general practice were often asked to assess aspects of health care such as accuracy, humaneness, informativeness and availability. Aspects such as professional competence, indication, empathy and accommodation were included less frequently. The following aspects were rarely asked about:

- effectiveness
- suitability, safety, hygiene, nutrition
- prevention of superfluous care and the effects of an illness on the patient's functioning
- mutual trust between the patient and GP
- accountability and autonomy – aspects concerning the patient's responsibility for his own life
- continuity, efficiency, integrated care

The authors commented significantly that in only five of 40 publications in research into patient judgements had patients been involved in selecting the aspects of care that were to be examined. They offered as a possible explanation that:

> 'patients (were assumed) not capable of passing a meaningful judgement on some particular aspects of care. This assumption may be true for medical/technical aspects … It seems that organisational aspects of care, for instance, lend themselves excellently for quality assessments by patients' (Wensing, Grol & Smits 1994).

Box 6.4

Aspects of Care (Health Research Council Netherlands, 1990)

■ Professional performance
  — effectiveness: actual improvement of the state of health
  — professional competence: availability of the necessary knowledge and skills
  — indication: insight into one's own competence and possibilities in relation to that of other professionals
  — suitability: physical and mental suitability to practise the profession
  — safety: risk minimization
  — accuracy: in the use of knowledge and skills
  — hygiene: minimization of the risk of iatrogenic infections
  — nutrition: quality and taste of diets
  — prevention of superfluous care
  — burden: consequences for the patient/consumer with regard to his or her total functioning
■ Attitude of the professional
  — humaneness: respect for the patient and his or her own responsibility
  — informativeness: willingness to provide the patient with information
  — mutual trust: respect for the personal privacy of the patient
  — cooperation: cooperation between the practitioner and the patient
  — accountability: ability of the practitioner to account for his or her actions and behaviour
  — empathy: ability of the practitioner to assume the role of the patient
  — autonomy (of the patient): whenever possible, active involvement of the patient in clarifying his or her problem
■ Organization of care
  — continuity: adequate transfer of treatment in case of more providers of care, substitution by a locum or retirement
  — availability: availability of the practitioner to potential patients
  — efficiency: right balance between input (money, means, time) and output (of care)
  — integrated care: tuning the care provided by different professionals to one another
  — material privacy: safeguarding the individual privacy of the patient or consumer by protecting physical data
  — accessibility: physical and geographical accessibility of the care, including the necessary equipment
  — financial accessibility
  — accommodation: physical suitability of the organization.

Levels of Participation

People who use health services can participate (in theory) at a range of levels. The fundamental building block is, however, the involvement by individuals in their own care and treatment. Many of the studies quoted have highlighted what are key aspects of care for users. Unless people are listened to by the primary health care team there will continue to be unplanned or unanticipated outcomes of treatment.

All people receiving secondary mental health services, the majority of whom are still receiving care from the GP or practice nurse, are required to have a care programme. This approach devised by the Department of Health in 1991 means that every person should have an assessment, a care plan, a review date and a key worker. Lamentably, many primary care workers are still unaware of this cornerstone of mental health care. Of even greater concern, however, is that many users and carers are unaware of it. People need to be active participants in their own care planning because they are the ones who are most intimately involved with their own bodies, beliefs and behaviour.

For many years, but particularly since the Community Care Act 1990, there has been a move to foster needs-led assessment. This is based on looking at the needs of the individual and separating these from the services and interventions required to meet those needs. Too often, even today, however, professionals of all types are service-led: they fit people into services available rather than fitting services to people. Thus we see people going to day centres or nursing homes because this is what is on offer and may minimize risk. This may not be what is needed by the individual who may want a break from carers or to remain in their own home.

General practitioners and practice nurses, along with other members of the primary health care team, contribute towards community care assessments. How many discuss these with the service users before completing the necessary forms?

To overcome the real problem of lack of needs-led assessment skills in staff, despite considerable training, a new initiative in mental health has taken place. Self assessment is a process facilitated with the support of an advocate or befriender whereby individuals complete their own assessment. A framework is used, for example, the Avon Mental Health Measure, through which a person can take an holistic view of their lives. Areas include housing, effects of medication, social support, community involvement, risk to self, income, etc., and a full personal profile is produced. Experience to date shows that service users feel more in control over their own lives in a way not previously possible. It is already beginning to impact on the style of services being provided in Avon (Avon Mental Health).

> **Box 6.5**
>
> **Community and Participation for General Practice (Brown 1994)**
>
> - Individual ethic
>   — exit/choice
>   — information
>   — consultation
>   — service provision
>   — voice
>   — organization
>   — groups and empowerment
> - Collective ethic

Moving then from the foundation stone of a person's involvement in their own care and on to what might be construed at a more community level, there are a number of ways to consider this. Brown (1994), with his individual versus collective ethic, mapped the factors listed in Box 6.5 in relation to general practice. In general practice the ultimate choice for users is to vote with their feet and change practice.

Information

This is an essential element of participation. It can be provided through noticeboards, leaflets, newsletters, open days and direct personal contact. Increasingly, the Internet can help people access information on their own health care needs.

Consultation

This is linked with market research and can happen through patient surveys, suggestion boxes, etc. These will tend to be one-off exercises based on specific issues.

Service Provision

Service provision can take the form of users and lay people providing a service such as visiting elderly people, providing transport or raising money for the practice. This was seen in Brown's study as the most legitimate activity for a patients participation group (Brown 1994).

Voice

This is more the equivalent of a housing tenants group. A forum for the community with some degree of independence can frame the questions and set the agenda.

Organization

Organization can be described as 'humanizing the process' within general practice and building links to the natural networks of

---

Box 6.6

User Involvement for Purchasers and Providers (Barker & Peck 1996)

- Purchaser
  - quality standards and monitoring
  - planning/strategy development
  - needs assessment
  - devising specification
- Provider
  - quality standards and monitoring
  - planning/service development
  - service management/board representative
  - recruitment of staff

---

local people. In this context, participation is a relationship as an organization with the community, not just with individuals.

Groups and Empowerment

This refers to work with groups with an explicit agenda of empowerment: community development with an emphasis on marginalized groups.

The higher the level of participation the greater the potential threat to the practitioner. Looking at levels from a different perspective Barker & Peck (1976) illustrated how user involvement can be achieved for both purchasers and providers (Box 6.6).

As general practitioners are both purchasers and providers and with the new primary care groups ultimately becoming primary care trusts, these two perspectives remain relevant to primary health care teams.

Quality Standards

Quality standards are fundamental for describing the aspirations of services and for auditing how far those aspirations have been achieved. In 1992 the Department of Health issued a 10-point guide that practices might give to their patients in their Executive Letter (92)88. Partnership, as with current guidance, was emphasized, but without clear ideas on how this might be achieved (Box 6.7).

Although it is helpful to have formal support for and guidance on user involvement, local situations vary. At the outset standards need to be shared and discussed to ensure there is common understanding of them. Areas that need improvement should be identified and a plan agreed on how to address them. Review and audit mechanisms need to be in place to ensure they are monitored. Service users should therefore form part of the standard setting and standard monitoring procedure.

Box 6.7

Users' Guide to Primary Health Care (EL[92]88 Annex D)

We are committed to giving you the best possible service. This will be achieved by working together. Help us to help you.

1. You will be treated as a partner in the care and attention you receive
2. You will be treated as an individual and will be given courtesy and respect at all times, irrespective of your ethnic origin, religious belief, personal attributes or the nature of your health problems
3. Following discussion you will receive the most appropriate care, given by suitably qualified people. No care or treatment will be given without your informed consent
4. You have the right to see your health records, subject to any limitations in the law, which will be kept confidential
5. We will give you full information about the services we offer. Every effort will be made to ensure that you receive the information which directly affects your health and the care being offered
6. People involved in your care will give you their names and ensure that you know how to contact them. Please let them know if you change your name or address
7. It is our job to give you treatment and advice. In the interest of your health it is important for you to understand all the information given to you. Please ask questions if you are unsure of anything
8. We need help too. Please ask for a night visit only when you feel it is truly necessary and home visits by the doctor only when patients are too ill to visit the surgery
9. Please do everything you can to keep appointments, tell us as soon as possible if you cannot and be ready to tell us details of your past illnesses, medication, hospital admissions and any other relevant details
10. We will provide you with information about how to make suggestions or complaints about the care we offer. We want to improve services, we will therefore welcome any comments you have

---

Planning, Strategy and Service Development

These are, only really meaningful if they involve all stakeholders, including users and carers. It can of course happen at the consultative level where people are asked to comment on the final draft of a document; more appropriately people can be involved at the outset, for example, through membership of a project group planning a health centre. There are now well-established principles on how to make planning involvement meaningful. These include ensuring that the individual is well prepared, making meetings more comfortable and accessible, providing all the necessary information in advance and paying reasonable expenses. Too often someone is dragged in at the last minute from a voluntary group without preparation. Equally, statutory services need to learn to be more imaginative on how planning is undertaken. Engaging with a number of users by going to their groups or setting up focus groups to elicit views are some of the options available.

Needs Assessment

Needs assessment is a complex area that commonly gets carried out without reference to the user perspective or experience. The care programme approach, if working properly, should highlight unmet need and therefore deficits in service. The Newcastle Mental Health Consumers Group was set up by Newcastle Health Authority and the NHS Trust with the support of Social Services Department. Member users were paid an honorarium and they contributed to needs assessment by telling their own stories of what they needed of services and where those services had succeeded and failed. Such anecdotal evidence brought epidemiological data to life and made it possible to understand not only qualified need, but also what would have helped. The latter point is of real importance because it is well known that even if there is agreement about deprivation and levels of need, priorities differ according to perspective. Smoking cessation may be the top priority for the practice nurse, but housing may be the priority for the same target user group. Real health improvements can only be really gained through community participation.

Service Management/Board Representatives

Service management and board representatives for users is unusual. However, some trusts, for example, have Community Health Council representatives as regular members at board meetings.

Devising Specifications

In Tamworth, people who have learning disabilities and their carers were full partners in drawing up a specification for a staffed home and participated in selecting the provider of the service.

Staff Recruitment

Involving users in the selection of staff is increasingly common. People who have physical disabilities, for example, regularly interview people who will be providing care for them, and they also have the capacity to employ them.

Returning our focus to methods for involving the public in health care decision making Jordan et al (1998) described the approaches to public consultation on health care priorities (listed in Table 6.1).

Table 6.1
*Approaches to Public
Consultation*

	Informed	Uninformed
Deliberated	Citizen juries User consultation panels	Focus groups
Undeliberated	Questionnaire surveys with written information	Opinion surveys of standing panels/one-off questionnaires

Citizen Juries

Participants are selected as representatives of public or local opinions. They sit for a specified length of time during which they are presented with information to help in decision making. Typically, experts give evidence and jurors have an opportunity to ask questions or debate relevant issues. This method is increasingly popular on television and radio (e.g. The Moral Maze).

User Consultation Panels

These consist of local people selected from representatives of the locality or population. Members rotate to ensure a broad range of views are heard. Based on available information topics are decided in advance and meetings are often facilitated by a moderator. An example of such a panel is the Droitwich Community Health Forum (Bunce 1997) where six people were selected from various local voluntary organizations. They were trained in research, report writing and evaluation techniques and they could call on specialists for expert opinion. They were asked to prioritize 17 proposed options for change by the health authority. They rejected ideas such as setting up baby equipment hire and health education books in libraries in favour of preventative coronary work and improving communication between hospital and community settings. The panel is seen to enable a wider debate about health care provision:

> 'Contrary to some of the fears that were expressed in the early days … the panel has not raised patients' expectations unreasonably. In fact, they now understand the problems the health service faces and accept that not everything is possible.' (Bunce 1997).

Focus Groups

These are typically semistructured discussion groups of between six and eight participants led by a facilitator, and focus on specific topics. A variation of the focus groups with links to the consultation panels is the 'single issue quality group' such as that used at Manor House Surgery in Glossop. Groups are made up of all members of the primary health care team and each group canvasses the views of patients to find out how or if the service has improved. All the practice's inhouse activities are being audited in this way. Once again, the key finding is that communication is of the foremost importance to patients.

Questionnaire Surveys

Questionnaire surveys can be postal or distributed at the surgery. This systematic data collection allows information to be collected from a large sample of people.

Opinion Surveys of Standing Panels

These are similar to audience groups for television in that they comprise large sociologically representative samples of a population in a health authority. Despite the multiplicity of options for community participation there is 'poor understanding' and limited uptake of local consultation within primary care (Jordan et al 1998). Their view is that this is due to lack of training of the necessary skills in health professionals. Local people are usually unused to being asked their opinion on health care, let alone taking on a more active role. They too require training as for citizen juries or patients' panels, and without this one-off consultations can have limited benefit.

What Can the Practice Nurse Do?

Practice nurses as part of the primary health care team are already in touch with local networks such as mother and toddler groups, schools and voluntary organizations. They are producing community profiles that can be used to develop stronger links with the community. The spread of appropriate knowledge and skills and the practical need to divide workloads make it vital that the whole primary health care team is involved in community participation. Such involvement is in line with the underlying general ethos of full participation in health care decision making.

Although the outcome of common participation in needs assessment can lead to conflicting needs and priorities, it nevertheless is likely to result not only in promoting good health, but also in reducing inequalities in its distribution.

Conclusion

In conclusion, it is fair to say that despite the burgeoning literature on user involvement and community participation and the Department of Health imperative of delivering to a user and carer agenda, the degree to which this occurs at practice level is disappointingly low. As a practice nurse you can have an impact on the patients' full involvement in their own care and on developing standards in the practice through a variety of methods, including a patients participation group. You can work with your primary care colleagues to use existing links with community networks to involve them in needs assessment and in delivering the health improvement programme. To do this you will need to be able to come to terms with a loss of power and find ways of working with your colleagues to share that perspective. In embarking on these approaches you will be making a significant contribution to the promotion of community health.

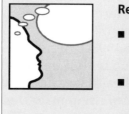

Reflection Points

■ Consider how you as a practice nurse can increase participation at both a collective and individual level
■ What or who are the barriers to participation within the community within which you work

References

Avon Mental Health 1994 Avon mental health measure: a user centered approach to assessing need. Avon Mental Health, Avon

Barker I, Peck E 1996 User empowerment – a decade of experience. The Mental Health Review 1:4

Britten N 1994 Patients' ideas about medicines: a qualitative study in a general practice population. British Journal of General Practice 44:465–468

Brown I 1994 Community and participation for general practice perceptions of GPs and community nurses. Social Science and Medicine 39(3):335–344

Bunce C 1997 Involving patients. Medeconomics August: 56–57

Department of Health 1990 NHS and community care act. HMSO, London

Department of Health 1991 Joint Health and Social Services, Health and Social Services develop caring for people, HC (90)23/LAFF 90: 11. HMSO, London

Department of Health 1992 Users guide to primary health care, executive letter, (92)88, Annex D. HMSO, London

Department of Health (1997a) The new NHS: modern, dependable. HMSO, London

Department of Health 1997b RCGP Primary Mental Health Toolkit. HMSO, London

Department of Health 1998 Modernising health and social services: national priorities guidance 1999/2000–2001/2002. HMSO, London

Gell C 1996 User involvement in primary care. The Mental Health Review 1:3

Jordan J, Dowswell T, Harrison S, Lilford R, Mort M 1998 Health needs assessment. Whose priorities? Listening to users and the public. BMJ 316: 1668–1670

Perkins R 1996 Seen but not heard: can 'user involvement' become more than empty rhetoric? The Mental Health Review 1:4

Pritchard P 1994 The patient's voice in primary health care. Primary Care Management 4(1)

Valori R et al (1996) The patient request form: a way of measuring what patients want from their general practitioner. Journal of Psychomatic Research 40(1):87–94

Wensing M, Grol R, Smits A 1994 Quality judgements by patients on general practice care: a literature analysis. Social Science and Medicine 3(1):45–53

Woloshynowych M, Bellenger N, Aluvihare V, Salmon P

PART **3**

Public Health – What Does It Mean for Nurses in Primary Care?

Maureen Morgan

INTRODUCTION

The launch of the Government's health strategy for England, Scotland, Wales and Northern Ireland in the late 1990s underpinned the importance of the role of public health in the NHS (Department of Health 1998c). Although previous initiatives such as the *Health of the Nation* set out the former Government's commitment to preventative health measures, public health, as a comprehensive strategy for addressing major health issues had until then failed to achieve national prominence. The appointment of a minister for public health signalled the re-emergence of one the most successful health disciplines, and one which arguably will need to be adopted and taken forward by nurses, if the opportunities it presents are to be fully realised.

With renewed emphasis on improving health, organized health care is set to go forward in the 21st century in the same manner in which it left the 20th, with public health strategies offering the best opportunities for impacting on the health of the population in the United Kingdom.

Key Issues

- Historical perspective of the public health movement
- Link between health strategy and public health
- Role of public health and its application to primary care nursing

---

The Public Health Movement – An Historical Perspective

The popular view of public health has largely been formed by the radical movement of the last years of the Victorian era. This so-called 'golden age' of public health is credited with bringing about a dramatic improvement in the health of the British people. The early pioneers of public health recognized that the poor health of a large section of the population had its roots in the poverty and appalling living conditions that shaped their lives. Action taken to improve

> **Box 6.8**
>
> **Key Strands Underpinning Public Health Work**
> - Health is influenced by social and material conditions
> - People have health needs as groups and communities
> - There is a need to harness the power of collective action

housing, provide sanitation and clean water, the regulation of food and workplaces, and the introduction of some rudimentary welfare provisions such as pensions, transformed mortality and morbidity rates for everyone, but especially for children. A century or so ago, only six babies out of ten survived to adulthood, and although scientific discoveries such as vaccinations have played their part, the decline in the mortality rate was well underway before these became widely available (Ashton 1988, DHSS 1976).

The success of early public health work was founded on strategies that identified the major causes of ill health in the population, and addressed them through large-scale measures. It was recognized that treating individual symptoms would not solve the health consequences of social problems. Instead far reaching action at the population level was required.

The examples of early public health successes offer an insight into the key strands that underpin public health work. (Box 6.8).

However, the development of effective medicines, such as antibiotics, and of improved surgical treatments, began a move away from population approaches and towards personal medical services (Ashton 1988). The emphasis on public health strategies diminished alongside a growing belief that advances in medical technology held the key to longer healthier lives. The term, public health, became more associated with public health medicine, epidemiology, infection control and promoting the health of individuals. Thus public health was robbed of its campaigning hallmark of earlier years.

Nevertheless, throughout the 1980s and 1990s studies such as the Black Report began to highlight the widening gap in the health experiences of the better off compared with those people in the lowest income group (Davidson et al 1986). This, coupled with a growing concern that unemployment and changes in the welfare system were pushing more people into poverty, served to reawaken interest in the social determinants of health. At the same time, the rising costs of health care began to fuel the debate about costs and effectiveness, thereby heralding a realization of the limitations of some modern medical interventions in bringing about overall improvements in health. The long-term love affair with 'high-tech' medicine began to cool. Many people looked again at what public health could offer to the NHS agenda.

Social Determinants of Health

The Black Report was the first major document to claim there were marked inequalities in health between the social classes in the United Kingdom. Using mortality rates as an indicator of health, the authors reported that the rates tended to rise inversely with falling occupational status for both sexes and at all ages.

The Black Report claimed that the weight of evidence supported the view that material deprivation played the major role in explaining the unfavourable health record of poorer sections of society, with biological, cultural and personal lifestyles being secondary contributing factors (Davidson et al 1986).

Townsend, Phillimore & Beattie (1988), in a later work on inequalities in health in a northern region, claimed that social class should not be regarded as another indicator of deprivation, but should be acknowledged as the social concept that is fundamental to the explanation of the distribution of health, to which all other indicators are secondarily related. Townsend et al (1988) also stated that the single most important component of social class with regard to health was income. An important finding of the study was that whereas poor health was related to material deprivation, the opposite was also true: good health correlated with material wealth (Townsend et al 1988). The findings from these influential studies in the 1980s, linking poverty and health, have been replicated in the 1990s, with several other researchers drawing the same conclusions – that although mortality rates have improved across the board, persistent health inequalities exist between social groups (Acheson 1998, Whitehead 1992). The Chief Medical Officer, presenting his annual report for 1998, noted that:

> 'social inequalities in death rates as judged by the
> gradient in mortality between the highest and lowest
> social groups do not appear to have decreased over the
> past forty years' (Department of Health 1998a).

In addition, some research studies have indicated that it is not simply material deprivation that needs to be considered. Instead relative poverty appears to be an important factor that can be more damaging to health than the absolute poverty of being without the basic necessities of life (Haines 1997). Relative poverty is defined as having an income that is significantly below the average for the society in which one lives (Blackburn 1991). Although estimates vary according to the definitions used, levels of relative poverty are generally assumed to be around one in four adults and one in three children (Wilkinson 1997).

The proportion of people whose income is below average has been at about 60% for the past 30 years. However, the proportion of people at below half of the average income (the European Union definition of poverty) has grown over this period from 10% in 1961 to 20% in 1991, although it did decrease in 1995 to 17% (Acheson 1998). In May 1993, 9.8 million people relied on income support for all or part of their income. Nearly one in three babies were born into families with income low enough to qualify for special payments from the social fund (Laughlin & Black 1995).

The most regularly reported effects of poverty on health include earlier death, increased rates of heart disease and strokes, mental illness, suicide in young men, low birth weight for babies and higher rates of accidents, ear and chest infections in children (Department of Health 1998a). In 1998, the Chief Medical Officer reported that half of the deaths of men aged between 25 and 34 years were from accidents, suicide and homicide, and these had strong social class gradients – over 40% could have been prevented if all men in this age group had had the same all-cause death rates as those in social classes 1 and 2 (Department of Health 1998a).

It is widely acknowledged that remedial action to reduce health inequalities permanently will require a comprehensive strategy incorporating all aspects of political, social, economic and environmental policies. In July 1997 Sir Donald Acheson, former Chief Medical Officer of Health, was invited by the Secretary of State for Health to prepare a report summarizing health inequalities and identifying priority areas for action. The report was published in September 1998 and is recommended reading for those wishing to further their understanding of all the issues (Acheson 1998).

For the NHS, the link between social group and health experience becomes of vital importance when we examine in detail the Government's health strategy and the targets that have been set for us to achieve in the early years of the 21st century.

Health Strategy and Public Health

The Government's health strategy for England is comprehensively laid out in two key documents: *The New NHS: Modern, Dependable* (Department of Health 1997) and *Our Healthier Nation* (Department of Health 1998c), each of which have similar counterparts for Wales and Scotland. The former makes it clear that the duty of the NHS is to improve health, reduce inequalities in health and include patients' experiences in measures of quality and effectiveness. The responsibility for achieving this rests with newly established primary care groups and with health authorities, who are required to set out a health improvement programme on an annual basis. *Our Healthier Nation* emphasizes the need for the NHS to take account of the

---

Box 6.9

Two Main Aims of *Our Healthier Nation* (Department of Health 1998c)

■ To improve the health of the population by lengthening life and increasing the number of years spent free from illness
■ To improve the health of the worse off in society and narrow the health gap

---

social determinants of health and to develop comprehensive strategies with other public sector departments such as education, housing and social services, to address the major health issues. The two main aims of *Our Healthier Nation* are clearly stated and are given in Box 6.9.

So that improvements can be measured, targets (each to be realised by 2010 for people under 65 years of age) have been set within the following four priority areas:

■ heart disease and strokes – the death rate is to be reduced by at least a further one-third
■ cancers – the death rate is to be reduced by at least a further one-fifth
■ accidents – to be reduced in number by at least one-fifth
■ mental health – to reduce the rate of suicide and undetermined injury by at least one-fifth.

In addition to the national targets, it is anticipated that local targets will also be set to reflect local need.

Achieving Health Targets

When considering action plans to achieve health targets it is reasonable to ask how realistic such targets are. Have we already reached optimum levels of health in the United Kingdom so that we could begin to witness the law of diminishing returns? Would the investment of resources needed to improve health even further be so great as to give a poor return when set against what else could be done with the same amounts of money? To answer this *Our Healthier Nation* draws comparisons with similar countries to suggest that we do have real room for improvement. For example, it says, we have one of the highest death rates from circulatory and coronary heart disease in the European Union. Our particular problem in the United Kingdom seems to be that although we achieve mortality rates to rival the best for certain groups in the population, we are not consistent. As we have seen there are wide variations in people's health in this country and these variations influence our overall performance. For example, an analysis of the death rates in men aged 20–64 years shows that if the death rates of all the men in this group equalled those of the well off, there would have been an estimated 17 000 fewer deaths for each year between 1991 and 1993 (Acheson 1998).

If we could achieve the health advances that have been gained by some people for everyone, we would more than succeed in reaching the Government's health targets. To make progress in improving mortality rates across the population we may now need to give priority to those at greatest risk, whose need is most profound. This will mean considering how the health service, particularly primary care, can develop strategies that effectively reduce mortality rates for those people adversely affected by their social and economic environment. Although improving how we provide health care, and making sure everyone has good access will undoubtedly have a positive effect on achieving targets, the suggestion in *Our Healthier Nation* and elsewhere, is that we should rediscover some of our public health skills and apply them to modern, socially derived health issues.

Adopting a Public Health Approach

As we saw earlier, a key principle of public health is collective action at the population level. The *Report of Emerging Findings* from the *Chief Medical Officer's Project to Strengthen the Public Health Function*, noted that 'better population health is the sum of the health of individuals, but needs more than individuals to achieve it' (Department of Health 1998a). This statement is evident in much of the work of public health departments, where measures are taken to control the spread of communicable diseases and to avoid large scale epidemics, or to alert us to new hazards, such as the emergence of methicillin-resistant *Staphylococcus aureus* and HIV infection and AIDS. In these situations it is clear that action involving whole populations is the key to effectiveness.

However, the renewed interest in public health, particularly public health in primary care, centres around taking the principles of working with populations and applying them to what has been hitherto, more or less exclusively, a medical model of health care focused on the individual, illness and risk. The new dimension has been best expressed by the Public Health Alliance, who said that 'within a public health model, the unit on which the attention of primary care is focused, is extended beyond the individual and family group, to include the community in its broadest social, economic and environmental sense' (Taylor 1998). In this way it is possible to include notions of wellbeing and positive health, and to identify those factors that are health enhancing as a alternative to being overly concerned with disease. The Public Health Alliance, in their publication *A Public Health Model of Primary Care – From Concept to Reality* (Taylor 1998), reminds us that the ability to make sense of our lives, having control over what happens to us and a dynamic approach to dealing with life challenges are three factors that help us to remain healthy in difficult life circumstances. Such factors occur more readily when the prevailing conditions generate equity, good social networks, social cohesion and empowered individuals and communities. These observations echo the World Health Organization's *Health for All Strategy*, which emphasized a model of primary care built on intersectorial partnerships, equity and community participation as a precondition to promoting health and reducing health inequalities (WHO 1978).

The notion of factors that offer a degree of protection from the health costs of poverty and deprivation helps us to understand the sorts of interventions that will contribute to reducing health inequalities. We also see another key principle of public health emerging: that of partnerships and collective action. It becomes clear that the kind of social structures that will protect health can only be created through the cooperation of everyone involved in providing public services in communities, including local people themselves. The health service cannot act alone.

This is no doubt why the Government, having stated its intention to tackle the root causes of ill health, has designed a new framework for the NHS with interagency partnerships at its core. Health policy now places a duty on all the agencies in the public sector to work together in several settings, for example, in health action zones, healthy living centres, and of course, primary care groups.

The challenge for the doctors and nurses in primary care groups will be to learn to work with groups and communities rather than just individual patients who present for care, and to develop productive partnerships with others locally, so that together they can maximize the conditions that protect health, even in adverse social circumstances.

Public Health: the Nursing Contribution

For nurses, the idea that they should play a prominent role in developing public health approaches was outlined in a report of the Standing Nursing and Midwifery Advisory Committee (SNMAC), published in 1995. Entitled *Making it Happen*, the report suggested that while some nurses, such as health visitors, school nurses, occupational nurses and those working in communicable diseases, had long traditions of public health work, many others were also ideally placed to increase their contribution to public health to the benefit of patients. The report urged nurses in every sphere of practice to become 'thoughtful in promoting public health strategies and interventions, working together with the people and communities they serve'. The report also claimed that mobilizing the nursing, midwifery and health visiting workforce within the public health arena would have a considerable impact on the nation's health. This, the authors said, was because as well as constituting the largest professional group in the NHS, nurses offered a variety of skills and had contact with a wide cross-section of society, in hospitals, homes, schools, workplaces and communal environments. Nurses were also trained to see patients and clients in their social context and so were more able to apply both social and medical models of health (SNMAC 1995).

Public Health Nursing Activities

Public health nursing covers a wide spectrum of activities, including infection control, health promotion, screening and carrying out immunization programmes. This type of work is familiar to most nurses and many will have found themselves involved in at least one or more of them at some time.

The remainder of this section describes public health nursing work which may be less familiar, particularly to non-health visitor readers, but is increasingly seen as being a key contribution that nurses in primary care can make to the public health agenda. The examples given (Box 6.10) demonstrate the principles of addressing determinants of health, working with populations and taking collective action.

Health Profiling

Hitherto, a criticism of medically focused primary care has been that it is limited by its failure to look beyond the individuals who present for care. Health profiling addresses this problem by enabling all health needs to be recognized, whether or not people seek out services. It forms a crucial stage in assessing the differing influences on health for individuals, groups and communities, and so helps in developing a picture of the major health issues facing local people.

The process of profiling involves gathering data from a variety of sources, including the Office for National Statistics for demographic and socioeconomic electoral ward-based information, mortality and morbidity data and other health statistics from the health authority, to

---

Box 6.10

The Key Activities of the Nursing Contribution to Public Health

- Health profiling
- Population-based approaches to meeting need
- Community development
- Working in partnerships

complement local information kept at practice and caseload level. It must also include methods of incorporating the views of local people, either by involving them in a systematic way or by collating evidence from the stories heard during their everyday work by members of the primary health care team in surgeries, clinics, homes, shops and schools. The completed profile will define the population served, help to determine the groups at risk and identify those who already have health problems. Analysis of the information must include comparisons with national and local norms to help teams decide which issues are important and should be given a high priority. Information must also be collected about what else is being provided in the neighbourhood so that best use can be made of all resources. Gaps in service provision must also be identified (Rowe et al 1997).

This combination of socioeconomic data, health statistics and personal knowledge of working with local people provides a rich seam of information, unrivalled by other official documents, making the health profile a powerful mechanism for recognizing trends and targeting health care to those who will benefit most. It also provokes consideration of different patterns of health action and interventions that may be more effective in meeting the needs of those who have the poorest health experience, than some of the more traditional ways of providing care.

A health profile can become the building block for developing public health approaches. It can help to move primary care nurses and GPs away from a simple concern for the patient in front of them and enable them to consider the health needs of the population as a whole.

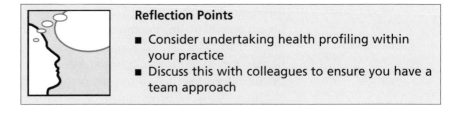

Reflection Points

■ Consider undertaking health profiling within your practice
■ Discuss this with colleagues to ensure you have a team approach

Population-based Approaches to Meeting Need

Compiling a health profile helps nurses in primary care recognize the patterns drawn by the individuals who make up the local community so that connections can be made between social or environmental conditions and opportunities for health. In public health terms, taking a population approach to meeting need also means considering whether interventions aimed at groups and communities will be more effective than dealing with people on an individual basis. This is because people for whom life is a day-to-day struggle of trying to make ends meet can find it impossible to achieve and maintain health on their own. Unsurprisingly, other concerns take precedence.

In the past, health promotion in primary care has focused most of its efforts on trying to persuade individuals to adopt healthier lifestyles. Although this can be a useful strategy, especially if offered at some critical points in peoples' lives, such as post-myocardial infarction, individual health promotion tends to be less successful for people living in difficult social circumstances who have more pressing concerns than the risk of hypothetical health problems in the future (Acheson 1998).

People make complex decisions about their health that can sometimes appear perplexing to the professional. However, persistent behaviours that are at odds with good health choices do become more understandable when seen within the context of people's lives and the competing demands on their resources. Although it is common for health professionals to speak of health choices, for poorer people it would often be more accurate to talk about health compromises. For example, cigarette smoking is cited by some people, particularly young working class mothers, as a coping strategy to help them deal with the stresses and hardships of their lives and as representing the only luxury available to them (Graham 1988).

The starting point for effective interventions must therefore deal with the issues that people themselves regard as priorities. Their concerns are frequently about shortage of money, unemployment, poor housing and lack of safe play areas for children, all of which may have little to do with their own individual behaviour and more to do with the political, economic and social framework within which they live. To respond to issues that cause concern for the majority of people in a neighbourhood or community, primary care nurses need to be willing to stimulate local action to improve the environment and increase resources for health. This may mean ensuring that there is easy access to welfare rights advice or to expert help in implementing crime or accident prevention strategies. It could also mean collaborating with others to devise projects to attract special government funds, such as those available for regenerating deprived areas.

Consideration may also need to be given to restructuring how health resources are used. For example, it could be more effective to set up self help groups instead of working with individuals. Public health nursing activity may also include making representations to local politicians to elicit their support in bringing about improvements in general conditions for the population as a whole.

Working within a public health and social model of health means accepting that personal behaviour is only one of the influences on health and, just as collective action was needed to establish an effective sanitary system, collective action will be needed to generate the kind of supportive environment and resources for health necessary to tackle health inequalities.

Community Development

Although the social problems prevalent in some communities can appear overwhelming, certain conditions can help to reduce the harmful health effects of deprivation. When people feel part of a supportive network and when they are encouraged to take some control over what happens to them, they are more likely to respond positively to health promotion messages.

Although not widely represented in the NHS, community development work is an effective means of engaging with people to help them achieve change for themselves. It is built on principles that hold that all people, despite any disadvantage, have skills they can draw on to help themselves, that people should be allowed to define the problems facing them for themselves without having unhelpful labels attached to them by others, and that they should not be prevented from taking action on their own behalf (Laughlin & Black 1995).

A key factor in community development is the recognition that people who lack power and influence in their ordinary lives can gain it by coming together in groups. Frequently such groups can be formed around small communities, such as exist on housing estates or even single streets or tower blocks. Other times they may constitute a community of interest, such as young unsupported mothers or women who are victims of domestic violence. The crucial concept is that people can gain strength from others in the same position as themselves and can learn from each other. This enables them to articulate their needs, decide for themselves which issues are most important and determine what actions or services will help them most. Taking control in this way, increases confidence and self esteem, and this is a key factor in helping people change.

The role of the professional is to create the networks to bring people together, provide the physical environment and resources, and facilitate group activity. Community development also requires a genuine attempt on the part of the professionals to understand how local people feel and a real willingness to share power and decision making.

Working in Partnerships

The twin themes of partnerships and participation figure highly in public health nursing in the community. Implicit in public health approaches is the need to work in collaboration with other agencies. This is because many people operating in the statutory or non-voluntary organizations, such as housing departments, have a great influence on health or health resources in the community. Some of the voluntary groups, such as those who cater for people who have severe mental health problems, provide day or drop-in centres or other community facilities:

'Working effectively with other disparate agencies, in recognition that they affect health and well-being, means working through others, sharing evidence of local needs, encouraging contributions and acting as a catalyst and taking a "whole systems approach"' (Department of Health 1997).

Nurses who develop their skills in working across organizational boundaries are able to influence the policies of other groups and agencies so that health features higher on their agendas. Working collaboratively makes it possible to organize coordinated approaches to issues such as accident prevention, which require intervention at several levels in the community to be really effective.

Case Study 6.2

Public Health in Primary Care – Supportive Social Network – Preventing Accidents to Children

Following completion of their health profile, primary health care team A wanted to reduce the number of accidents to children as one of their objectives. Although it was difficult to get an absolutely accurate picture of the number of accidents involving children, because the team served a population in which there were high levels of deprivation and they were aware that the children most likely to suffer accidents are in low-income families, they were not surprised that anecdotal evidence from GPs and health visitors indicated that rates locally were high. They were also aware that accident prevention was one of the Government's targets for health improvement so it seemed reasonable to include accidents as one of their three main priorities for the forthcoming year. Their action plan had several strands:

- First, to be able to evaluate their performance in future years they needed to ensure they kept better statistics within the practice. This meant agreeing terminology: for example, they agreed to define their group at risk as being all children aged 14 years and under. They then had to design a computer code for recording accidents that could be used by everyone. They also decided to include a category to indicate the degree of severity. To obtain more complete data they linked with the paediatric liaison health visitor at the accident and emergency department and determined to encourage parents to record accidents that needed home treatment in the parent-held record
- Raising awareness in the community – to raise awareness of accidents locally, data were depicted on the information boards in the health centre and members of the primary health care team visited groups such as the mother and toddler clubs to talk about local accidents. Volunteers were also sought to join in to map local

Case Study 6.2   Cont'd

accident danger zones. The results of the mapping exercise would be presented to the local council for their consideration, as well as to all local people. First aid classes were also to be offered to parents in the schools as a means of raising awareness as well as improving knowledge and treatment

■ Ensuring a safer environment – this comprised working with other local agencies to develop safe play areas for children as well as setting up a safety equipment loan scheme for items such as fire, stair and cooker guards. The team also linked with the local fire brigade who were keen to extend the use of smoke detectors in homes and to talk to people about how to use them successfully

■ Improved treatment – here the team agreed to update their own skills and knowledge in respect of first aid treatment. The reception staff and practice manager were included in these sessions to increase the level of expertise in the team and in recognition that occasionally, non-clinical staff were the only people present in the health centre when accident victims arrived

■ Evaluation – an evaluation of the accident action plan was included at the beginning of the programme. This was to include an audit of the completeness of accident data on the practice computer at the year end, as well as an audit of all childhood accidents to highlight trends. The first aid sessions for parents were to be evaluated at the end of the programme. The team also expected to have produced a joint accident prevention plan with all local agencies and aimed to audit the resources for home safety that had been supplied to determine the percentage of households that had safety equipment

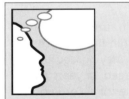

Consider this case study in relation to your own practice. What strategies would you use to adopt a public health perspective within your practice?

Conclusion

John Ashton states that the starting point for public health action is the recognition that most health is gained or lost in everyday life through the environments that determine exposure to hazard or shape lifestyle (Ashton 1988). Practice nurses are only too well aware of this. The evidence greets them each day in their working lives. Their future position in primary care groups offers them the potential to take part in planning, delivering and commissioning health care that accepts people's health as the product of the conditions that surround them. They will have the opportunity to develop strategies that acknowledge this, and can create a future in which health care professionals work alongside people, taking part in health care activities with them rather than 'doing things' to them. A public health way of thinking will allow them to plan, provide and commission health services that place an emphasis on protecting and sustaining health as well as offering care and treatment.

This chapter has highlighted the knowledge and skills associated with public health practice. Although knowledge and skills are necessary precursors to public health action, public health is also about a way of thinking that looks beyond the individual and does not separate them from their social and economic circumstances. Public health is therefore more than public health medicine. It combines scientific, biomedical and social models of health to address the most pressing health issues. And crucially, as the Alliance for Public Health argues, public health is about how communities can use medicine, and other sciences, political developments and processes to achieve health gain for themselves (Taylor 1998).

References

Acheson D 1998 Independent inquiry into inequalities in health report. Department of Health, London

Ashton J 1988 The new public health. Open University Press, Milton Keynes

Blackburn C 1991 Poverty and health: working with families. Open University Press, Milton Keynes

Davidson N, Townsend P, Whitehead M 1986 Inequalities in health: the Black report. Penguin, Harmondsworth

Department of Health and Social Security 1976 Prevention and health: everybody's business. HMSO, London

Department of Health and Social Security 1980 Inequalities in health: a report of a research working group. HMSO, London

Department of Health 1997 The new NHS: modern, dependable. HMSO, London

Department of Health 1998a Chief medical officer's project to strengthen the public health function. HMSO, London

Department of Health 1998b On the state of public health. HMSO, London

Department of Health 1998c Our healthier nation: a contract for health. HMSO, London

Graham H 1988 Women, health and the family. Health Education Council, London

Haines A 1997 Working together to reduce poverty's damage. British Medical Journal 314:529–530

Laughlin S, Black D 1995 Poverty and health, tools for change. Public Health Alliance, Birmingham

Rowe A, Mitchinson S, Morgan M, Carey L 1997 Health profiling: all you need to know. A practical guide for primary health care teams. Liverpool JMU and Premier Health, Liverpool JMU Enterprise Unit, Liverpool

SNMAC 1995 Making it happen. HMSO, London

Taylor P 1998 A public health model of primary care – from concept to reality. Public Health Alliance, Birmingham

Townsend P, Phillimore P, Beattie A 1988 Health and deprivation in a northern region. Croom Helm, London

Whitehead M 1992 The health divide. In: Townsend et al (eds) Inequalities in health: the Black Report and the health divide, 2nd edn. Penguin, London

WHO 1978 Primary health care Alma-Ata 1978. Report on the international conference on primary health care, Alma-Ata, USSR, 6–12 September 1978. WHO, Geneva

Wilkinson RG 1997 Health inequalities, relative or absolute material standards. British Medical Journal 314:591–594

7 *Mental Health – does the Practice Nurse Have a Role?*

Mick McKeown

INTRODUCTION

Mental distress is common in contemporary society and the most usual point of contact for people seeking treatment or health advice is general practice. Nurses, among all health professionals working in this area, are likely to be in a prime position to engage effectively with people who have a range of psychic or emotional problems. A person's mental health may be the principal reason for seeking a consultation or problems may be secondary to, or associated with, a physical complaint. Contrary to popular misconception, the majority of people who have mental health problems, including many who present the severest need, are treated in general practice without the intervention of specialist psychiatric services.

The prevention or minimization of mental ill health, with a special emphasis upon reducing the number of suicides, is a major strand of government health policy, with mental health constituting one of the four key primary care foci. Both mental health and primary care provision are high on the agenda of NHS research priorities. This welcome move to giving primary care a lead role in the modern NHS, together with the established process of deinstitutionalizing mental health care, raises expectations for the treatment, care and support of mentally distressed people within the context of general practice.

Given the constellation of factors coalescing to raise the profile of mental health issues in primary care, it is arguable that practitioners are inadequately prepared to meet the demands placed upon such services. The numbers of registered mental nurses employed as practice nurses or nurse practitioners remains proportionally tiny in relation to those holding general nursing qualifications. Despite the prevalence of mental health problems in community populations and the consequential pressure upon general practice consultations, the subject has received scant attention to date in texts, other than those written specifically for mental health nurses and other specialist practitioners. With the notable exception of Armstrong's work (1995, 1997) little has been written directly for practice nurses. Given the thrust of policy towards community care and preventative initiatives, these omissions are in need of remedy if practice nurses are to be in a position to answer the titular question posed here.

Mental health problems are common, representing a major fraction of overall health demand and resulting in significant costs to the economy as a whole. Although official figures are widely considered to underestimate the situation, the Health Education Authority (HEA 1997) compiled a sobering collection: population studies suggest that at any one time, one in four adults will experience a mental health problem. Coroners' statistics record over 3500 suicides per year, approximating to ten such deaths every day. The overall annual cost of mental health problems was estimated in 1997 to be £32 billion, and NHS spending on mental health was £1.93 billion in 1992–1993, accounting for nearly 5% of all inpatient expenditure. In the latter period spending on psychiatric medication alone totalled over £201 million, and has been estimated as rising by around 25% year on year. Local authority social services spending for mental illness in 1994–1995 was £311 million. In terms of employment, at least 80 million working days are lost annually as a result of anxiety and depression, with other stress-related sickness accounting for half of all absences.

Key Issues

- Impact of government policy
- The range of mental health problems and needs
- Involvement of service users and families
- Challenging stigma and negative stereotypes
- Suggested features of role for practice nurses in mental health
- Balancing inputs between primary care and specialist services

---

Policy

The half century since the establishment of the NHS has also coincided with the drawn out process of retracting the Victorian psychiatric asylum system. In the latter decades of this project mental health services have become almost the paradigm case of a wider set of policy aims known as 'care in the community'. Driven by pointed and well-founded criticism of the wholly unacceptable institutionalizing, and often abusive, regimes, the large asylums have been slowly decommissioned since the 1950s. Almost contemporaneously, advances in psychotropic medication helped to further expedite this project and added to the optimism that community care could be managed effectively.

However, the representation of the mentally disordered as individuals worthy of the care and compassion of the community has shifted to fears and anxieties expressed by communities. The issue of public safety has fuelled the promise of legislation and reorganization targeting the community supervision of the severely mentally ill. These policy concerns have been framed amidst a backdrop of lurid and sensationalist media attention, putting the spotlight on grave shortcomings in the provision of systematic care and support. Several catastrophic failures of community care resulting in homicide or high-profile exhibitions of vulnerability raise misgivings for a system deemed to be in crisis. However, the recent confidential inquiry (Steering Group of the Confidential Inquiry into Homicides and Suicides by Mentally Ill People 1996) into homicide and suicide among people with mental disorder correctly reaffirms all the earlier studies into these matters, which have consistently exploded the myth that the mentally ill pose a higher than average risk of committing murder or that such murders are on the increase. This is neither to argue that the issue of mentally disordered offenders is unimportant nor to be disinterested in learning lessons from the various cases when they occur. Rather we should be careful about generalizing from the small numbers of high-profile cases presented in the media, and be clear what the actual lessons to be learnt are.

Has Community Care Really Failed?

Despite the undoubted mistakes made and repeatedly illustrated in successive inquiry reports, it is worth pointing out that typically they have resulted from failures in the systematic management of care and need not be interpreted as damning the entire notion of care in the community. The crucial features of effective risk management (applying equally to other areas such as child protection), are systematic, multiprofessional, multiagency coordination and communication, and are built into the case management models envisaged under the care programme approach (CPA) (Department of Health 1990).

Less prominent in public consciousness, yet nonetheless visible, have been the numbers of mentally ill homeless, either inhabiting substandard or temporary accommodation, or quite literally on the streets, or those currently detained in prison. Indeed, the increase in the provision of penal accommodation in recent years almost exactly matches the reduction in beds in mental institutions. Taken with the national scandal of the figures for suicide rates among the severely mentally ill, all these factors have contributed to a sense of pessimism that community care is not working. It is perhaps more realistic to view the delivery of care in the community as problematic, yet envisage practical solutions to these problems rather than jettison the whole idea.

Future Prescriptions

The government's blueprint for modern, clinically effective mental health services promises to make progress with respect to a number of key policy strands (Department of Health 1999a, 1999b). These will include a general focus upon primary care, enhanced involvement of service users and carers in the commissioning, planning and delivery of services, a continuation of emphasis towards prioritizing the needs of the severely mentally ill and systematic attention to the supervision and management of risk. Given that at least some of these are seemingly contradictory, a degree of confusion may extend into the operationalizing of policy at service level.

For those practitioners working towards meeting the needs of mental health service users within primary care, the most obvious contradiction in policy to date has been the emphasis upon specialist secondary psychiatric services and their liaison with local social services, to the relative neglect of primary care. This has happened despite the fact that most people who have mental health problems receive their care from a mixture of primary care and community services (Goldberg & Huxley 1992). A major policy theme in mental health has been around the organizational configuration of services and how these can ensure optimum standards, effective interagency communication and systematic coordination of care delivery and accountability. Notably, this focus has resulted in the adoption of the Care Plan Approach. Butler and colleagues' (1997) call for a recognition of the extensive role played by professionals in primary care in the provision of mental health services, should be coupled with mechanisms to ensure improvements in communications between this sector and specialist services in the interests of better treatment and management. In effect, what is urged is that mental health policy objectives are compatible with the broader NHS policy of prioritizing primary interventions (Butler et al 1997).

What do Service Users Want?

When people who have mental health problems are asked which aspects of their lives they would most wish to improve, clinical concerns (the concerns of clinicians) seldom feature prominently. These are usually secondary to four main social wants: namely, housing, employment, money and friendships. Peck (1997) makes the insightful observation that mental health services cannot continue tinkering around the edges of these concerns without attempting to link mental health policy to broader social policy. The idea that all aspects of government policy development could be informed with recourse to a mental health template, such that mental health policy becomes focused upon the mainstream, with the aim of 'mainstreaming' service users, is an ambitious yet, nonetheless, laudable aim. Indeed, it would seem to be neatly compatible with New Labour's oft repeated rhetoric of implementing social justice by eradicating social exclusion. It is to be hoped that the real implications of this grand claim to be against marginalization extend to the specifics of key policy directives, apply to the mentally distressed as a socially excluded group and are not compromised by a heavy handed emphasis on assuaging misplaced public fears of dangerousness. Despite the relatively easy political capital that can be accumulated by playing up to heightened public fears and damning the previous administration for the imperfections of community care, it is worth remembering the continued validity of care in the community as a worthwhile and worthy objective. In this context, the future success of mental health policy, to be measured in the quality of lived experience for the users of our services, will to a large extent be played out in the field of primary care.

Mental Health Problems and Needs in Primary Care

In many respects the United Kingdom's primary care services have an enviable and deserved international reputation. Upwards of 98% of the population are registered with a GP, with an average list size comprising approximately 2000 patients. In any one year 60% of those patients registered will consult their GP and between one-fifth to one-quarter will have a mental health problem either as a sole reason for attending or as major feature of their presentation (Shepherd et al 1981, RCGP et al 1995). Jenkins (1992) has claimed that ten times as many people consult their GP for mental illness than attend psychiatric outpatient clinics. On top of this it has been estimated that many GP consultations, perhaps as many as 90%, are taken up with stress-related complaints.

Psychiatry and general practice have been in the vanguard of those health care specialisms developing new approaches to their work, especially in the context of team working. Notwithstanding such developments, it would be fair to say that the national picture concerning integration between primary care and secondary care services is variable. Care in the community policies have placed an increased burden on GPs and primary care teams (Thornicroft & Bebbington 1989), with reductions in overall hospital bed numbers adding to the difficulties. Those areas without adequate provision of crisis care or respite facilities or a well-developed and robust CPA have particularly acute problems.

The range of recognizable mental disorders likely to be engaged within primary care is typically referred to as spanning the less severe neuroses to the more severe psychoses; from the so-called 'worried-well' to the chronically debilitated severely mentally ill. Platitudinous demarcations such as these can act to mask the complexity of an individual's problems or to unnecessarily minimize either the subjectively distressful experience of those at one end of the divide or the therapeutic optimism of practitioners with regard to those at the opposite end. Paradoxically, patients who present with mainly emotional or psychological problems may receive treatment for a perceived physical problem instead, whereas patients known to have severe mental health problems fail to have their real physical problems detected. Notwithstanding problems in identifying the actual extent of mental ill health, various social factors, most notably the negative effects of stigmatizing attitudes, can dissuade people from seeking help in the first place. Taken together there is a resultant 'iceberg' effect where a great deal of societal mental distress remains hidden and hence does not attract professional help, support or treatment. Although this state of affairs is worthy of our concern it ought to be tempered with a recognition of the possibly undesirable consequences of an unfettered medicalization of hitherto untouched aspects of personal or interpersonal upset.

The majority of patients who attend general practice complaining of mental distress have depression or depression-like symptoms; other important presenting diagnoses include anxiety, schizophrenia and dementia. Studies of numbers attending general practice suggest that in a typical practice population 20% will have symptoms of depression, amounting to 300–400 individuals in total, with a quarter of these having a major depressive illness. Figures for people who have psychotic problems are much lower, usually no more than 4–12 persons in any practice (Strathdee & Jenkins 1996). This variation largely depends upon location, with a higher incidence in inner cities, but the GP's affinity for mental health work can be influential (Armstrong 1998).

A matter of concern for health practitioners is the fact that people who have severe mental health problems have a significantly greater risk of committing suicide than the general population. A notable subgroup among those who have low mood and depression are women immediately following childbirth. Another major client group often referred to under the remit of mental health services, even though their problem is probably better defined as a social problem, are people with substance use problems, whether street drugs, alcohol or misuse or dependency upon prescribed medication.

Usually people concerned about their mental health will report a complex mixture of symptoms and problems, some of which are distinct to a given diagnostic category, some of which are common to a number of psychiatric diagnoses. Confusion can occur because problems such as sleep disturbance or sexual dysfunction may arise directly as a symptom of mental ill health or as a consequence of prescribed medication. It may often be the case that such physical complaints first bring people to the attention of their family practice. Alternatively, the first point of contact with services for a person with mental distress may be an upset family member reporting strange or incomprehensible behaviour.

Limits of space preclude detailed discussion and description of a range of specific mental health problems. Practitioners interested in such information will find the main mental health problems likely to be encountered in primary care, together with information on screening tools, and the role of practice nurses dealt with in Armstrong's (1997) *Primary Mental Health Care Toolkit* (published by the Royal College of General Practitioners with the support of the Department of Health), schizophrenia and psychosocial interventions in McKeown, McCann & Cooper's (1998) distance learning pack, and numerous information booklets, leaflets and videos produced by a variety of sources such as MIND.

The attachment of a diagnosis may be welcomed by service users and their families as an explanation for seemingly incomprehensible problems. On other occasions service users may reject a diagnostic label, perhaps because of its stigmatizing effects. Either way it can often make most sense to engage where possible in a problem-focused way that is not dependent upon acceptance or otherwise of a diagnosis, and may enable more active participation of the service recipient in agreeing how to address the specific problems for which help is sought. An important dimension of effective interventions for mental health problems can be the involvement of family and friends in the delivery of care, or indeed, recognizing the distinct needs of informal carers for their own emotional and practical support in this context. A neglect of these concerns can mean that the carers themselves seek a practice consultation for physical or mental health problems of their own.

Severe Mental Health Problems in Primary Care

Current policy, practice and research trends urge practitioners and services to prioritize the needs of people who have the most severe mental health problems. The rise to prominence of terms such as 'severe mental illness', 'severe and enduring mental illness', 'serious mental health problems' and other variations on the same theme, has not been matched by precision in definition. This can cause problems in reading research reports and policy recommendations if the particular group in question is poorly defined or not made explicit. Similarly, various therapeutic interventions may demonstrate clinical effectiveness for a specific client population (e.g. those who have schizophrenia), but applicability within a more broadly defined 'severe' grouping may be open to question. Conversely, too rigid an approach to definition, or attempts to impose particular definitions across the board, can pose difficulties for personnel attempting to develop services that match local circumstances. Repper & Brooker (1998) point out that whichever definition is employed, there is consensus that this priority group contains those people who, despite heterogeneity of diagnoses, exhibit high levels of need resulting from problems that seriously limit their everyday lives.

In practice, the group of people most usually referred to in this context have received a diagnosis of schizophrenia. Indeed, many texts use the term severe mental illness as a virtual synonym for schizophrenia. Although the actual numbers of people who have serious mental health problems in any practice may be relatively small, the allegation that GPs only concern themselves with patients who present with anxiety and depression has been strongly challenged (King 1992). Reports have consistently demonstrated that up to 25% of patients in the community who have schizophrenia and are discharged from mental health facilities are managed only by their family doctor. The most recent of these reports, carried out by the mental health charity SANE (1997), showed that 55% of people who had been diagnosed with schizophrenia saw their GP regularly, and for 6%, the GP was the only professional they reported any contact with.

Getting the Balance Right

Despite policy pronouncements and various critical reviews of services, community mental health teams (CMHTs) and community psychiatric nurses in particular have been accused of neglecting the needs of people who have severe and enduring mental health problems (Gournay 1994). Where attempts have been made to shift the balance toward prioritizing the severest need, this has been resisted as tantamount to dismissing the needs of other mentally distressed service users (Barker 1993). This counterargument highlights the practical and moral folly of excluding those labelled as 'worried-well' from a roll-call of the 'needy' merely because they are not suffering from psychosis. People complaining of anxiety and depression are often described as 'less seriously ill', but may nevertheless experience levels of distress and curtailment of ordinary social activity that most people would find intolerable. The dilemmas raised in this debate highlight how the laudable desire to prioritize services can result in the unwholesome demarcation of potential service users into the deserving and undeserving. These issues will be most acute at times of limited investment in service infrastructure and staff development – unfortunately a typical state of affairs in recent decades.

Notwithstanding such concerns, it is essential that services are prioritized. Such priority setting should be about altering the balance of existing resources and redeploying them for the maximum collective benefit. Resource allocation will always be an issue. The challenge for mental health services is to achieve the appropriate balance in provision of services for the whole range of severity of mental health problems in the community. This may involve developments where specialist secondary services prioritize their work towards people who have serious and enduring mental health problems, while the primary care team focuses on the treatment of less severe mental health problems with the support of their local CMHT. Such a division of labour would not imply, however, that practitioners in primary care would abrogate all input to people with the severest problems. Rather, a range of meaningful activity would preferably continue; what would be at stake is the allocation of key responsibilities within systems of case management, and the delivery of particular specialist interventions by the appropriately skilled personnel.

The Practice Nurse's Role

A comprehensive role for practice nurses and other colleagues in primary care towards meeting the complexity of need presented by people who have mental health problems in their practice can be envisaged as having a number of key dimensions (Box 7.1). In many

---

Box 7.1

Dimensions of Mental Health Role for Practice Nurses

- Screening for emotional and psychic distress; both as a primary problem or associated with presenting physical complaint. Important role in screening for suicide risk. Early warning signs of psychotic breakdown
- Provision of supporting interventions within bounds of competence
- Detection and management of physical problems in people who have severe mental illness
- Detection and management of the mental distress associated with physical illness
- Engagement and support of service user's family members or significant others in their social network
- Mental health promotion initiatives
- Liaison and shared care with specialist services
- Establishment and maintenance of nondiscriminatory practices towards those who have mental health problems generally, and specific minority or marginalized groups
- A systematic approach to identifying and meeting relevant professional training needs across the team
- Evaluation and audit

respects these involve the traditional concerns of nurses working in primary care, but with a mental health focus, and, as such, would not necessarily be a radical departure from the typical practice nurse role. Such features would include health promotion, preventive measures at different levels, concern for individuals within a wider social network, aspects of physical care and liaison across the primary and secondary care interface.

At the level of values and attitudes, which can have a powerful impact upon the delivery and organization of care, important issues of equity arise if services are not to offend or discriminate against potentially marginalized and stereotyped groups. Contemplation of specific helping interventions may raise issues of competency, necessitating further training, operation within agreed protocols or referral on to other agencies. Indeed, the entire range of role development in relation to mental health generates its own training implications and also raises specific issues of evaluation and audit.

When contemplating these issues it is worth noting that several of the potential developments in the practice nursing role outlined here are already within the compass and practice of many nurses in primary care. Others may be taken on by other members of the primary care team, or be offered elsewhere, either by community mental health teams or various external agencies, following referral from the practice nurse. Alternatively, the intervention may take place within the general practice setting, but be delivered by specialist practitioners on a sessional basis. Extensions to role are best thought of as possibilities, with actual developments in any individual practice likely to depend upon a number of factors, not least the willingness of particular practitioners or teams to take on the role. Mead, Bower & Gask (1997) raise the salutary caution that it is often commentators outside of general practice who generate seemingly endless lists describing the tasks that are 'ideally suited' to primary care practitioners. Speculation over ideals must take place side by side with a realistic appraisal of total resources, including the competing demands on staff time.

Notwithstanding the need for prudent examination of the contingencies of taking up aspects of a mental health role, there are good reasons why nurses are well placed to do so. A number of studies have reported people's preferences to talk about their emotional or psychological problems with the practice nurse rather than the GP, seeing the nurse as more approachable and understanding in such matters (Stilwell 1988). Furthermore, there are other factors in favour of people having their mental health problems dealt with in general practice. It is less likely that a person's psychosocial problems will be stigmatized, assisting in the normalization of mental distress (Wilkinson 1992). There is also evidence that people have more confidence in a continuity of treatment, from reporting the problem through therapeutic intervention, from the practitioner with whom they have their initial contact (Johnson & Courtney 1993 unpublished, cited in Mead et al 1997). The general philosophical aim advocated could be reduced to a plea for holism. The notion of holistic care ought to be complementary and compatible with the practice of all nurses, and present few problems of acceptance. However it is worth reflecting upon Armstrong's (1998) cautionary note that the rhetoric of holistic care often masks a reality wherein the physical is emphasized.

Mental Health Screening

It is widely acknowledged that much mental disorder goes unrecognized in primary care populations. Some of the hidden mass of mental distress is due to the disinclination for people themselves to recognize or acknowledge a mental component to their problems, or even where this is recognized, a reluctance to admit this to professional staff. However, the inability of GPs to detect mental ill health is also important. It seems that GPs across Europe and America have difficulties in recognizing or treating the extent of mental health problems in their practice populations (Higgins 1994, Joukamaa, Lehtinen & Karlsson 1995, Ormel et al 1991, Tiemens, Ormel & Simon 1996, Vazquez-Barquero et al 1997). Few studies have examined the abilities of other primary care staff in the detection of mental disorder, but Thomas & Corney (1993) report that practice nurses assess large proportions of their patients as having 'psychological distress'. It is difficult to draw meaningful comparisons because the nurses in this study saw people who did not see the GP; however, Mead and colleagues (1997) contrast the lack of sensitivity in the GP assessments with a possible lack of specificity among the nurses. A number of factors apparently interact to confound the ability of practitioners to accurately detect mental ill health (Box 7.2), suggesting the need for training to raise awareness and specific and systematic methods of assessment.

Although surveys of practice nursing workload suggest that many practice nurses are active in picking up the emotional problems of their clients (Atkin & Lunt 1993, Greenfield, Stilwell & Drury 1987), a more systematic approach to screening would improve general practice recognition and treatment of mental distress. Effective screening is commensurate with a preventative health approach to mental health problems and of particular importance in suicide prevention. Similarly, focused screening initiatives can act as a precursor to measures aimed at preventing relapse in severe psychotic conditions. Armstrong (1997) offers a semistructured interview schedule, together with guidance for practice nurses in incorporating questioning

---

Box 7.2

Confounding Factors in Detection of Mental Health Problems

Patient factors

■ Gender – women are more likely to attend and more willing to discuss psychological problems
■ Marital status, middle age, unemployment – these groups are more likely to be identified with mental health problems by GP
■ Ethnicity – certain ethnic groups may more readily somatize problems (see below)
■ Coexisting social problems – facilitates recognition of mental health problems
■ Physical illness – hinders detection
■ Old age – underdiagnosis of depression
■ Previous psychiatric history – more likely to be identified as having current problems
■ Education over age 23 – less likely to be detected

Practitioner factors

■ Communication skills – poor engagement skills create barriers to disclosure; practitioners may be reluctant to delve into emotional distress because they lack the skills to respond
■ Attitudes/stereotyping – relevant to much above
■ Personality – may result in presenting a brusque and mechanical manner; antithetical to the task
■ Cultural insensitivity – problems across mental health services in over representation of ethnic groups in particular diagnoses
■ Interviewing skills – inability to effectively elicit necessary information to detect mental health problems
■ Transference and countertransference
■ Reliance on intuitive judgement over use of systematic assessment tools
■ Lack of relevant training and experience – especially in specialist mental health issues and services
■ Pressure of time

---

about mental health problems, especially depression, into routine health checks, such as initial registration interviews and well-woman or well-man clinics. Given the tendency to miss depression in the elderly it makes sense for practice nurses to incorporate systematic eliciting questions for depressed mood into their routine screening of older people. Mottram and colleagues (1996) argue that such an approach ought not to be restricted to the over-75 year age group. Whatever the severity of mental health problem, screening can be allied to attempts to avoid deterioration or help target conditions that may benefit from early intervention. Outreach screening can help

> **Box 7.3**
>
> **Examples of Systematic Assessment Tools Appropriate for Screening in Primary Care (Armstrong 1997)**
>
> - The General Health Questionnaire (GHQ) (Goldberg & Williams 1988)
>   — target group: general mental health screening
> - Hospital Anxiety and Depression Scale (HAD) (Zigmund & Snaith 1983)
>   — target group: anxiety and depression
> - The Geriatric Depression Scale (GDS) (Sheikh & Yesesevage 1986)
>   — target group: depression in the elderly
> - Edinburgh Postnatal Depression Scale (EPDS) (Cox et al 1987)
>   — target group: postnatal depression
> - Beck Depression Inventory (BDI) (Beck et al 1961)
>   — target group: depression; some use in suicide screening
> - Abbreviated Mental Test Score (Hodkinson 1972)
>   — target group: dementia screening

encourage GP registration among socially marginalized groups, such as the homeless or illicit drug users.

A number of structured systematic assessment tools are well suited to screening for mental health problems in primary care. The benefit of such tools is their reliability as an aid to diagnosis; many can be administered either as an interview or given to people to complete as a self report questionnaire. Systematic assessment data can be used to monitor the effectiveness of any subsequent intervention in terms of individual progress, or can be used in wider audit. In the *Primary Mental Health Care Toolkit*, Armstrong (1997) advocates the use of a limited battery of assessment tools as a first line in mental health screening of particular at-risk groups (Box 7.3). Other tools can be employed in assessing people who have psychotic problems, associated social functioning, and the side effects of antipsychotic medication; these include the Manchester scale also referred to as the KGV (Krawiecka, Goldberg & Vaughan 1977), the social functioning scale (SFS) (Birchwood et al 1990), and the LUNSERS (Day et al 1995), respectively.

Although formalizing assessment and screening is intended to offer greater accuracy in detection than simple reliance on the experience or intuition of the practitioner, some consider that their use constitutes a deskilling of expert practitioners (Barker 1998). Undoubtedly, unskilled or merely mechanical administration of structured assessment interviews is likely to be unproductive. However, skilled employment of formal assessments and screening in conjunction with other equally important communication skills would appear to be the best way forward.

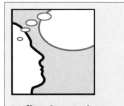

Reflection Point

What are your own education needs with respect to the use of these, or other, systematic assessment tools?

Risk and Vulnerability

It is important that primary care teams are both involved in and supported in the assessment and management of risk and vulnerability in this client group. It is not uncommon, with hindsight, to be able to point out deficiencies in the management of risk and vulnerability in the community. A typical shortcoming is lack of appropriate liaison and exchange of information between interested professionals and agencies. Just as important has been the lack of involvement of families as valuable informants about deteriorations in mental state and worries about possible consequences. It is essential that the concerns of family members who seek help regarding concerns about suicide risk or potential for other harms, are taken seriously. This ought to involve specialist services as appropriate.

The consequences of suicide or violent incidents in the community are devastating for all concerned – the victims, families and professionals concerned. Minimization of these risks is in everybody's interests and is a priority area of current health policy. Of course, not all serious risk can be predicted. As such, primary care services may, from time to time, be necessarily involved in coping with the aftermath of awful and distressing events. These can range from providing bereavement support for the families of suicide victims or caring for the victims of serious crime and their families. It is important to remember that the families of mentally disordered offenders in this context can assume a status similar to that of victims and will also require our support (McCann, McKeown & Porter 1996).

Suicide

Suicide is a major cause of death in this country. Often people who have established mental health problems are at greatest risk, and it is difficult to imagine what somebody who contemplates suicide must be going through. Although not everyone who thinks about suicide or attempts it succeeds in ending their life, the aftermath of a person taking their own life can devastate close family and friends.

Suicide is most common among young men (Jenkins 1994). Overall it accounts for about one in every hundred of all deaths, but it is preventable. It can be helpful for suicidal people if their problems are listened to and engaged with by others. They often have unbearable feelings of helplessness and hopelessness, but can be helped to gain hope and think about other ways of taking control of their lives. Talking about suicidal ideas can help; doing this will not plant the idea of committing suicide in people's minds or increase the risk of them acting upon such thoughts. It is important that people who need such help are taken seriously. Often the degree to which a person is at risk can be weighed up on the basis of the sort of things they say and this can be systematically screened for in primary care. The BDI is a useful first screening tool for suicidal

> **Box 7.4**
>
> **Risk Factors in Screening for Suicide Risk**
>
> ■ People who say they currently want to kill themselves
> ■ People who have made a specific plan of how to do this
> ■ People who have made active preparations, such as buying tablets
> ■ People who have already made suicide attempts
> ■ Increased risk if the previous attempts were recent (in the last month), or if the means chosen was considered by the person to have had a good chance of being lethal
> ■ People who are depressed or recovering from a depressive episode
> ■ People who are psychotic, particularly if they hear voices telling them to harm themselves
> ■ People who have problems of drug use, including alcohol
> ■ People who have experienced a significant bereavement

thoughts; other tools more specific to assessing suicide include Beck's Suicide Inventory (BSI) (Beck, Kovacs & Weissman 1979) or the relevant subsection of the KGV. There are some general risk factors, but they will not apply to every person. High-risk groups are listed in Box 7.4. The risk factors can be explored by sensitive questioning of people considered to be especially vulnerable.

Relapse Prevention Screening

In some mental health disorders, particularly schizophrenia, manic depressive psychosis and severe depression, the pattern of illness may involve repeated episodes. The individual might be completely well or have few symptoms in between episodes, but from time to time becomes unwell. The periods of acute illness are called relapses. Relapses themselves are distressing, but it is also thought that the frequency with which a person relapses might have an overall negative effect upon a person's long-term mental health. For these reasons it is important to avoid relapses, making this area of tertiary prevention a suitable focus for screening for signs of continued wellness or deterioration in mental state.

A feature of psychotic relapse for many people is the occurrence of a prodromal period immediately before relapse. During this time the person experiences a number of symptom-like phenomena, which typify this phase and are sometimes referred to as the prodromal signature. An important way of helping people to avoid relapse is to aid them in recognizing these 'early warning signs' so that action can be taken when they begin to occur. The length of this prerelapse period will be idiosyncratic for each individual, as will the prodromal signs experienced; importantly, not everyone will be able to identify a set of early warning signs. An individual's particular early warning signs might be less severe versions of the

> **Box 7.5**
>
> **Early Warning Signs of Psychotic Relapse**
>
> - Spending more time alone in the bedroom
> - Becoming more irritable, perhaps with specific people
> - A particular idea keeps coming into the individual's mind
> - Certain objects or people seem to assume a special significance or meaning
> - Laughing out loud for no apparent reason

full-blown symptoms that occur when they are ill, or they might be more vague sensations, thoughts or feelings. (Examples of early warning signs are given in Box 7.5.) The important thing is that they typically form the experience that the individual goes through just before a relapse. Family, friends and professionals can help to identify early warning signs and work out an action plan to use if these occur.

Interventions at Practice Level

Depending upon whatever arrangements have been made in terms of shared care or liaison with secondary services or other agencies (see below), a number of possible therapeutic interventions might be appropriate to consider in general practice settings. It is likely that these would mostly target those people who have less severe or relatively short-lived problems, typically the range of emotional distress, minor anxiety and depression, but certain work is possible with people who have more severe problems and their families. Mead and colleagues (1997) have reviewed the extent to which primary care nurses are already active in the care of people who have emotional problems, and the potential for role development in the field. They outline a possible role for practice nurses involving a range of primary, secondary and tertiary interventions.

Primary Interventions

Following screening for people at risk of developing mental health problems, early interventions include support and counselling, possible onward referral to the GP and the provision of information about self help strategies or details of alternative helping agencies, and health promotion measures (see below). Armstrong (1997) suggests that practice nurses could teach and support people in practising simple problem solving techniques. A trial of such an approach in Oxford showed that although this problem solving approach was costlier to deliver than standard GP consultations it was ultimately cost-effective given the significant reductions in medication costs and working days lost to sickness (Mynors-Wallis et al 1997). A variety of stress management or relaxation strategies could be advised upon or delivered in general practice settings, either individually or in groups. A number of commercially produced packages, including audiotapes or videos are available to aid in supporting such work.

Secondary and Tertiary Interventions

Psychotherapy and counselling have proliferated in primary care in recent years, driven by a growing demand for nonpharmacological approaches to emotional disorders and the provision of reimbursement for the costs of counsellors. However, this growth has not been accompanied by an evaluation of effectiveness, perhaps because of difficulties in researching outcomes in psychotherapy in general practice (King 1997). A survey of counselling in primary care in Southampton revealed that 39% of practices employed at least one counsellor, and that most of the therapeutic work was short term and focused upon relationship difficulties, anxiety, depression and bereavement (Clark, Hook & Stein 1997). Again, with appropriate training, there are possibilities for the practice nurse to take on this role. Alternatively, a need has been expressed within practices that employ a counselling service for the provision of less specialized levels of counselling, ideally accessed by self referral (Corrie 1992 (unpublished), cited in Mead et al 1997).

A particular focus for such therapeutic intervention is following bereavement. This has typically been seen as a traditional role for the GP, though what is actually done tends to vary between practices. Woof & Carter (1997) suggest a number of ways in which the bereaved might be helped in general practice (Box 7.6).

Other secondary prevention has included provision of support and regular monitoring of people prescribed antidepressant medication (Jenkins 1992, Wilkinson 1992, Wilkinson et al 1993). A

Box 7.6

Bereavement Follow-up in General Practice (Woof & Carter 1997)

- Efficient means of notifying practice team of death
- Routinely record death in the bereaved's notes
- Letter of condolence
- Written information about grief and the services available
- Practical advice
- Bereavement visit soon after the death
- Use of risk assessment in planning care
- Follow-up visit at 6–10 weeks
- Links with other bereavement services
- Professional bereavement counselling within practice
- Psychologist-led group bereavement therapy within practice

similar role could be envisaged for people who have more severe mental health problems. Lang, Johnstone & Murray (1997) reported that only 8% of GP consultations with this client group were solely due to mental state. Lack of time in general practice was seen to limit the role for medical practitioners, leading to the suggestion that the role of practice nurses could be developed with further training.

For those people who have been newly diagnosed with serious mental health problems, the initial engagement of the client and their family is crucial, and is perhaps the best place for practice nurses to develop their role. This group of service users will need information about psychotic problems, the role of stress, medication and side effects, and the provision of practical and emotional support for the whole family. Importantly, families should be actively involved in participative therapeutic alliances rather than thought of as passive recipients of care. Some specific approaches to working with families and carers are outlined in a later section.

Most of the effort in working with people who have severe long-term mental health problems is targeted at relapse prevention; however, it is equally important to consider how best to achieve agreed goals that address quality of life issues. Some measures aimed at relapse prevention are listed in Box 7.7. These

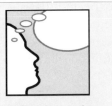

Reflection Point

In your view, how appropriate is the suggestion that practice nurses develop the role discussed above in secondary prevention?

Box 7.7

Measures for Avoiding Relapse of Serious Mental Health Problems

General measures
- Long-term use of medication
- Learning to manage and cope with stress
- Working together with family and friends on ways of communicating needs and feelings, and how problems are solved at home
- Looking after physical health
- Keeping in touch with health care staff
- Keeping active socially or at work, but balancing this against pressure and stress
- Recognition and monitoring of early signs of relapse

Examples of early interventions
- Adjusting medication
- Crisis counselling
- Support with stress management and relaxation
- Involvement of family and friends
- Identifying any specific stressors and working on how to cope or avoiding the factor that is causing too much stress at this time
- Enhancement of general coping strategies

interventions are split into general measures and early interventions to be employed on the recognition of early warning signs of impending relapse

Once a set of early warning signs has been identified the signs can be documented for reference and should be recorded in case notes and incorporated into any interagency care plan. Relapse prevention and close monitoring are especially crucial for those clients deemed to be at serious risk to themselves or others. It is expected that such risks would be identified by specialist services before discharge from hospital and may result in an individual being formally placed on the local supervision register. If this is the case the GP should be informed as matter of course.

Meeting Physical Health Needs

Services have been criticized for failing to meet the physical health needs of people who have serious mental health problems (Clinical Standards Advisory Group 1995). Many physical health problems go undetected despite relatively high consultation rates (Brugha, Wing & Smith 1989). Morbidity rates are higher for people who have long-term mental health problems than for the general population, and these individuals have higher rates of attendance with physical complaints, even compared with people who have other chronic conditions (Lang et al 1997, Nazareth & King 1992). Standardized mortality rates are of serious concern, being more than double overall (Allebeck 1989). These startling figures are partly accounted for by suicide and accident rates, but also include significantly higher mortality rates from respiratory disorders and cardio-vascular disease (Burns & Kendrick 1997). Meeting the physical health needs of this group of individuals is important, not just because of the higher incidence of treatable physical condi-tions, but also because the physical problems are likely to have a nega-tive impact upon the course of the individual's mental health problems (Kisely & Goldberg 1997). Despite relatively frequent contact with this client group, Lang and colleagues (1997) found that primary care records contained very little information relat-ing to these consultations, often failing to note the reason for attending.

Reviewing the primary care of people who have schizophrenia, Burns & Kendrick (1997) suggest a mixture of reasons for their gen-erally poor physical health and the relatively low rates of detection and intervention. The higher rates of physical ill health may be con-tributed to by long-term use of antipsychotic medication, higher con-sumption of cigarettes and generally higher rates of hypertension and obesity. Despite widespread awareness of these as risk factors for various serious physical illnesses, GP case records show little evidence that appropriate interventions are carried out with this group. Specific characteristics of the client group may also militate against detection of physical health problems or the uptake of helpful interventions. People who have negative symptoms, such as apathy and motivational problems, or problems with confidence and self esteem, may be ill-equipped to seek appropriate help or even raise their physical health in discussions with practitioners. Conversely, the lack of confidence may lie with professionals who feel unprepared to engage with this client group (Kendrick, Burns & Freeling 1995).

Perhaps unsurprisingly, most commentators recommend that the route to improved standards of physical health care for people who have serious mental health problems is in establishing a more systematic approach to the issues (Burns & Kendrick 1997, Clinical Standards Advisory Group 1995). Lang and colleagues (1997) suggest, furthermore, that the appropriate practice personnel to take up this role would be the nurses. Suggested initiatives include the estab-lishment of appropriate quality standards linked to written protocols for case management, regular physical health checks (including equality of access to typically routine screening initiatives), improvements in record keeping and the introduction of a disease register. The deleterious consequences of long-term medication ought to be prominent in the minds of prescribers, and a regular review of prescriptions in terms of balancing symptom control against side effects ought to be undertaken, hopefully leading to an optimum (minimum) therapeutic dose.

Mental Health Problems Resulting From Physical Illness

Many physical health problems have emotional sequelae, for example any chronic or disabling physical condition, acute or chronic pain, life-threatening conditions or terminal illness (Mead et al 1997). All of these can adversely affect other family members or carers. Physical illness has been noted to be a trigger for depression or a factor in maintaining depressed mood, and this may be particularly true in the elderly (Mottram et al 1996). People who have conjoint physical and emotional problems, especially depressed elderly clients, have worse outcomes, respond more slowly to their treatment or fail to comply with it (Mottram et al 1996). All of these points add weight to the case made previously for effective screening of mental health problems in tandem with physi- cal health checks. As in the previous section, the suggested role for practitioners is essentially a plea for holistic care, which ought to be compatible with the philosophy and practice of nurses.

Families and Carers

Practitioners in primary care settings may be ideally placed to help and support the families of people who have severe mental health problems. Surveys of the needs of carers invariably report that what they most wish for from services are quality information, involvement in packages of care and emotional and practical support. The weight of research evidence into the course of psychotic mental disorder emphasizes the importance of psychosocial stress in the exacerbation of symptoms and the precipitation of relapse. A significant breakthrough has been the recognition of the stress that can arise in the interpersonal relationships of people in close social networks, the deleterious effects this can have upon psychotic problems, and ways in which such stress can be minimized to everyone's benefit. Importantly, a focus upon social networks has typically involved working with families, nonjudgementally, in a spirit of therapeutic alliance. Such an approach ought to be well suited to the general practice setting, where the idea of offering services to support whole families has long been a feature.

The specialist services may offer a family therapy service. The most effective of such therapies are behaviourally orientated and attempt to address the needs of whole families, providing education and a focus upon interpersonal communication, aiming towards independent problem solving skills (Falloon et al 1988). Close liaison with secondary care providers allows such interventions to be supported by the efforts of the primary care team. Similarly, knowledge of the type and style of communication skills addressed in family therapy can help interested practitioners improve their own communications with service users. The initial identification and preliminary attempts at engagement of families who might benefit from more structured interventions might take place in general practice through contact with any of the family members.

Aside from the need for structured programmes of family therapy, there is a much more general need to support informal carers. The carers of any chronically ill person will undoubtedly be in need of varying degrees of support, some of which could be facilitated within GP practices. Support groups for carers need not be organized around specific conditions. If the focus is on the shared experiences and needs of carers, regardless of their relative's particular problems, this may be a route to dismantling forms of stigma associated with mental health problems. Various community groups, such as MIND, the Hearing Voices Network or Making Space, may provide local support for carers, as may the local community mental health team. It must also be recognized that the need for such support also extends to professional carers across the range of community-based residential facilities.

Case Study 7.1

The Roberts Family

John Roberts has had a schizophrenia diagnosis for about 1 year, during which time he has had two lengthy hospital admissions. His mother has attended for a routine health check with the practice nurse, Julie. At this consultation Mrs Roberts reports a range of stress-related problems relating how difficult she is finding it coping with her son's problems. She describes a picture of chronic tension and arguments at home, together with intense worries about John's wellbeing when she is not there to keep an eye on him. She is thinking of leaving her part-time job to spend more time at home.

In Julie's practice there is a good relationship with the local CMHT – they have developed a small resource directory for mental health problems and Julie herself has attended some awareness raising training sessions around serious mental health problems. She recognizes that this consultation might be an appropriate juncture to attempt to engage the Roberts family with more structured support. She expresses her understanding about how difficult it must be for the whole family and attempts to normalize these experiences by explaining that they are typical of other people's in similar circumstances. Julie is aware that there is a local family therapy service, and informs Mrs Roberts of this together with some simple information on its purpose. This is supported with a leaflet from the resource directory, produced by the family therapy practitioners. Julie offers to make the introduction to this team if Mrs Roberts and her family wish, and also offers to stay in touch for ongoing support if needed.

The Roberts family discuss this and accept the offer of family therapy. This occurs in their home over the next 2 years, with the frequency of appointments becoming less intensive over time. During this period the practice are kept informed of progress, and Mrs Roberts occasionally meets with Julie to tell her how things are going from her perspective. John also makes some appointments, both with his GP and hospital consultant, where he takes up issues about his medication and side effects. Mrs Robert's minor physical complaints subside and the family become much better able to manage their own stress and solve problems between themselves. John does not require hospitalization at any time during the 2 years.

In the course of the family therapy, it becomes clear that much of the tension at home arises because of their close relationships; because they care for each other, and are distressed and upset about how things have changed. It is pointed out that when the atmosphere at home does become quite emotionally charged, one thing that can happen is that people lose sight of positive things that happen, focusing just on the negative things. This can lead to people being hostile and critical to each other, and finding it difficult to solve problems among themselves. So the family worked on ways to focus on good things done or said, making a point of paying compliments.

Case Study 7.1   Cont'd

Another thing they looked at was the need to express upsetting or negative feelings, but without doing this in a way that causes more upset. This was important so as not to avoid difficult issues or bottle up feelings. Rather, the family practised telling each other how they felt in clear and unambiguous language, offering a way of sorting out the thing that had caused the upset. The family found that clearly and calmly letting each other know when they had made each other feel good or bad, helped to reduce tensions and stress at home, making it easier to avoid arguments.

A particularly stressful problem for Mrs Roberts was when John would lie in bed most of the morning. Initially she could not do anything about this without John complaining he was always getting nagged. Whatever she did, he did not get up any earlier. Mrs Roberts remembered being surprised to find out that this behaviour of John's could be caused by a symptom of schizophrenia, and not just laziness. The family also learned ways of asking each other to do things that were more effective over time and less stressful all round. They also practised how to listen to each other's points of view, even if they disagreed. Eventually, as they began to employ these new ways of communicating more consistently there was much less stress in their relationships, and some of their problems resolved or became less acute. The family therapy concluded with the family being able to discuss their problems in a quite structured way, working together towards agreed solutions. Mrs Roberts identified how useful the family therapy had been, despite misgivings about it initially.

Julie was impressed by the progress that Mrs Roberts reported and has herself become much more knowledgeable about the needs of people who have serious mental health problems and their families. The practice resource directory and materials have been added to and kept current, and Julie has begun to provide simple, but accurate information to other families in the practice. She sees the need for a practice-based support group for families and elicits Mrs Roberts' help in setting it up.

The group talk about problems and coping in their own families, and share helpful solutions. People are reassured by the expressions of common experience and a nonjudgemental philosophy of understanding people's difficulties. Julie is on hand to help with information or find things out for following meetings, but the group members themselves are rightly seen as experts in living with schizophrenia.

Some time later, the CMHT and the primary care team decide to organize some joint training for staff. The support group is invited to contribute to one of these sessions and Mrs Roberts agrees to talk to staff about their experiences and how best to help.

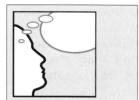

Reflection Point

In what ways could the Roberts' family case study and the experiences of Julie, the practice nurse, have relevance to your current or future practice?

Mental Health Promotion

Mental health promotion ought not to be seen as distinct or separate from general health promotion, just to be practised in mental health centres or only offered to people already diagnosed as mentally ill (Armstrong 1993, HEA 1997). In effect, the need for mental health promotion is universal, although initiatives ought to reflect diversity among the practice population (HEA 1997). Specifically, given the recognized deficits in physical wellbeing of people who have severe and enduring mental health problems, there must be an effort to improve access for this group to general health promotion clinics.

The idea that mental health can be promoted raises the question of what exactly is a positive sense of mental health or mental wellbeing. Clearly, attempts at defining this specifically raise all the acknowledged problems with finding a satisfactory definition of health generally. However, in the often contested domain of mental health, the definition of what precisely is, or is not, mentally healthy can raise important political or ethical concerns. There is a need to view society as a whole as an important target for health promotion activity because of some of the more unfortunate mechanisms of marginalization and social exclusion to which the mentally ill are subject, and the relative powerlessness of some individuals to effect lifestyle changes on their own. Most urgently, this must involve challenges to the social stigma of mental health problems, at both an individual and societal level. Attempts at delivering effective mental health promotion need to be based upon evidence and subject to ongoing review and evaluation.

An important concept in mental health promotion is that of vulnerability. People may be especially at risk of developing mental health problems because of their social circumstances or life history, and it is possible to identify risk factors or vulnerable groups and target these for health promotion initiatives. Similarly, other factors may be identified as protective against threats to mental ill health, and these may be actively supported or promoted. The HEA (1997) presents a number of important determinants of mental health status, dividing these into internal and external protective and vulnerability factors, respectively. Examples of internal protective factors include adequate physical health and emotional resilience stemming from a good sense of self-esteem. External protective factors include having positive educational experiences, especially preschool, and a supportive social network. Various vulnerability factors include social isolation, poverty, unemployment, poor housing and threats to emotional resilience, such as a lack of self-worth or autonomy, and the experience of stigma or discrimination. Box 7.8 summarizes key features that are known to be effective in promoting mental health (HEA 1997).

> **Box 7.8**
>
> **Effective Mental Health Promotion Activity (HEA 1997)**
>
> - Promoting social relationships
> - Developing coping skills
> - Providing social support, either directly or by focusing on important people in a person's social network
> - Bringing together mass media campaigns with local community activity

Challenging Stigma

A major focus for health promotion activity, and a feature of the professional role more generally, ought to be a concerted challenge to damaging stereotypical images and representations of people who have mental health problems, and the inevitable discrimination that ensues. The stigmatization of people who have mental health problems increases stress and reduces quality of life, adding to the social isolation that often accompanies a serious mental illness. The development of mental health prevention and promotion work at primary care level can be an important contribution to dismantling such attitudes. This must include reflection upon one's own attitudes as practitioners within a team. When we come across the effects of stigma or people who rely upon it, they can be confronted and resisted.

Stigma and social exclusion can be sad facts of life for many people who have mental health problems. They are stereotypically represented in many ways, by both individuals and the media, with recourse to a variety of pejorative and demeaning labels. Despite reported improvements in people's attitudes generally, 'nimbyism' is rife when the location of community mental health facilities is considered, and one specific stereotype – that the mentally distressed are violent and dangerous – has proved to be most enduring. Research by the Glasgow Media Group has shown how such unfounded fears are so strongly held they are not even affected by personal experience; which is normally the case with respect to other stereotypical attitudes (Philo et al 1994). Jodelet (1991) argues that what is at stake is a set of representations of 'madness', which set up a social demarcation between the lives of the sane and insane: a world in which people who have severe mental health problems is constructed as 'alien' or 'other' based on deep rooted prejudices akin to the fear of contagion, leading to prohibition of contact and the creation of hierarchies. This implies that negative personal attitudes probably say more about the holders of these attitudes and their own fears and insecurities than about the reality of experiencing mental health problems.

Nurses whose practice involves health promotion or the support of clients in the community should have particular interest in the mechanisms by which popular images of mental illness and media influences are generated and how these affect people's everyday lives. Interestingly, it is possible to find more positive images of people who have mental health problems presented by the media, with service user groups and organizations such as MIND bringing pressure to bear. Nurses and other interested practitioners can play their part, both in their routine professional practice and involvement in the broader politics of health equality. Various national and international initiatives have addressed stigma and mental health: the World Psychiatric Association is developing an educational programme to 'fight schizophrenia and its stigma' (Sartorius 1997) and MIND (1997) has initiated the 'Respect' campaign to resist discrimination on mental health grounds. Six national mental health charities have joined forces to form *Mediawatch*, calling on people to challenge stigmatizing publications and broadcasting (Mental Health Foundation et al 1998). At the practice level this can involve efforts to enhance the involvement and participation of service users, and the promotion of positive images of mental health at work. Wider action can involve participation in organized local action against examples of stereotyping or discrimination.

Liaison with Specialist Services, Case Management and Organizational Issues

In whichever way primary care practitioners and services develop a role in mental health care, liaison with specialist mental health services, specifically CMHTs, will be important. It is likely that there will be contemporaneous interest among CMHTs in developing primary care initiatives of their own. It is paramount to consider channels of communication and support, and integration of services such that nonsensical and wasteful duplication is avoided, and gaps in provision are minimized. This will ideally involve an agreed division of labour and responsibilities, and, with respect to meeting the needs of people who have serious mental health problems, an active role for primary care practitioners in the CPA. Innovative examples of joint practice can be envisaged, including models of liaison psychiatry and shared care initiatives, with the possibility of radical local service configurations such as the Buckingham model of family care (Wilkinson et al 1995).

Armstrong (1998) has pointed out how particular practices have different needs and requirements when deciding linkages between primary and secondary care services. For instance, practice populations will vary with respect to potential demand for mental health care, and among the primary care team the

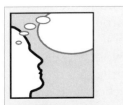

Reflection Point

What sort of measures could you take in your own practice to promote positive mental health and challenge stigma?

practitioners' skills, qualifications and levels of training will be diverse.

Case Management and the CPA

Involvement of the primary care team with the care programme in their practice and locality has benefits for GPs and their patients and carers, and ought to be a key development for CMHTs. The CPA was initiated as a framework for ensuring quality case management of community care, and is intimately bound up with the desired aim of prioritizing the needs of people who have serious mental health problems, particularly aiming to avoid loss of contact with the services by vulnerable or dangerous people. The key features of the CPA are systematic assessment of needs, a multidisciplinary and multiagency package of care, negotiated and agreed with service users and providers (including in primary care), a key worker to ensure regular contact and, crucially, identified accountability and regular monitoring and review. The CPA is meant to be applied to all patients involved with specialist psychiatric services or discharged from hospital, not just the severe and enduring group; however national implementation has been variable, raising concern that people who have disabling, but nonpsychotic problems will be denied access to services (Armstrong 1998).

Practitioners within primary care may be concerned about the potential for them to be expected to be involved in the delivery of care, but find themselves effectively excluded from CPA decision making and review meetings. Armstrong (1998) notes that although it is a responsibility for CPA key workers to work closely with primary care and make sure service users are registered with a GP, many members of CMHTs give general practice little consideration. She especially criticizes published descriptions of CPA implementation which describe cursory communication with GPs, limiting the information passed on to care plan summaries and reviews on spurious grounds of confidentiality. A common excuse for failing to include primary care practitioners in CPA meetings is to blame them for unavailability. Armstrong (1998) suggests that this could be resolved by the simple expedient of calling meetings outside of the busiest surgery times. Notwithstanding this, bodily attendance at every possible CPA meeting may not be wholly appropriate for every practitioner. It may be more practicable that efforts are made to canvass their views, and regardless of actual attendance, have these articulated when the relevant decisions are made.

It is axiomatic that the quality of written communications is of equal importance in ensuring smooth liaison between primary and secondary services; this is a two-way equation. Various commentators have summarized the flaws in such communications, both in referral letters from GPs and replies or discharge summaries from

---

Box 7.9

Primary and Secondary Care Expectations of Written Communication (Armstrong 1998, Strathdee & Jenkins 1996)

What GPs want

- Clear guidance on management
- Indication of suicide risk
- Individual's knowledge of their condition
- Prognosis and effect on lifestyle
- Expectations of general practice input
- Continued role of specialist team
- Division of responsibilities (e.g. who will undertake prescribing)

What the CMHT wants

- Background information about the family
- Social history
- Identified problems relating to the referral
- Interventions already tried and outcomes
- Reason for the referral
- Does the GP intend to continue involvement in the care, and to what extent?

---

specialists (Armstrong 1998, Strathdee & Jenkins 1996). Ideal expectations of the appropriate content of written communications for both parties are listed in Box 7.9.

Liaison Psychiatry and Specialist Attachments

Liaison psychiatry or other specialist attachments, in which psychiatrists or other mental health practitioners, notably CPNs, work directly within general practice settings saw rapid expansion before the early 1990s. The advantages of such arrangements are ease of access for patients to information and review. However, the role of CPNs in particular was subject to critique with the shift in priorities to the care of people who have serious and enduring problems. A succession of reviews of CPN activity highlighted the excessive demands on their time taken up with less severe cases, to the relative neglect of those with the severest need (Gournay 1994). As a consequence of this many CPNs were drawn back into specialist teams against the wishes of GPs, further damaging liaison between primary and secondary services (Armstrong 1998). With the advent of the CPA, some CPN attachments are being reinvented around more clearly defined roles in the care of people who have serious mental health problems. Such practitioners are ideally placed to take on liaison work, either informally or more explicitly as a practice facilitator (Armstrong 1998).

Liaison psychiatrists spend a portion of their time working directly in primary care. The number of such posts is increasing, but the national picture is variable. Strathdee & Kendrick (1996) point out the advantages for the practice in assessment, short-term treatment and improved communications. Conversely, particularly for GPs who are relatively well versed in mental health, it may be more important that their referrals are seen by specialists with more clinical expertise than their own, regardless of where the consultation takes place (Strathdee & Jenkins 1996). The most obvious advantages of specialist attachments, particularly those with an explicit facilitation remit, is the opportunity for access to a named link person to secondary services, who is likely to be sensitive to the contingencies of primary practice when calling liaison meetings for instance (Armstrong 1998).

Shared Care

Shared care involves a division of labour in the care of individuals between practitioners working for different organizations. The importance of shared care was recognized in the joint report of the Royal Colleges of Psychiatrists and General Practitioners (1993). This consensus statement recognized that both secondary and primary services share an interest in treating the whole person, and that organizational developments in both sectors had increasingly blurred boundaries between practitioners. The implementation of shared care arrangements would seem to be most appropriately envisaged in relation to people who have serious mental health problems (Armstrong 1998). Such developments in the coordination of disparate activity and inputs to care ought to be compatible with both the philosophy and practice of CPA developments.

Most commentators agree that the integrated care system developed by Ian Falloon and colleagues in Buckinghamshire represents the most comprehensive attempt to systematically implement shared care in the UK (Armstrong 1998, Pullen 1995, Wilkinson et al 1995). This system, based largely upon the delivery of behavioural family therapy and support in people's own homes, is claimed to have fundamentally changed local structures; such that inpatient beds, day hospitals, and outpatient clinics have been more or less dispensed with. However, the project is not without its critics. Kendrick (1995) speculates that the reliance on specialist teams may serve to exaggerate the exclusion of GPs from the care of this client group, serving to deskill primary care practitioners.

Organizing Effective Liaison and Joint Working

From the above discussion it is clear that effective liaison or joint working will not occur without a number of organizational developments. Key items for the attention of primary care practitioners are summarized in Box 7.10.

> **Box 7.10**
>
> **Organizational Issues (Armstrong 1998, Royal College of Psychiatrists/Royal College of General Practitioners 1993, Strathdee & Jenkins 1996)**
>
> - Alignment of catchment areas between agencies/coterminous boundaries
> - Specialist attachments in primary care and named link personnel
> - Clearly defined roles and delineation of clinical responsibilities
> - Joint audit – based on needs assessment
> - Practice-based disease or case registers – especially important for severest need
> - Local resource directory and library of information materials
> - Close integration of training

Developing a Mental Health Resource Directory

It is extremely unlikely that any single practice or, for that matter, associated specialist mental health team, will be in a position to directly meet all of the complex needs that may arise for mentally distressed service users. Specific mental health problems or attendant social problems may be best addressed by recourse to more focused initiatives, specializing in meeting the needs of people who have particular problems or disorders, or of different groups, carers for example. If practitioners are to effectively help individual service users and their families they need to be in a position to offer information that is informed, accurate and as comprehensive as possible regarding available resources for support. A varied range of statutory and voluntary agencies or self-help groups offers an equally diverse range of support, intervention or information services, which can be invaluable in helping to meet specific needs. Similarly, more general agencies may have specific departments or identified personnel for dealing with the particular needs of people who have mental health problems. It can be extremely helpful to have easy access to an up-to-date directory of such resources at local, regional and national levels. Examples of items for inclusion are listed in Box 7.11.

Entries would record clear local information and description of the service, who can access them, and how. Recorded details would include full address, telephone numbers and contact person, and specifics of public transport access. Ideally the collation of information would take place in liaison with colleagues in CMHTs, who will likely have first-hand knowledge of the range and quality of local resources or have already established a resource directory of their own. Similarly, a wealth of relevant information may be held by active local service users groups, local MIND for instance.

> **Box 7.11**
>
> **Examples for Inclusion in Local Resource Directory**
>
> - Anger/aggression management therapies
> - Befriending services/support workers/home help
> - Bereavement support
> - Counselling services
> - CRUSE
> - Depressives Anonymous
> - Domestic violence/refuges
> - Drug/alcohol services
> - Employment networks
> - Hearing Voices Network
> - Housing offices
> - MIND – national and local
> - National Schizophrenia Fellowship
> - Psychotherapy services
> - Specialist mental health social services
> - Women's/men's support groups

Depending upon the extent to which local progress has been made towards establishing a directory will make the task within individual practices more or less onerous. Regardless of the ease with which a resource directory can be drawn up, it is crucial that the information contained is kept up to date. Different groups or agencies can come and go, or established services can change their focus, their address, or key personnel.

The best directory will be a 'live' entity that is constantly updated and accessed, with attention paid to feedback from service users in relation to the quality and use of specific entries with respect to particular needs. Such feedback can help in avoiding giving inappropriate advice, and, where possible, and with regard to confidentiality, can be passed on to different service providers with a view to improving matters. An effective resource directory can also assist in directing people who have less severe mental health problems towards appropriate community support, helping to priortize interventions, and reduce the number of inappropriate referrals to the CMHT over time.

A useful resource that could be developed alongside the directory would be a practice 'library' of information materials relevant to a wide range of mental health and related problems, issues, agencies and services. Such resource materials could be available on request in the context of individual consultations, loaned out to service users as appropriate, or relied up on to support psychoeducational work or health promotion with users or carers.

Practice Registers

A practice register for people who have severe mental health problems is an effective device for aiding the management of this client group and targeting resources (Strathdee 1992). A typical register would:

- record sociodemographic information
- record clinical information
- record service contacts
- provide for regular review (e.g. of medication)
- facilitate practice policy on recall

The case registers held within each practice are essential to the maintenance of a prioritized focus upon those who have serious mental health problems, ensuring that those who are in contact with secondary care are supported by the CPA, while identifying those who are provided for in primary care settings. A functioning register would identify due dates for review meetings, prescribing monitoring and a variety of health checks (importantly physical health checks).

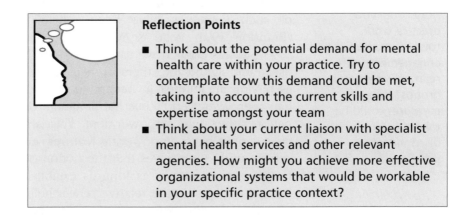

Reflection Points

- Think about the potential demand for mental health care within your practice. Try to contemplate how this demand could be met, taking into account the current skills and expertise amongst your team
- Think about your current liaison with specialist mental health services and other relevant agencies. How might you achieve more effective organizational systems that would be workable in your specific practice context?

Nondiscriminatory Practice

Health services in general need to be sensitive to the issue of equity in access and delivery of care and treatment. In this respect, psychiatric services, in particular, have had a chequered history, especially in terms of anomalies in the treatment of ethnic minority groups and women. The evidence of less than objective reasoning creeping into clinical judgement around mental health screening, for instance, suggests that such concerns are not only the prerogative of secondary services. Similarly, a number of marginalized and socially excluded groups, the homeless or illicit drug users for instance, find themselves at greater risk of worsened mental health, and simultaneously are relatively less likely to be actively engaged with by practitioners in primary care, not least because they are not registered as patients in the first place.

Given the fact that primary care services are the usual first point of contact for service users, whatever the health problem, it is most important that individual practitioners and teams address such concerns, both from the perspective of their own attitudes and practices, and the material and political structures, locally and nationally, that might affect the attainment of nondiscriminatory services. This could involve training initiatives, the sort of wider political activity suggested in relation to challenging stigma, and concerted efforts to make contact with marginalized groups, engage them in valued health care activity and maintain them within primary services.

Service User Involvement and Participation

Models of collaborative and participatory care are becoming increasingly more routine within modern health services, not least because of the welcome agitation and persuasion of service user groups. It has become clear that both professionals and service users have a mutual interest in grappling with issues such as advocacy, empowerment, rights and partnerships. The compelling arguments in favour of such initiatives have been rehearsed at length elsewhere (Brandon 1991, Read & Wallcraft 1992, Rogers, Pilgrim & Lacey 1993). In this context we can conceive of both mental health service users and significant others in their social network, usually families, as having an interest in becoming more involved in services. Care has been exercised to use the language of involvement and participation rather than empowerment. This is not to say that such initiatives cannot have empowering features; rather it is often thought by service users themselves that the notion of empowerment in mental health is a misnomer as long as established structures of inequity persist, not least in the relative power held by practitioners over service users in the context of their interpersonal relations, whatever the intentions of individual practitioners (Morrall 1996).

Practice Training Needs

Perhaps the most obvious factor to take into account when addressing the training needs of practice nurses in particular, and the primary care team more generally, is that it will be rare for them to have undertaken training that equips them to be a specialist mental health practitioner of any discipline. Overwhelmingly, practice nurses are general nurses, with less than 2% holding a mental health nursing qualification (Atkin et al 1993). However, this does not necessarily imply that these staff do not possess skills and knowledge appropriate to mental health care or deny that many have undertaken relevant post-basic training, in for example, therapeutic communication skills. Practitioner training courses that incorporate

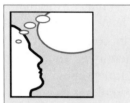

Reflection Point

How could your practice work towards maximizing engagement with relatively marginal groups? What measures could be taken to avoid discriminatory practice?

problem-based learning, ideally with the opportunity of shared learning across disciplines, are a further positive development.

It is likely that in any given practice the training needs of individual members of the team will vary. It is therefore important to review current levels of knowledge and expertise, and target mental health education based on the perceived needs of the whole team. That said, it is worth noting that the team's own assessment of what is desirable for their professional development may be at odds with the training they may actually need (Turton, Tylee & Kerry 1995).

A systematic approach to meeting learning needs should include multidisciplinary training and involve all team members, including reception and administration staff. In practices working to develop systems of liaison with secondary services there is the possibility to participate in or organize shared learning initiatives. Current evidence in terms of effectiveness of clinical training suggests that the best initiatives ought to be aimed at whole teams, with the training taking place in the practice environment, allowing the practitioners themselves to modify the taught knowledge and skills so that it can impact upon their routine practice (Corrigan & McCracken 1995). In districts that have a progressive approach to the development of mental health care in general practice key personnel may be employed to facilitate practice-based training and joint activity with specialist practitioners (Armstrong 1998).

Training is also a good place to attempt to involve service users, if possible. The content of training packages should reflect the identified needs of the practice personnel and be explicitly commensurate with attaining the aims of the practice in meeting the needs of its specific population of service users. The items of practice nurse role development highlighted in Box 7.1, could be used to help identify training needs appropriate to anticipated extensions of role and service developments across the team.

The main barrier to addressing training needs appears to be lack of funding. Armstrong (1998) bemoans the lack of appropriate training courses for primary care teams, making the powerful observation that what is available is paid for and delivered by pharmaceutical firms. The other major barrier to practice nurse training is the attitude of some GPs, who may undervalue the relevance of training to the development of the practice nurses role or simply fail to see specific training packages as a priority (Robinson, Beaton & White 1993, Ross 1992).

Audit and Evaluation

Any modification in health care practice or implementation of new systems of working must be monitored and evaluated systematically. This might simply involve auditing activity levels with respect to the provision of services for specific groups. More sophisticated is the evaluation of clinical effectiveness. Clearly there is merit here in not restricting outcome measures to singularly clinical concerns and trying to reflect some alternative measures of effectiveness voiced as desirable by service users themselves.

A variety of tools are available for assessing outcomes concerning the relative amelioration of symptoms and problems, quality of life measures and satisfaction with specific aspects of services. A starting point for auditing primary care services in relation to mental health should be some form of systematic needs assessment and outcome measures. The CMHT may employ tools such as the *Camberwell Assessment of Need* (Phelan et al 1994) or the *Health of the Nation Outcome Scale* (Wing et al 1998) as a matter of routine practice in the context of the CPA. Broad local needs in mental health may also have been evaluated by the public health consultant. Such broad measures will give the practice an idea of mental health need or psychiatric morbidity in the catchment area of the practice and surrounding areas for comparison.

Conclusion

A primary care-led NHS has been promised and only time will tell if it is to be realized effectively. Within such a vision, mental health care should figure prominently. The wider focus upon primary care and the anticipated innovation promised via the primary care groups ought to encompass novel developments in the delivery and commissioning of health and social care for mental health service users. The challenge will be to ensure consistency and systematization across the range of mental health care provision, but not at the expense of local flexibility. All too often in the past access to high-quality user-friendly care has been an accident of geography rather than a guaranteed minimum expectation. Past models of competitive management and organization have further contributed to the isolation of examples of excellence in practice. The current stress on evidence-based practice should raise questions about the content of mental health services, not just their configuration (Butler et al 1997). Although this is to be welcomed, the enthusiasm for evidence ought to be tempered with a critical disposal towards whose outcomes are presented as paramount. The case of counselling in primary care is noteworthy in this respect, being valued by both GPs and service users, yet failing to prove its clinical effectiveness (Peck 1997).

Practice nurses should not see themselves as passive recipients of policy flux or organizational changes in this field: they have an exciting opportunity, together with other colleagues in primary care, to be in the vanguard of shaping the new NHS. Practitioners should not feel that they are being asked to develop quality services from scratch. In this respect, Kerwick & Goldberg (1997) must be correct in arguing that:

> 'There is no shortage of activities that can be locally implemented in primary care to enhance the delivery of (mental health) care ... More resources are just one part of an agenda that has been established for some time now. The messages need to be repeated again and again until they are taken up or facilitated into practice.'

In terms of the specific roles taken on by practice nurses it is worth remembering that many of the developments advocated here may already be undertaken by practice nurses. It is likely that particular practices will have made variable progress toward implementing a comprehensive range of nursing care in mental health. The elements of a mental health role described here are simple in structure and compatible with both broader philosophies of primary care nursing and organizational developments among CMHTs. The assumption of such a role may depend upon specific local circumstances, notably the level of support from key practice personnel, especially the GP, and colleagues in specialist mental health services. Crucially, the disposition of practice nurses themselves towards the provision of care and support to mental health service users will be of fundamental importance in the development of new initiatives and their ultimate quality. In this sense, the answer to the question of whether practice nurses do have a role in mental health may, ultimately, be in their own hands.

References

Allebeck P 1989 Schizophrenia: a life shortening disease. Schizophrenia Bulletin 15:81–89

Armstrong E 1993 Promoting mental health. In: Dines A, Cribb A (eds) Health promotion: concepts and practice. Blackwell, Oxford

Armstrong E 1995 Mental health issues in primary care: a practical guide. Macmillan, Basingstoke

Armstrong E 1997 The primary mental health care toolkit. Royal College of General Practitioners Unit for Mental Health Education in Primary Care & Institute of Psychiatry Section of Epidemiology and General Practice, London

Armstrong E 1998 The primary/secondary care interface. In: Brooker C, Repper J (eds) Serious mental health problems in the community: policy, practice and research. Baillière Tindall, London

Atkin K, Lunt N 1993 A census of direction. Nursing Times 89(42):38–41

Atkin K, Lunt N, Parker G, Hurst M 1993 Nurses count. A national census of practice nurses. Social Policy Research Unit, University of York

Barker P 1993 Squaring the circle. Nursing Times 89(49):38–40

Barker W 1998 Let's trust our instincts. Community Practitioner 71(9):305

Beck A, Ward C, Mendelson M, Mock J, Erbaugh J 1961 An inventory for measuring depression. Archives of General Psychiatry 4:561–571

Beck A, Kovacs M, Weissman A 1979 Assesment of suicidal intention: the scale for suicidal ideation. Journal of Consulting and Clinical Psychology 47:343–352

Birchwood M, Smith J, Cochrane R, Wetton S, Copestake S 1990 The social functioning scale: the development and validation of a scale of social adjustment for use in family intervention programmes with schizophrenic patients. British Journal of Psychiatry 157:853–859

Brandon D 1991 Innovation without change? Consumer power in psychiatric services. Macmillan, Houndmills

Brugha T, Wing J, Smith B 1989 Physical health of the long-term mentally ill in the community: is there unmet need? British Journal of Psychiatry 155:777–781

Burns T, Kendrick T 1997 The primary care of patients with schizophrenia: a search for good practice. British Journal of General Practice 47:515–520

Butler T, Glendinning C Gask L, Rummery K, Rogers A, Lee J, Bower P 1997 Mental health and primary care: an alternative policy agenda. Journal of Mental Health 6:331–334

Clark A, Hook J, Stein K 1997 Counsellors in primary care in Southampton: a questionnaire survey of their qualifications, working arrangements, and casemix. British Journal of General Practice 47:613–617

Clinical Standards Advisory Group 1995 Report of a CSAG committee on schizophrenia, vol. 1. HMSO, London

Corrigan P, McCracken S 1995 Psychiatric rehabilitation and staff development: educational and organisational models. Clinical Psychology Review 15:699–719

Cox J, Holden J, Sagovsky R 1987 Detection of postnatal depression: development of the Edinburgh Postnatal Depression Scale. British Journal of Psychiatry 150:782–786

Day J, Wood G, Dewey M, Bentall R 1995 A self rating scale for measuring neuroleptic side effects: validation in a group of schizophrenic patients. British Journal of Psychiatry 166:650–653

Department of Health 1990 The care programme approach for people with a mental illness referred to the specialist psychiatric services [HC(90)23]. HMSO, London

Falloon I, Mueser K, Gingerich S, Rappaport S, McGill C, Hole V (1988) Behavioural family therapy: a workbook. Buckingham Mental Health Services, Buckingham

Goldberg D, Huxley P 1992 Common mental disorders: a biosocial approach. Routledge, London

Goldberg D, Williams P 1988 A user's guide to the general health questionnaire: GHQ. NFER-Nelson, Windsor

Gournay K 1994 Redirecting the emphasis to serious mental illness. Nursing Times 90(25):40–41

Greenfield S, Stilwell B, Drury M 1987 Practice nurses: social and occupational characteristics. Journal of the Royal College of General Practitioners 37:341–345

HEA 1997 Mental health promotion: a quality framework. HEA, London

Higgins E 1994 A review of unrecognised mental illness in primary care. Archives of Family Medicine 3:908–917

Hodkinson H 1972 Evaluation of a mental test score for assessment of mental impairment in the elderly. Age and Ageing 1:233–238

Jenkins R 1992 Developments in the primary care of mental illness: a forward look. International Review of Psychiatry 4:237–242

Jenkins R 1994 The prevention of suicide. HMSO, London

Jodelet D 1991 Madness and social representation. Harvester Wheatsheaf, London

Joukamaa M, Lehtinen V, Karlsson H 1995 The ability of general practitioners to detect mental disorders in primary health care. Acta Psychiatrica Scandinavica 91:52–56

Kendrick T 1995 Peer commentaries on 'an evaluation of community-based psychiatric care for people with treated long-term mental illness'. British Journal of Psychiatry 167:38–40

Kendrick T, Burns T, Freeling P 1995 Randomised controlled trial of teaching general practitioners to carry out structured assessments of their long term mentally ill patients. British Medical Journal 311:93–98

Kerwick S, Goldberg D 1997 Mental health care in the community: what should be on the agenda? British Journal of General Practice 47:344–345

King M 1992 Management of patients with schizophrenia in general practice. British Journal of General Practice 4.2:310–311

King M 1997 Brief psychotherapy in general practice: how do we measure outcome? British Journal of General Practice 47:136–137

Kisely S, Goldberg D 1997 The effect of physical ill health on the course of psychiatric disorder in general practice. British Journal of Psychiatry 170:536–540

Krawiecka M, Goldberg D, Vaughan M 1997 A standardised psychiatric assessment scale for rating chronic psychiatric patients. Acta Psychiatrica Scandinavica 55:299–308

Lang F, Johnstone E, Murray G 1997 Service provision for people with schizophrenia II: the role of the general practitioner. British Journal of Psychiatry 171:165–168

McCann G, McKeown M, Porter I 1996 Understanding the needs of relatives of patients within a special hospital for mentally disordered offenders: a basis for improved services. Journal of Advanced Nursing 23:346–352

McKeown M, McCann G, Cooper B 1998 Psychosocial interventions for severe and enduring mental health problems in primary care settings. Liverpool John Moores University, Liverpool

Mead N, Bower P, Gask L 1997 Emotional problems in primary care: what is the potential for increasing the role of nurses? Journal of Advanced Nursing 26:879–890

Mental Health Foundation, Manic Depression Fellowship, National Schizophrenia Fellowship, Mind, Mental After Care Association, Mental Health Media 1998 Mediawatch [pamphlet]. Mental Health Foundation, London

Mind 1997 Respect: time to end discrimination on mental health grounds [pamphlet]. Mind, London.

Morrall P 1996 Clinical sociology and the empowerment of clients. Mental Health Nursing 16(3):24–27

Mottram P, Hamer C, Williams J, Wilson K 1996 Long-term agreement. Nursing Times 92(49):40–41

Mynors-Wallis L, Davies I, Gray A, Barbour F, Gath D 1997 A randomised controlled trial and cost analysis of problem solving treatment for emotional disorders given by community nurses in primary care. British Journal of Psychiatry 170:113–119

Nazareth I, King B 1992 Controlled evaluation of management of schizophrenia in one general practice: a pilot study. Family Practice 9:171–172

Ormel J, Koeter M, van den Brink W, van de Willige G 1991 Recognition, management, and course of anxiety and depression in general practice. Archives of General Psychiatry 48:700–706

Peck E 1997 The future and the past. Journal of Mental Health 6:321–325

Phelan M et al 1995 The Camberwell assessment of need: the validity and reliability of an instrument to assess the needs of people with severe mental illness. British Journal of Psychiatry 167:589–595

Philo G, Secker J, Platt S, Henderson L, McLaughlin G, Burnside J 1994 The impact of mass media on public images of mental illness, media content and audience belief. Health Education Journal 53:271–281

Pullen I 1995 Peer commentaries on 'an evaluation of community-based psychiatric care for people with treated long-term mental illness'. British Journal of Psychiatry 167:38–40

Read J, Wallcraft J 1992 Guidelines for empowering users of mental health services. COHSE/Mind, London

Repper J, Brooker C 1998 Serious mental health problems in the community: the significance of

policy, practice and research. In: Brooker C, Repper J (eds) Serious mental health problems in the community: policy, practice and research. Baillière Tindall, London

Robinson G, Beaton S, White P 1993 Attitudes towards practice nurses – survey of a sample of general practitioners in England and Wales. British Journal of General Practice 43:25–29

Rogers A, Pilgrinm D, Lacey R 1993 Experiencing psychiatry: user's views of services. Macmillan/MIND, Houndmills

Ross F 1992 Barriers to learning. Nursing Times 88:(38):44–45

Royal College of General Practiners, Office of Population Censuses and Surveys, Department of Health 1995 Morbidity statistics from general practice. Fourth National Study, 1991–1992. HMSO, London

Royal College of Psychiatrists, Royal College of General Practiners 1993 Report of a joint working group on shared care. Occasional paper 60. RCGP, London

SANE 1997 Schizophrenia: the sufferer's point of view. SANE, London

Sartorious N 1997 Fighting schizophrenia and its stigma. British Journal of Psychiatry 170:297

Sheikh J, Yesesevage J 1986 Geriatric depression scale: recent findings and development of a shorter version. In: Brink T (ed) Clinical gerontology: a guide to assessment and intervention. Howarth Press, New York

Shepherd M, Cooper M, Brown A, Kalton G 1981 Psychiatric illness in general practice, 2nd edn. Oxford University Press, Oxford

Steering Group of the Confidential Inquiry into Homicides and Suicides by Mentally Ill People 1996 Report of the confidential inquiry into homicides and suicides by mentally ill people. Royal College of Psychiatrists, London

Stilwell B 1988 Patients' attitudes to the availability of a nurse practitioner in general practice. In: Bowling A, Stilwell B (eds) The nurse in family practice. Scutari Press, London

Strathdee G 1992 The interface between psychiatry and primary care in the management of schizophrenic patients in the community. In: Jenkins R, Field V, Young R (eds) The primary care of schizophrenia. HMSO, London

Strathdee G, Jenkins R 1996 Purchasing mental health care for primary care. In: Thornicroft G, Strathdee G (eds) Commissioning mental health services. HMSO, London

Strathdee G, Kendrick T 1996 The regular review of patients with schizophrenia in primary care.

In: Kendrick T, Tylee A, Freeling P (eds) The prevention of mental illness in primary care. Cambridge University Press, Cambridge

Thomas R, Corney R 1993 The role of the practice nurse in mental health: a survey. Journal of Mental Health 2:65–72

Thornicroft G, Bebbington P 1989 Deinstitutionalisation: from hospital closure to service development. British Journal of Psychiatry 155:739–753

Tiemens B, Ormel J, Simon G 1996 Occurrence, recognition and outcome of psychological disorders in primary care. American Journal of Psychiatry 153:634–644

Tully C, Watson C, Abrams A 1998 Postnatal depression: training health visitors to use the EPDS. Community Practitioner 71(6):213–215

Turton P, Tylee A, Kerry S 1995 Mental health training needs in general practice. Primary Care Psychiatry 1:197–199

Vazquez-Barquero J, Garcia J, Simon J et al 1997 Mental health in primary care: an epidemiological study of morbidity and use of health resources. British Journal of Psychiatry 170:529–535

Walls K 1998 Family therapy: different approaches in practice. Community Practitioner 71(9):294–296

Wilkinson G 1992 The role of the practice nurse in the management of depression. International Review of Psychiatry 4:311–316

Wilkinson G, Allen P, Marshall E, Walker J, Browne W, Mann A 1993 The role of the practice nurse in the management of depression in general practice: treatment adherence to anti-depressant medication. Psychological Medicine 23:229–237

Wilkinson G, Piccinelli M, Falloon I, Krekorian H, McLees S 1995 An evaluation of community-based psychiatric care for people with treated long-term mental illness. British Journal of Psychiatry 167:26–37

Wing J, Beevor A, Curtis R, Park S, Hadden S, Burns A 1998 Health of the nation outcome scales (HoNOS). British Journal of Psychiatry 172:11–18

Woof W, Carter Y 1997 The grieving adult and the general practitioner: a literature review in two parts, Part 2. British Journal of General Practice 47:443–448

Zigmund A, Snaith R 1983 The hospital anxiety and depression scale. Acta Psychiatrica Scandinavica 67:361–370

8 Clinical Supervision – What Will It Offer to the Development of Practice Nurses?

Sylvina Tate   Sue Dobson

INTRODUCTION

The concept of clinical supervision is not new. It has been a feature of midwifery, mental health nursing and counselling practice for many years (Butterworth & Faugier 1992). The transference of the concept to general nursing was clearly identified in the implementation of the *Vision for the Future* document (NHS Management Executive 1993). This document recommended the exploration and further development of the concept of clinical supervision:

> 'so that it is integral throughout the lifetime of practice, thus enabling practitioners to accept personal responsibility for and be accountable for care and to keep that care under constant review' (NHS Management Executive 1993, p. 15).

Given the direction set by Yvonne Moores, clinical supervision is increasingly recognized as a fundamental issue for nursing practice. Indeed, much has been written about clinical supervision (Butterworth & Faugier 1992, Faugier & Butterworth 1994, Johns 1993, Kohner 1994a) with the development of appropriate models for different areas of practice being the focus of investigation (Faugier & Butterworth 1994, King's Fund Centre 1994). This development has led to the belief among 'clinical supervision experts' that before the introduction of clinical supervision, nurse leaders in each area of specialist practice need to consider the context and constraints impacting on their nurses to adopt the model that is most appropriate. This chapter will explore the adoption of a model of clinical supervision used with one group of practice nurses in Wirral, Merseyside. The project, together with its evaluation and the views of the practice nurses involved, will be the focus of this chapter.

> **Key Issues**
>
> - A description of clinical supervision.
> - The exploration of training needs prior to the introduction of clinical supervision
> - Details of the project to introduce clinical supervision into practice nursing within one Health Authority
> - Examples of how clinical supervision has impacted on practice nurses

What is Clinical Supervision?

There continues to be much confusion, particularly among nurses who are not receiving supervision, about what constitutes clinical supervision. It is not unusual to find nurses who have the misconception that clinical supervision is 'someone coming into the practice to watch me doing my work' (Bishop 1998, Bond & Holland 1998).

Butterworth (1994) defines clinical supervision as:

> 'an exchange between practising professionals to enable the development of professional skills' (p. 1).

This simplistic definition allows contextual interpretation, enabling professionals to decide what is most appropriate within their specific work arena. Wright's earlier definition (1989) is more comprehensive. He states:

> 'supervision is a meeting between two or more people who have a declared interest in examining a piece of work. The work is presented and they will together think about what was happening and why, what was done or said, and how it was handled – could it have been handled better or differently, and if so how'?

Within both these approaches to supervision the authors highlight the use of reflective practice and critical incident analysis as useful tools to analyse professional practice. In contrast to Butterworth and Wright, Worsley (1994) incorporates outcomes within his definition of supervision. He claims that:

> 'Supervision is a mandatory or negotiated contractual relationship between a supervisor and supervisee in which the worker gives an account of his or her work with the express purpose of developing their competence in providing the highest quality of service to the client or customer.'

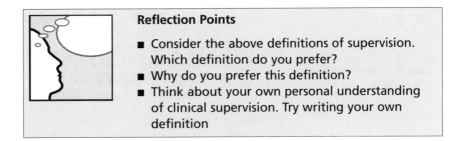

Reflection Points

■ Consider the above definitions of supervision. Which definition do you prefer?
■ Why do you prefer this definition?
■ Think about your own personal understanding of clinical supervision. Try writing your own definition

Why is Clinical Supervision Important?

Health care has been subject to a great deal of change over the past few decades, particularly in practice nursing, mainly as the result of changes in government policy (Department of Health 1990). As a result of this change, practice nursing has developed greater autonomy and accountability for its practice. Sheppard (1992) reports that the number of nurses employed within general practice rose from an estimated 3700 in 1986 to 18 000 by 1991. Atkin & Lunt (1995) found that practice nurses undertook:

'a broad range of work with varying degrees of responsibility; it included performing delegated clinical activities as well as work that required independent judgement and action. Most practice nurses felt they had considerable autonomy in organising their work. GPs usually issued general guidelines, leaving the practice nurse to work out the specific detail' (p. 5).

Other changes impacting upon the role of the practice nurse have included the introduction of the *Code of Professional Conduct for Nurses, Midwives and Health Visitors* (UKCC 1983). This resulted in practitioners becoming accountable for their own practice (UKCC 1983). Hall in her opening address, stated that:

'the underlying philosophy of the professional conduct function is to protect the public, to promote high standards of professional practice and conduct of nurses, midwives and health visitors, to ensure that justice is being done, and seen to be done, in respect of those who are brought within this function...'.

(Heywood Jones 1990 p. 7)

The publication of the *Scope of Professional Practice* (UKCC 1992a), further enabled nurses to extend their practice to enhance patient care, provided that they had achieved a level of competency related to the specific role expansion. Practice nursing is arguably one branch of nursing that has fully embraced the opportunities presented. This is confirmed by Atkin & Lunt (1995) who reported the following view, held by practice nurses, of practice nursing:

> 'Although they accepted the importance of treatment room work, practice nurses emphasised how their role had developed beyond treatment room tasks. Other work included chronic disease management, health promotion, and less frequently family planning. Chronic disease management, as defined by amendments to the GP contract in 1993, highlights four conditions – asthma, diabetes, coronary heart disease and stroke' (pp. 5–6).

The impact of the changes has led to a situation where nurses are embracing new practices, and they are individually accountable for the outcomes, sometimes with devastating results. This extension and expansion of practice is not without its conflict for nursing, for as Butterworth (1995) suggests, the Allitt enquiry in the 1990s 'crystallised a number of concerns about the supervision of safe and accountable practice' (p. 1).

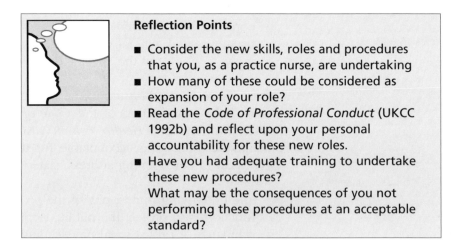

Reflection Points

■ Consider the new skills, roles and procedures that you, as a practice nurse, are undertaking
■ How many of these could be considered as expansion of your role?
■ Read the *Code of Professional Conduct* (UKCC 1992b) and reflect upon your personal accountability for these new roles.
■ Have you had adequate training to undertake these new procedures?
What may be the consequences of you not performing these procedures at an acceptable standard?

Aim and Purpose of Clinical Supervision

Anecdotal evidence suggests that there is much confusion and misconception about the aim of clinical supervision (Castledine 1994) Butterworth & Faugier (1994) state that clinical supervision:

> 'should not be confused with simple managerial oversight. Its purpose is to facilitate reflective practice and push forward a patient-centred focus' (p. 1).

Guidelines issued by the King's Fund Centre (1994), the UKCC (1995) and the University of Manchester (Butterworth & Faugier 1994) have attempted to define the process, purpose and benefits of clinical supervision. They suggest that the process is a formal arrangement between two professionals, involving 'reflection on practice in order to learn from experience and improve competence' (Kohner 1994b, p. 1). The purpose is 'to improve the quality of patient care' with benefits accruing for patients, professionals, the organization and the profession.

As such clinical supervision may serve a number of functions for the practitioner. Proctor (1986) identifies these as 'normative, restorative and/or formative'. The normative function refers to the managerial and quality control aspects of professional practice; restorative to the supportive help for professionals constantly working with stress and distress; and formative to the educative process of developing skills, knowledge and behaviour (King's Fund Centre 1994).

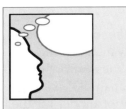

Reflection Points

- What do you think is the purpose of clinical supervision?
- Make a list of at least five reasons for undertaking clinical supervision

Approaches to Clinical Supervision

There are no hard and fast rules about how supervision must be undertaken, but it is important to recognize the principles presented by Butterworth (1995) and the King's Fund Centre (1994). How clinical supervision is implemented will depend upon first identifying its purpose, process, content and focus as well as clarifying the relationship between supervision and management. It is important that all grades of staff are involved at this stage to avoid the perception that this is a topdown imposition. There needs to be a balance between the needs of the individual and the needs of the organization.

There are a variety of ways of organizing clinical supervision (Box 8.1).

Box 8.1

Ways of Organizing Clinical Supervision (Butterworth 1995)

- Regular one-to-one sessions with an expert supervisor from your own discipline
- Regular one-to-one sessions with a supervisor from a different discipline
- One-to-one peer supervision (working with people of a similar grade and expertise)
- Group supervision (shared supervision by teams)
- Network supervision (a group of people with similar expertise and interests who do not necessarily work together on a day to day basis)

None of the approaches listed in Box 8.1 is superior to the other. Each has its own advantages and disadvantages. What is more important is the matching of the approach to the needs of the organization.

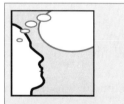

Reflection Point

Can you list the possible advantages and disadvantage of each of the above approaches?

Models of Clinical Supervision

There are number of clinical supervision models and Faugier & Butterworth (1994) suggest that these 'fall into three major categories:

- those which describe supervision in relation to the supervisory relationship and its main constituents;
- those which describe the elements of the main function or role of supervision; and
- developmental models which emphasise the process of the supervisory relationship.'

Details of the models can be obtained from the original source, but again each model has advantages and disadvantages. An analysis of each model identifying the strengths, weaknesses, opportunities and threats of each approach (SWOT analysis) will help practitioners to identify the appropriate category of model for their clinical setting.

Reflection Point

Think about your own situation. What would be the best model for your supervision?

Recognizing the Outcomes of Clinical Supervision

In arguing for clinical supervision the King's Fund Centre (1994) points out that there are clear benefits for the individual, the organization and the service. It claims that it will improve the quality of patient care, improve staff performance, reduce staff stress and increase their confidence and competence through increased support, and be a means of professional development through supervised reflection on practice. Supporting this, Tingle (1995) suggests that clinical supervision can be an effective risk management tool with the potential to reduce clinical complaints and litigation.

However, there is currently no nationally recognized tool to evaluate the outcomes of supervision. Claimed outcomes of clinical supervision are therefore theoretical and have yet to be proven. However, the results of a large evaluation project examines whether existing evaluation tools are indeed appropriate for measuring the effectiveness of clinical supervision (Butterworth et al 1997). Concurrently, both Brocklehurst and Fowler (PhDs in progress) are working to develop evaluation tools that are specifically designed to measure aspects of clinical supervision.

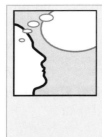

Reflection Point

Consider your own practice. Can you list five potential positive outcomes of clinical supervision for each of the following:

■ yourself
■ your practice
■ the patient
■ practice nursing

Introducing Supervision for Practice Nurses: A Case Study of Clinical Supervision in Wirral

Background

Although practice nurses working in Wirral are employed by individual GPs, professional advice, support and guidance are provided through senior nurses employed by Wirral Health. The role of the health authority includes the provision of training to meet the needs of practice nurses. This is coordinated through a training group, which consists of practice nurses, GPs and senior nurses. This group, anxious to introduce clinical supervision for practice nurses, but aware of the need to justify the costs, obtained the finances to fund an implementation project (Box 8.2). This was based upon the guidelines identified by Kohner (1994a). She suggests the following 10-point guideline for the implementation of supervision:

■ decide on its purpose
■ involve staff in its planning and introduction
■ consider the qualifications, skills and experience required of supervisors
■ provide appropriate educational opportunities for supervisors and supervisees
■ provide supervision for the supervisors
■ provide supervision for all grades of staff

Box 8.2

Specific purposes of the Wirral project

■ To identify a model of clinical supervision relevant to practice nurses
■ To provide suitable education and training for the preparation of supervisors of practice nurses
■ To provide suitable education and training for the preparation of practice nurses undergoing supervision
■ To evaluate the initiative in terms of the experiences of both the supervisors and the supervisees

- define the content, boundaries and process of supervision
- formally constitute the supervisor/supervisee relationship
- decide how to monitor and evaluate the process
- seek employing authority support

Seeking Support for Clinical Supervision

Atkin & Lunt (1995) reported that:

> 'community nursing providers and, to a lesser extent
> purchasers, questioned whether practice nurses have
> adequate supervision especially given the degree of
> autonomy they exercise. In particular, providers thought
> that some practice nurses performed work without
> recognising the extent to which they were professionally
> accountable for their actions. They felt that practice
> nurses would benefit from closer supervision, believing
> GPs were not capable of offering this. Certainly, practice
> nursing does seem to raise specific difficulties for the idea
> of clinical supervision. Practice nurses work outside
> traditional nursing hierarchies. They are not obliged to
> attend study days or demonstrate formally their
> competence in any task. Further, the person from
> whom they could receive clinical support is also their
> employer and may be less aware of the nursing code
> of conduct' (p. 8).

Atkin & Lunt (1995) further suggest that 'an educative aspect of supervision was not a common feature of their relationship with the GP' and 'the supportive aspect of supervision was an even rarer feature of the practice nurses' relationship with their employing GP'.

Aware of this situation, the health authority in Wirral was eager to offer support to the practice nurses working in their area and to this end obtained the funding for the project. They were aware that they needed to demonstrate the benefits of clinical supervision to both employers (GPs) and employees (the practice nurses) and viewed an evaluation project as the most appropriate method.

It is fair to conclude that the support of the employing authority was an implicit part of this project.

Recruiting Practice Nurses to the Project

It was considered important that the principles of good supervision should not be compromised even though we were balancing the demands to meet project objectives and a tight time schedule. The need to model good supervision during all stages of the project was considered to be vital. Therefore as part of the project, four awareness sessions were held in a variety of locations at lunch times and in the evening, to which all practice nurses were invited.

At the awareness sessions two members of the project team explained the project, and the concept of clinical supervision was clarified. Following discussions, application forms to take part in the project were distributed to all who attended. To ensure equity of opportunity, application forms were also posted to all nurses who could not attend the awareness sessions. Nurses were asked to volunteer to be trained as supervisors and/or supervisees and to nominate the person they would most like to have as their supervisor.

Having completed the negotiations, Wirral Health was only involved in a supportive and monitoring capacity. Initially the project was lead by the research team. Following completion of the project, the development and cascading of clinical supervision has very much been led by the practice nurses who were part of the project.

Identifying the Qualifications, Skills and Experience required of Supervisors

It is generally accepted that professional grade should not be equated with having the skills required to act as a supervisor. The role of clinical supervisor requires particular skills. Fowler (1989), through focus group discussions identified three themes: relevant knowledge, supervisory/teaching skills and personal relationship skills. More recently, Bishop (1998) suggested:

> 'there are three types of credibility required by the supervisor in order to achieve effective clinical supervision: personal, organisational and clinical' (p. 16).

Following completion of the awareness sessions, eight nurses identified their willingness to be considered for the role of clinical supervisor, and 15 for the role of supervisee. Those nurses who wished to act as supervisors were invited to attend a short selection process to determine their desire and suitability to undertake the role. It was considered that the role of the supervisor was a key role within the project. Although all practice nurses were employed at the same grade it was important that those accepted for training possessed appropriate 'personal characteristics' and the potential to develop supervisory skills. Therefore criteria for the role of clinical supervisor were drawn up to aid the selection process (Box 8.3).

Due to financial constraints it was only possible to select six practice nurses to train as supervisors. The selection process was undertaken by the project leader and evaluator. As a resulted five nurses who had attended the awareness sessions and one who did not were accepted to undergo training.

Box 8.3

Clinical Supervisor Person Specification

- A skilled and experienced practitioner (a minimum of 2 years' experience and evidence that skills and knowledge have been updated in the clinical setting)
- Has basic common sense
- Can provide constructive feedback
- Objective
- Good listener
- Generous in time and spirit
- Honest about their own limitations
- Open, trustworthy and honest
- Willing to learn
- Self-motivated, enthusiastic and flexible
- Prepared to invest in others, showing patience, concern and tolerance

Box 8.4

Content of Clinical Supervisors' Training

- The need for clinical supervision in practice nursing
- An introduction to clinical supervision
- Law and accountability
- Self awareness
- Team building
- Reflective practice
- Nursing knowledge
- Supervision skills
- Supervision practice
- Developing documentation and contracts
- Rights and responsibilities of supervisors
- Evaluation

Educational Opportunities for Supervisors and Supervisees

As practice nurses work in isolation with very little support (Atkin & Lunt 1995), it was considered appropriate to incorporate team building into the supervision training. This would ensure that the supervisors would have a source of mutual support, regardless of the outcome of the project.

Training the supervisors

Ideally supervisors should have received supervision themselves, giving them some insight to what it was like to be supervized. However, the concept of clinical supervision was new to all of the practice nurses and was an issue that needed to be addressed in the training (Box 8.4).

The supervisors received 5 days of training. The first 2 days were residential. One person, who had not attended the awareness sessions dropped out after the residential days for personal reasons. The remaining five supervisors received a further 3 days of training over the next month. The training was evaluated using Nominal Group Evaluation Technique. The results are presented in Box 8.5.

Box 8.5

Nominal Group Evaluation of the Supervisor Training (Dobson 1996)

Negative aspects

- Initial communication was poor
  - there was very short notice about the residential days of the course, leading to the members having to rapidly organize/reorganize their personal and working lives to accommodate it (this was caused by the tight time schedule)
- Residential venue was poor
  - the group members found the bedrooms very cold throughout their stay (the residential venue had been used previously with no problems)
- Little flexibility
  - the same days of the week were designated for the teaching sessions. This resulted in the same clinics etc. having to be cancelled each time and this was considered to be unfair to the patients and clients and potentially disruptive to relationships with the GPs (this resulted from the availability of the facilitator)

Positive aspects

- Teaching methods
  - the teaching sessions were enjoyable, well planned and learning objectives were explicit. The fact that more intense theory was done in the morning and 'games' played in the afternoon was seen as important. The atmosphere generated encouraged learning and empowered the participants
- Tutor's knowledge
  - the fact that ... really 'knew her stuff' came over. She was very genuine in her approach and this was appreciated. She is perceived as an enthusiastic and excellent teacher. The group was concerned that sometimes they were too 'raucous' to control, but overall it was felt that this approach has helped the group to 'gel'
- Self awareness
  - the process of undergoing the sessions had resulted in self awareness. The group members appreciated the opportunity to 'look at themselves'. It was also valuable to gain awareness of others in the group as individuals and of how the group functioned

---

Box 8.5 Cont'd

- Groupwork
  - the group work was excellent and could not have been done better. Many of the sessions were described as a 'revelation'. The group enjoyed the fact that the sessions were fun and encouragement was given. Surprise was expressed that after what were often long days, they felt soothed and relaxed instead of worn out as they would have expected
- Humour
  - the fact that humour had played a large part was seen as beneficial. There was plenty of it and it was felt that it helped being able to laugh at themselves and each other during the course of the sessions

---

Box 8.6

Content of Supervisee Training

- Introduction to clinical supervision
- Self awareness
- Reflective practice
- Nursing knowledge
- Setting contracts
- Supervisee rights and responsibilities

Training the Supervisees

Initially it was planned that all supervisees should receive 2 days of training (Box 8.6). However, it was only possible to recruit 10 supervisees who could manage to attend two consecutive days of training. This problem was addressed by modifying the project and a second group of five supervisees received 2 hours of training. The content was the same, but the depth was more superficial. Their experiences were compared through focus group evaluations.

Provision of Supervision for all the Supervisors

At the beginning of the project there were no available supervisors who could act as supervisors to the supervisors. This was recognized as a problem in the planning stage. To overcome this, one of the project team agreed to act as clinical supervisor for the six supervisors. Recognizing the need for mutual attraction to exist between supervisors and supervisees this was made explicit in the awareness sessions. Supervisors received 2 months of supervision before they started supervising their own supervisees.

Defining the Content, Boundaries and Process of Supervision

As part of the supervisor training, the content, boundaries and process of clinical supervision were discussed and explored, resulting in a supervision contract being devised and agreed (Box 8.7). Contracts are fundamental to the supervision process making explicit the rights and responsibilities of both supervisor and supervisee. The contract should:

'relate to expectations, goal evaluation, boundaries, rights and responsibilities; issues of self disclosure, dependency and anxiety; note taking, methods of recording; anticipating the need to share issues relating to unsafe or unprofessional practice and identifying appropriate action' (Butterworth 1995, p. 2).

Box 8.7

The Supervision Contract

WIRRAL PRACTICE NURSES ONE-TO-ONE CLINICAL SUPERVISION CONTRACT

Introduction
The purpose of supervision is to facilitate the development and growth of the practitioner to become increasingly effective in his/her work. It follows therefore, that the emphasis within supervision sessions will be on the practitioner's work rather than the practitioner themselves.

The Contract
To initiate and sustain the supervision relationship the following contract was negotiated on March 1st 1996. However, it is important to remember and recognize that as we participate in and experience supervision, needs and expectations will change. So, getting it right usually means evolving the interaction rather than restricting it. The contract is therefore an important foundation rather than a permanent 'prescription'. In one-to-one supervision the roles and expectations will be reviewed 6 monthly or earlier by negotiation.

Supervision will occur monthly for the first 6 months and will consist of 1 hour of one-to-one supervision.

It needs to be emphasized that the supervisor/supervisee relationship is nonjudgemental and one of equality.

Shared Responsibilities
- Agreeing the venue for supervision
- Ensuring attendance and punctuality
- Maintaining confidentiality
- Regularly reviewing the usefulness of the supervision
- Knowing and clarifying the boundaries of supervision
- Accepting responsibilities if boundary infringements occur

Supervisor Responsibilities
- For ensuring a safe place for professional issues to be raised
- To enable the supervisee to explore and clarify their thinking, feelings and beliefs about actual and potential professional issues
- To stimulate discussion about professional issues with the purpose of sharing information
- To facilitate reflection on clinical practice aimed at refining the supervisee's skills and understanding

> **Box 8.7   Cont'd**
>
> - To challenge perceived professional and personal blind spots. This must be done in an acceptable and helpful way.
> - To challenge practices that we judge to be ethically unacceptable, clinically unsound and/or professionally unwise
> - To provide clear feedback
> - To recognize and clarify organizational, professional and educational constraints that impact upon the supervisee and their clinical practice
> - To encourage the supervisee to maintain a personal reflective diary
>
> **Supervisee Responsibilities**
> - To identify issues in their professional practice which could benefit from being reviewed and discussed in supervision
> - To ask for the kind of response and feedback that is both useful and appropriate to their clinical situation and development requirements
> - To inform their supervisor of any organizational constraints on their work
> - To develop and seek support from their supervisor in confidently sharing professional practice issues
> - To be open to feedback from their supervisor
> - To identify and communicate when this is difficult (e.g. by justifying and/or defending actions or rejecting feedback)
> - To inform their employer of their supervision arrangements
> - To inform clients, peers and those to whom they act as clinical supervisor that they are in supervision (to seek their permission to discuss practice issues in supervision – it is important that they stress that identifiable biographical material will not be shared)
> - To bring to each session prepared written notes about issues that have occurred in practice and how they felt about them, for discussion
>
> The boundaries of confidentiality within supervision are anything that is illegal, breaks the code of conduct, or infringes employment contracts and policies.
>
> Supervisee signature_____
>
> Supervisor signature_____
>
> Date_____
>
> A copy of this contract should be retained by both parties and the supervisee's employer.

The contract was used as the basis of all supervisor/supervisee relationships.

It was agreed that, at least for the duration of the project, a record of the supervision sessions would be kept by the supervisor and the supervisee. A recording sheet was devised for the purpose (Figure 8.1). It was the responsibility of the supervisee to complete the record. Some chose to complete it with their supervisor at the end of the session. Others chose to complete the form at home following

Figure 8.1 *The Clinical Supervision Recording Sheet*

Wirral Practice Nurses' Clinical Supervision Recording Sheet*

Name of supervisee: ....

Name of supervisor: ....

Date of session: ....

Venue of session: ....

Duration of session: ....

Identified aims (Were these identified at the beginning of this session or the end of last session?): ....

....

....

Were these aims adhered to?   YES/NO

If not, why? ....

....

Please identify any skills and/or knowledge obtained from this session: ....

....

How will this help inform your practice? ....

....

Agreed plan of action and time scale: ....

....

Please categorise the content of your supervision session.

Items for discussion/aims:	Points for practice/actions:
Clinical issues	
Role reflection/support	
Professional/leadership/educational/research activities	
Workload/management issues	
Clinical supervision contract	

Signature of supervisee: ....

Signature of supervisor: ....

Date of next session: ....

---

* Note that the recording sheet is larger in practice.

a period of personal reflection. The purpose of the form was to provide evidence of development for personal professional portfolios. Following the project some chose to discontinue record keeping.

Formally Constituting the Supervisor/Supervisee Relationship

The relationship between the supervisor and the supervisee was formally constituted through the supervision contract. The contract was introduced to each supervisee during their training sessions when they had the opportunity to discuss and explore their rights and responsibilities. The responsibility for matching supervisees to supervisors was undertaken by the trainer. Supervisees were given information about the supervisors and requested to give a first, second and third choice and given no guarantee that they would receive their first supervisor of choice. It was considered important that the supervisors also had choice in whom they supervised. While maintaining confidentiality, the first-choice supervisors were approached by the trainer and asked if they wished to act as a supervisor to the supervisees who had chosen them. Supervisors were chosen for a variety of reasons. Examples of reasons were: they were known to the supervisee, they were not known to the supervisee, they lived in close proximity, they worked in a similar practice. At the end of the negotiation process, each supervisee had been matched up with their first-choice supervisor.

Evaluating the Project

The evaluation process had been agreed before commencement of the project, and therefore information relating to the evaluation process was given during the awareness sessions. The evaluation was undertaken by a third member of the project team who had no contact with the supervisors or supervisees other than to evaluate their experiences. The reasoning behind this was to increase the validity of the evaluation. It was hoped that participants would be more honest with an independent evaluator.

The project was evaluated using a qualitative technique to explore the practice nurses' perception of clinical supervision and its effect on their role. The 20 participants were allocated, by type of training, into three groups: one group of supervisors and two groups of supervisees. Data were collected during nine focus group interviews. The nine focus group interviews, three with each group of supervisors and supervisees, were conducted at the beginning, middle and end of the project. Topics for the interview guides for the first set of interviews were generated after a review of the literature. Interview guides for the other sets of interviews were modified according to emerging issues in previous interviews so that insight could be obtained into the participants' perceptions of clinical supervision as time progressed. The interviews were recorded using audio-tapes, to which all participants agreed, following an explanation relating to confidentiality and anonymity.

A method of thematic content analysis, as described by Burnard (1991) and adapted from Glaser & Strauss (1967), was undertaken. Open coding produced many categories, which were placed together in list form. The list was then scrutinized and the number of categories 'collapsed' resulting in the identification of four main themes, which are discussed below.

Feeling Safe

Feeling safe referred to issues that were perceived as crucial components in developing an atmosphere for clinical supervision to function effectively.

At the start of the project the practice nurses perceived the term 'clinical supervision' as something of an enigma, having associated connotations of being scrutinized from a 'big brother' or managerial perspective. Following the awareness sessions and study periods the participants' perspective was altered. Individuals appeared to be clear that this was not a management exercise and that the model of supervision adopted encouraged individuals to focus on their practice in dialogue with their supervisor:

> 'I felt at first that it was people coming in and actually watching you work and that put me off but when I went to the first meeting I was genuinely surprised at what it really meant, an innovative idea, and I wanted to be involved in it' (Focus Group 1).

As clinical supervision progressed the respondents felt strongly that for the process to be meaningful, confidentiality was a key issue. Central to the issues of desiring confidentiality was a 'fear of exposure'. From the participants' perspective, fear of exposure was concerned with preservation of the image individuals portrayed to the world. In some cases it was felt that issues raised in supervision would not have been raised in an informal relationship 'just in case it's something stupid' (Focus Group 2), whereas in other cases more potentially threatening situations were envisaged. It appeared that overcoming their 'fear of exposure' would ensure that the respondents' practice could truly be examined in such a way as to allow them to admit areas of weakness or concern. The idea of dialogue with another professional seemed central to their ability to examine their own practice and respondents recognized that the situation before supervision did not present this opportunity.

None of the supervisors in the project was in a managerial relationship and all supervisees had chosen their supervisors. Being allowed to choose their supervisor was seen as important. Some chose a person they knew and 'got on with' or who they perceived as an experienced practice nurse, whereas others deliberately chose someone they did not know. The key issue appeared to be personal choice. In the main, participants felt safe in the supervision relationship because the ground rules on confidentiality were laid down and the supervisees put their trust in their supervisor.

Shifting Perspectives

Shifting perspectives comprised of participants' perceptions that the supervision process had influenced their view of themselves and their practice.

In undergoing clinical supervision the practice nurses identified that their perspectives with regard to their work practices had changed. The development of self awareness appeared to be the starting point for this change to happen.

> '... it has made me look at myself totally differently and actually go down roads now that I wouldn't have thought of doing previously and that to me has been a big change from a couple of months ago' (Focus Group 2).

For the participants the development of self awareness was thought to have facilitated the development of reflective practice. It was felt that previously, in their busy working life, there was pressure to get things done and to 'give out to other people' (Focus Group 2) so that reflection, if known about, remained in the theoretical rather than the day-to-day practical domain. Reflective practice was not a new concept to some of the participants; however, it appeared that knowledge or use of reflective practice had previously been on a theoretical or academic level:

> 'I think I've tried to be a bit more reflective on every thing. I'd done reflective practice in an academic situation, you do it but you only do it when you have to, but it's been easier than in an academic situation' (Focus Group 1).

The isolated nature of practice nursing was perceived as problematic in identifying good practice. It was felt that individuals were 'not getting a lot of feedback' (Focus Group 1) and concern was expressed that there was little way of knowing if they were on the 'right track' (Focus Group 1) or 'who would be there to tell you' (Focus Group 2) if you were. Clinical supervision, with its focus on self awareness and reflective practice, appeared to go some way to offset the feeling of isolation, and provided reinforcement and encouragement:

'It's reinforcing the good practices that you've got. It's
telling you "yes carry on, that's the way to do it, there's
nothing wrong with what you are doing"' (Focus Group 2).

As well as acquiring positive feedback on current good practices, the
participants were also, by way of reflection, gaining differing insights
or views of what had been habitual practice. There was a feeling
that supervision, in requiring the nurses to undertake preparation or
identify incidents to take to the session, had empowered or encouraged them to view their situation from a different perspective. For
many of the respondents clinical supervision had been an eye opening experience, which may, in part, have been linked to the fact that
nursing in the past encouraged individuals to 'obey instructions'
rather than to conceptualize the whole process of nursing:

'... I think as nurses, we're used to being asked or told
what to do. I think nursing's changed very much and you
actually, perhaps, need to be quite courageous and brave
and go to your GPs and say "you can't ask me to do this
and I can give you a valid reason why, and it might be that
you haven't had sufficient training"...' (Focus Group 1).

The practice nurses felt that the supervision sessions had encouraged them to take a broader view. This was perceived to have
engendered an expansion in outlook and to have facilitated their
ability to take on new approaches. It could be argued that talking
things over in an informal way with another practice nurse or nursing colleague could have achieved the same outcome. The participants, however, did not perceive this to be the case; rather it was
thought that the focused and structured nature of supervision and
the safe environment had been contributing factors:

'Its nice to have a fellow professional to talk things over
with ... to have somebody else's slant on a problem ... I
mean you can talk them through with a colleague you
work with but it's not the same' (Focus Group 2)

Expanding Horizons

Expanding horizons encompasses the participants' perceptions of
the impact that clinical supervision has had on their professional
identity and methods of working.

Respondents clearly identified that as practice nurses they felt isolated, practice nursing being perceived as 'quite lonely' (Focus
Group 3) and that practice nurses were a 'bit out on a limb' (Focus
Group 1). Although the 'practice nurse group' was perceived as a
network that existed, this was felt to be more of a 'social setting'

(Focus Group 1) that allowed neither the time nor the opportunity to speak to someone in confidence about problems or concerns. It was perceived that clinical supervision would reduce isolation by providing a forum for discussing their roles with other colleagues. The strength of their isolation was illustrated by the metaphors used by some nurses to describe how they felt about clinical supervision:

> 'Its almost like a safety valve really because if you've got no-one to discuss with, no-one at all ... that's quite hard going ...' (Focus Group 1).
> 'I like to think that I've got my supervisor as a life-line' (Focus Group 1).
> 'I feel as though I've been thrown a life-raft and I've climbed on board and it's going quite nicely' (Focus Group 2).

Reducing isolation, however, was not merely perceived as having someone to talk to, but afforded some kind of strengthening of group identity. It was as though, having worked in isolation, they did not feel affiliated to a strong professional group, but that clinical supervision was helping to generate a shared identity. It is during training and education that individuals learn the values and standards of the occupation (Holloway & Penson 1987). There has, until recently, been no recognized statutory training or education for practice nursing and most practice nurses have been appointed with little specific training. Supervision had enabled participants to feel part of a community that was described as 'more of a friendship' (Focus Group 1) or 'a kinship' (Focus Group 1) that afforded insights into the other practice nurses' situations.

From the start of the project there had been an awareness of how the practice nurse role and the delivery of health care were continually responding to change. Clinical supervision was seen by the respondents as a major way of coping with this change. Respondents identified that their self perception had altered during the project. Many felt more confident in themselves or could identify increased confidence in others. This increased confidence often appeared to be associated with the fact that they had sounded out ideas or had been encouraged to gain further information on a topic of concern. This had impacted upon their assertiveness in interactions with other health care professionals and was perceived as having had an impact on patient care:

> 'because it effects an expanded knowledge base and you've got more confidence in your knowledge and your own abilities, that you will stand your ground and practice your patient advocate role ...' (Focus Group 3).

Some respondents gave accounts of things they had been prompted to do by their supervisor that had directly impacted on patients:

'I did a survey of what my patients expected … I was amazed that I actually got responses' (Focus Group 2).
'She (supervisor) prodded me into doing something and I approached the doctors …' (Focus Group 2).

In other cases the supervisor had provided contacts for the supervisees who were starting new techniques (e.g. group sessions) in their practice. It was felt that this line of communication would not have been available but for supervision.

Emerging Issues

Emerging issues referred to the participants' perception of issues pertinent to the implementation and organization of clinical supervision. Throughout the period of supervision there were several emergent issues that pertained to the organizational, administrative and supportive aspects of the project. These issues were relevant to the smooth running of clinical supervision in the future.

The overwhelming feeling from the respondents was that the model of clinical supervision should continue. The practice nurses found it hard to identify disadvantages; most people praised it: 'it's marvellous, I can't speak too highly (of it)'. As the project progressed, myths had been dispelled about its purpose and method of working; a consequence of this was that other practice nurses, not currently involved in the project, were reported to be interested.

The respondents hoped that supervision would be 'here to stay' (Focus Group 3), but were concerned that it was not 'going to last' (Focus Group 2) and that it would just 'become a fad' (Focus Group 2). For some the fact that it was a pilot project and was under the scrutiny of evaluation had helped a momentum to be maintained and had encouraged people to 'stick to it' (Focus Group 3).

The clinical supervision sessions had all taken place in the practice nurses' own time; this had resulted in the perception that clinical supervision was not viewed by others as legitimate work. In addition, it was perceived that inequality existed because district nurses and health visitors were thought to have supervision in their work time. The practice nurses, however, were concerned that their employers (the GPs) would not allow them to take time 'away from the practice' (Focus Group 2).

The venue for the supervision meeting was deemed important, although finding a suitable venue was often difficult. It was generally felt that confidentiality and safety were of prime importance and therefore a room in the GP practice was not suitable because dialogue could be overheard or interruptions might occur:

'Even though we said "please don't disturb us it is out
time (lunch hour) and we're having a meeting" the doctor
came in, the receptionist came in, all with valid queries
... but I thought to myself I wouldn't have it here again'
(Focus Group 1).

The supervisees perceived that the supervisors had had some good
training and were well prepared for their role and the supervisors
were satisfied with their preparation. Those supervisees who had
had only 2 hours' preparation, however, generally felt overwhelmed
and confused by the amount of information given at the start of the
project. Some supervisors, after the first session of supervision with
their supervisees, had noticed a difference between those who had
had 2 hours and those who had had 2 days of preparation, whereas other supervisors had not noticed a difference. For all participants
the first session of individual supervision was akin to stepping into
the unknown, but it appeared that as the project progressed, their
apprehension was relieved.

Clinical Supervision – Support or Practice Development?

The respondents perceived that supervision had engendered self
awareness and that this had facilitated reflective practice. The supervision process, in encouraging reflection, had provided the opportunity, which had not otherwise been available, for affirmation of or
feedback on good practices. Furthermore, the respondents identified
that they were able to question habitual practices and to seek a
broader view.

The practice nurses perceived that their feelings of isolation were
reduced and that their group identity was strengthened. Clinical
supervision was enabling them to cope with change and increase
their confidence. It was felt that these circumstances would impact
positively on patient care.

Participants' perceptions of supervision within Wirral are
described in Box 8.8.

The experiences of the two practice nurses suggest that supervision
is both supportive and developmental.

Future Challenges

Clinical supervision has now been part of nursing's agenda since
1993. However, despite the fact that in 1994, 86% of trusts reported
that they were exploring appropriate models of clinical supervision
(Department of Health 1994), anecdotally it would appear that many
staff do not receive supervision in any form. Bishop (1998) suggests
that staff are under tremendous stress and that clinical supervision

Box 8.8

The Reality of Clinical Supervision

Practice nurse 1

Before becoming involved in clinical supervision, I often felt very isolated in my work. Although I regularly attended the local Practice Nurse Association meeting, this was not always the right arena for in-depth discussion regarding problems at work with staff or patients and clinical management of particular patients or diseases. Partly because of lack of time and also lack of privacy, these issues were never satisfactorily resolved at such meetings. I therefore welcomed the opportunity in supervision to have protected time, privacy and confidentiality to discuss issues which were pertinent to me.

I also felt that in the supervision sessions no judgement was made, which is one of the reasons why I was reluctant to speak to colleagues. Some of the issues I brought to supervision were quite personal and sensitive and I appreciated a nonjudgemental discussion, which helped me to see a way forward.

In working as a practice nurse, one can sometimes remain unaware of the standards of other nurses, alternative ways of delivering care and there is a lack of objective feedback of one's own work. Supervision enabled me to access more information, explore alternatives and obtain feedback which has greatly helped in developing my own practice and increased my confidence in the way I do my job.

On a practical level, I had one particular problem with a colleague which I was unsure how best to deal with. After exploring various options with my supervisor I felt able to take this to a higher authority, and having made them aware of the situation, felt that I had adhered to the UKCC *Code of Conduct* and had not let the matter remain unresolved. The support from my own supervisor and other practice nurse supervisors was invaluable at this time and I am sure that without supervision I would not have felt able to speak out.

Practice nurse 2

My personal experience of clinical supervision has definitely been positive. I have become more assertive in the work situation, whereas before my involvement in clinical supervision, it could be said that I was a 'shrinking violet' in some situations and would back down although I thought another course of action may have been needed. While in supervision I have been able to positively challenge the decisions of other professionals leading to more positive outcomes for patients.

could help staff to manage and deal with their stress. The question to be answered is why is this not happening. In practice nursing there are three sources of obstruction; GPs, nurse management and the practice nurses themselves.

Practice nurses may be disadvantaged in relation to clinical supervision because they are directly employed by their GPs. Without intending any direct criticism, it must be acknowledged that doctors and nurses belong to different 'tribes'. This results in each having differing professional agendas. GPs may therefore be unaware of nursing issues. However, because of the nature of practice nurse employment, any training requires locum cover or the cancellation of clinics. This, together with tight budgets and the need to meet specific health targets, may mitigate in GPs being unaware of or reluctant to fund nurses' need for supervision (Atkin & Lunt 1995). The evidence suggests that this approach is short-sighted.

Nurse advisors employed by the health authority are the source of professional advice and guidance for practice nurses. Yet, the quality of this advice and guidance varies dramatically between organizations, as Atkin & Lunt (1995) discovered:

> 'at one extreme there are those authorities which have minimal involvement and take little interest in practice nursing, believing it to be the responsibility of the employing GP. At the other end of the scale are those which take a more proactive role and directly intervene by attempting to target their resources, thus ensuring a more equitable distribution. The most usual pattern is somewhere between these two extremes' (p. 10).

The lack of direct line management from the same profession results in many practice nurses receiving little direction and support. For clinical supervision to be successful, nurse advisors employed by the health authority will need to acknowledge the benefits it can offer to practice nurses and be proactive in educating and influencing both GPs and practice nurses to change current attitudes to clinical supervision. From the Wirral study the most important change currently required is the acknowledgement that supervision is 'legitimate work' that can take place during the hours of employment. It is also necessary for the nurse advisors to provide training for supervisors and supervisees and to set up confidential systems to match supervisees with supervisors.

As for nurses from all paths of the profession, even when opportunities are available, there is a reluctance by a percentage of practice nurses to participate in clinical supervision. Many excuses emerge, with nurses viewing it as threatening, a management tool to 'beat them', not necessary for them, or they do not have the time. This is not an unusual response to new initiatives, as Plant (1987) suggested 'the important fact to remember is that resistance to change is a natural phenomenon' (p. 29). The reason for this may be that (practice) nursing is an apolitical genderized occupation (Howkins 1995) resulting in a reluctance to be challenged or to challenge. From our study it would appear that all those nurses who participated, together with those who entered clinical supervision subsequent to the project, have come to view supervision as a tool to help them. Practice nursing as a profession needs to take the responsibility for demanding that clinical supervision is available for all practice nurses, changing attitudes of individuals and auditing the availability and quality of clinical supervision.

When supervision is introduced it is vital that appropriate training is given to those who are entering supervision. Subsequent to our study, new supervisees now receive 1 day of training, and supervisors, as well as being required to be receiving supervision, receive a further 4 days of training. Anecdotally, we are unaware of any other health authority that provides such comprehensive clinical supervision training to all participants. We applaud and support the initiative, which hopefully will minimize the potential for supervisors to develop powerful or abusive relationships with their supervisees. It also clarifies the ethos around supervision and defines boundaries related to confidentiality. The challenge to the profession is to formalize the training requirements of those who enter supervision in either role.

Conclusion

Clinical supervision has the potential to be the most positive new concept to be introduced into the nursing profession, offering support, education and guidance in an increasingly stressful and constantly changing environment. However, this will only occur if nurses view the concept positively and make it work for them in their own environment. It will also require management to recognize the potential benefits of the process and invest in their staff. This is particularly so for practice nursing, which is an expanding, challenging and dynamic branch of community nursing, with many practitioners working in isolation with little support.

Acknowledgement

Special thanks to those nurses who contributed and participated in the Wirral Practice Nurse Clinical Supervision Project.

Further Reading

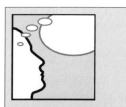

Reflection Point

Consider at this point the possible constraints and opportunities you might experience in your own area if you were asked to introduce clinical supervision

- Butterworth CA, Carson J, White E, Jeacock J, Clements A, Bishop V 1997 It is good to talk. An evaluation study in England and Scotland. The University of Manchester, Manchester

- Bishop V (ed) 1998 Clinical supervision in practice. Some questions, answers and guidelines. Macmillan/NT research, London

- Bond M, Holland S 1998 Skills of clinical supervision for nurses. Open University Press, Buckingham, Philadelphia

- Fowler J (ed) 1989 The handbook of clinical supervision: your questions answered. Mark Allen Publishing, Dinton

- Hawkins P, Shohet R 1989 Supervision in the helping professions. Open University Press, Milton Keynes

References

Atkin K, Lunt N 1995 Nurses in practice. The role of the practice nurse in primary health care. Social Policy Research Unit, University of York, York

Bishop V (ed) 1998 Clinical supervision in practice. Some questions, answers and guidelines. Macmillan/NT Research, London

Bond M, Holland S 1998 Skills of clinical supervision for nurses. Open University Press, Buckingham, Philadelphia

Burnard P 1991 A method of analysing interview transcripts in qualitative research. Nurse Education Today 11:461–466

Butterworth CA 1994 A Delphi survey of optimum practice in nursing, midwifery and health visiting. The University of Manchester, Manchester

Butterworth CA 1995 Clinical supervision in nursing, midwifery and health visiting: information for chief executives, purchasers and providers of services. The School of Nursing Studies, The University of Manchester, Manchester

Butterworth CA, Faugier J (eds) 1992 Clinical supervision and mentorship in nursing. Chapman & Hall, London

Butterworth CA Faugier J 1994 Clinical supervision in nursing, midwifery and health visiting. A Briefing Paper. The School of Nursing Studies, The University of Manchester, Manchester

Butterworth CA, Carson J, White E, Jeacock J, Clements A, Bishop V 1997 It is good to talk. An evaluation study in England and Scotland. The University of Manchester, Manchester

Castledine G 1994 What is clinical supervision? British Journal of Nursing 3(21):1135

Department of Health 1990a General practice in the NHS: a new contract. HMSO, London

Department of Health 1994 Testing the vision. HMSO, London

Dobson S 1996 Nominal group evaluation of clinical supervision. Unpublished, John Moores University, Liverpool

Faugier J, Butterworth CA 1994 Clinical supervision: a position paper. School of Nursing Studies, The University of Manchester, Manchester

Glaser BG, Strauss AL 1967 The discovery of grounded theory. Aldine, New York

Hall C 1983 An opening address as cited in Heywood Jones I 1990 The nurses' code. A practical approach to the code of professional conduct for nurses, midwives and health visitors. Macmillan Press, Basingstoke

Heywood Jones I 1990 The nurses' code. A practical approach to the code of professional conduct for nurses, midwives and health visitors. Macmillan Press, Basingstoke

Holloway I, Penson J 1987 Nurse education as social control. Nurse Education Today 7:235–241

Howkins E 1995 The political imperatives in community nursing. In: Cain P, Hyde V, Howkins E (eds) Community nursing. Dimensions and dilemmas. Arnold, London, ch 9

Johns C 1993 Professional supervision. Journal of Nursing Management 1:9–18

King's Fund Centre 1994 Clinical supervision: an executive summary. The King's Fund Centre, London

Kohner N 1994a Clinical supervision in practice. King's Fund Centre, London

Kohner N 1994b Clinical supervision: an executive summary. King's Fund Centre, London

NHS Management Executive 1993 A vision for the future. HMSO, London

Plant R 1987 Managing change and making it stick. Fontana, London

Proctor B 1986 Supervision: a co-operative exercise in accountability. In: Marken M, Payne M (eds) Enabling and ensuring. Leicester National Youth

Bureau and Council for Education and Training in Youth and Community Work, Leicester

Sheppard J 1992 The clinical task. British Medical Journal 89:288–290

Tingle J 1995 Clinical supervision is an effective risk management tool. British Journal of Nursing 4(14): 794–795

UKCC 1983 The code of professional conduct for nurses, midwives and health visitors. The United Kingdom Central Council for Nursing, Midwifery and Health Visiting London

UKCC 1992a The scope of professional practice of nurses, midwives and health visitors. The United Kingdom Central Council for Nursing, Midwifery and Health Visiting, London

UKCC 1992b The code of professional conduct for nurses, midwives and health visitors. The United Kingdom Central Council for Nursing, Midwifery and Health Visiting, London

UKCC 1995 Clinical supervision for nursing and health visiting. Registrar's letter 4/1995. The United Kingdom Central Council for Nursing, Midwifery and Health Visiting, London

Worsley P 1994 Clinical supervision. Organisation and personal development consultants, Somerset

Wright H 1989 Groupwork: perspectives and practice. Scutari Press, Oxford

9 *Nurse Prescribing*

Mark Jones

INTRODUCTION

'Nurse prescribing' is a topic that regularly appears as the heading of many journal articles and conference papers as we move forward in the new millennium. The future certainly demands a radical review of historical modes of practice – nurse prescribing as a concept is 20 years old, and its time must surely have come?

This chapter explores the evolution of the nurse prescribing debate, and moves to consider the relative success the nursing profession has had in securing, albeit limited, rights to prescribe. Prescribing has been linked to professional status and power, and until the early 1990s practice nursing was most certainly absent from consideration. Recent moves to categorize nursing by level of expertise – novice, expert, specialist – have provided the entry point for practice nurses to articulate their right to prescribe. This chapter follows the arguments put forward by practice nurses as they engage in the quest to attain a right and privilege that is ostensibly necessary to deliver the highest quality patient care.

> **Key Issues**
>
> - Nurse prescribing has a 20 year history
> - The right to prescribe is linked to professional identity
> - The right to prescribe is limited by political forces
> - The lobby in favour of nurse prescribing has been successful to a point, but thwarted by political vested interest

The Case for Nurse Prescribing

From their earliest recorded history at the beginning of the 19th century, practice nurses (then labelled the 'doctors' ladies') have not only fulfilled the role of secretary and accountant as well as actually nursing, but have been seen as the linchpin of the practice and ultimate ancillary assistant (Fry 1988, Lane 1969). Today, practice nurses are considered to have a central role in the delivery of care in general practice, but rather than being seen in the subservient role of their predecessors, modern day equivalents are partners and experts in their own right.

This recognition of practice nursing expertise is obvious when it comes to deciding on which particular medicine is relevant to the needs of a patient. A survey undertaken by the RCN asked a sample of 471 GPs to determine the extent to which practice nurses influenced their prescribing decisions when selecting therapy for patients who had asthma, diabetes or hypertension. The majority of respondents believed that 80–85% of relevant scripts across these therapeutic areas were produced as a result of the practice nurse's decision and recommendation with little or no decision making by themselves (RCN 1995). This may seem to be simple logic to the reader today – of course practice nurses have a proven expertise in chronic disease management, so why should GPs not turn to them for prescribing advice? Furthermore, is it then such a big step for practice nurses who are working to provide care for patients who have conditions for which they have a proven expertise to prescribe appropriate medicines for them?

Although such an analysis seems straightforward in the present, in the early 1980s when nurses first began to explore the potential for them to prescribe certain items this was radical thinking. Jones & Gough (1997) indicate that, just as with the practice nurses in the 1995 RCN survey, district nurses were well aware that on a daily basis they were deciding that patients required a particular dressing, appliance or adjustment to medication, but had to find a GP to sanction their decision and prescribe the items needed. As with the practice nurse survey, the GP simply endorsed the nurse's decision without question. In many cases the district nurse was simply frustrated at having to spend time making seemingly unnecessary trips between the patient's home and the GP practice, and some patients suffered as a result of the need to seek medical endorsement. For example, specialist community nurses with responsibility for palliative care described situations where they could not increase the dose of an analgesic or administer it before the time for which it was exactly prescribed because to do so would be to prescribe a prescription-only medicine in breach of prevailing legislation. This resulted in patients being left in pain with their relatives watching the clock while the nurse tried to contact a doctor to authorize the medication change (Jones & Gough 1997).

These arguments about the nurse having the specialist knowledge base to make prescribing decisions yet having to find a GP to action the decision, leading to time wasting on the part of both nurse and doctor, plus the more serious factor of denial of immediate care to patients, became the key points for a campaign to extend prescribing rights to nurses. Fortuitously, just as the awareness of this whole issue was growing within the nursing profession, the government commissioned a review of community nursing provision by a team of health experts and economists under the chairmanship of Julia

Cumberlege. The review team was asked to consider community nursing provision in England, and make recommendations for the future of that provision. The RCN saw this as an excellent opportunity to bring forward the arguments for amending legislation to allow nurses to prescribe (Jones & Gough 1997).

What About Practice Nurses?

At this point we need to summarize the essential arguments for prescribing rights for nurses, and consider the position of practice nurses. The nurse prescribing 'movement' began in the early 1980s. Even though there is a massive workforce in excess of 17 000 practice nurses today, there were fewer than 3000 employed at this time and practice nurses as a group were far less influential (Atkin et al 1993, Evans 1992, Jones 1996, Stilwell 1991). Additionally, the nurse prescribing debate focused on the time being wasted by district nurses as they travelled between their base, the patient's home, the GP practice and pharmacy, to obtain the items they knew were required. Although it was possible to identify inefficiencies in practice nurses not being able to prescribe today (RCN 1995) it was assumed that the proximity of practice nurses to GPs did not make this an issue. Other reasons for omitting practice nursing from the prescribing quest emerge later, but suffice to say in the opening rounds of the debate practice nurse prescribing was not an issue.

The final report of the Cumberlege review team both acknowledged the arguments for prescribing, and continued to deny any relevance to practice nursing. Cumberlege readily accepted the point that experienced district nurses were wasting their time and that of patients and doctors, and recommended that qualified community nurses should be able to prescribe from a limited range of medicines, appliances and dressings (Department of Health and Social Security 1986). As every practice nurse knows, however, the report also suggested that the system whereby GPs receive reimbursement for a large proportion of the costs of employing a nurse should be brought to an end. It is worth analysing this a little further if only to try to minimize any paranoic assumption that Cumberlege was 'out to get' practice nurses! The review team's view was simply that district nurses and health visitors were being stifled in their roles, and that GPs and community nurse managers should have a more constructive working relationship to allow nursing care to develop to offer a more comprehensive system meeting both the needs of patients and general practice. If this were to happen, GPs would not need to employ their own practice nurses.

With Cumberlege therefore, we see the first moves toward a system of 'occupational closure' operating against practice nurses that would eventually deny them access to prescribing rights. For what they believed were good reasons the Cumberlege team set in motion a wave of discontent among practice nurses, which would eventually lead them to becoming one of the strongest forces in community nursing, if not the whole profession. As noted by key commentators at the time (Allen 1991, Crawford 1991a), rather than sound the death knell of practice nursing, Cumberlege galvanized practice nurses into action. From the time of Cumberlege to the present, 'practice nursing' would engage on a quest for professional recognition, including rights and privileges such as a qualification and the ability to prescribe as examined in more detail below.

An Alliance Forms

Thankfully (for nurse prescribing at any rate) the Cumberlege Report was positively received by the Government, and in 1987 the House of Commons Social Services Select Committee supported the specific call for prescribing rights for community nurses (HC 37 Social Services Committee 1987). Buoyed by their success at achieving recognition of the prescribing issue, the RCN began to gather support for putting the Cumberlege and Select Committee recommendations into practice (Jones & Gough 1997). The RCN took its case

Reflection Points

It is worth taking a 'time out' here to consider where practice nurses featured in the ongoing chronology of the nurse prescribing campaign. Note that in 1988 the RCN were arguing for 'community nurses' to be able to prescribe – this translated to mean health visitors and district nurses – practice nurses were not given a specific mention. From the author's personal experience and perspective, the RCN was still reeling from outburst among its practice nursing membership as a result of the resounding endorsement the RCN had given to the Cumberlege Report. Similarly, practice nurses themselves were seemingly caught up in the struggle for their own survival and the quest for professional security through a recognized qualification. Arguing the right to prescribe for practice nurses was peripheral to both the RCN agenda to achieve those rights for community nurses, and to that of practice nurses themselves searching for more global recognition from the nursing profession. The nurse prescribing campaign moved on therefore, with practice nursing still not being given any real consideration.

and arguments for nurse prescribing along to what it considered to be at one and the same time their potential allies and opponents – the British Medical Association (BMA) and the Royal Pharmaceutical Society of Great Britain (RPSoGB). After much initial posturing and a good deal of negotiation, a tacit agreement was reached in late 1988 that the case for nurse prescribing was justifiable and sustainable, and that the Government should be petitioned to sanction this initiative (BMA 1988, RCN 1988, RPSoGB 1988). The RCN then began a concerted push for the implementation of the Cumberlege recommendations. In particular, it campaigned for the right of community nurses to be able to prescribe any medicines they needed to deliver nursing care and draw up agreements with doctors (later to be known as 'protocols') under which they could supply and administer a range of prescription–only medicines.

The Crown Report

With support from the BMA and RPSoGB, the RCN was successful in persuading the Government to take seriously their case for extending prescribing rights to nurses, and Dr June Crown was asked to lead an advisory group to report by October 1st 1989. The group was given the responsibility of advising:

> 'the Secretary of State, after consultation with the Standing Medical Advisory Committee, the Standing Nursing and Midwifery Committee and the Standing Pharmaceutical Committee, how arrangements for the supply of drugs, dressings, appliances and chemical reagents to patients as part of their nursing care in the community might be improved by enabling such items to be prescribed by a nurse, taking into account where necessary current practice and likely developments in other areas of nursing practice' (Department of Health 1989, p. 3).

Clearly the RCN was correct in forming an alliance with pharmacists and doctors, given that together these three professional interest groups were to be the focus of Crown's consultation process. The terms of reference went on further to echo much of the case that had already been made by the RCN for nurse prescribing to become a reality. The Crown group was specifically asked to make recommendations on:

> 'i. the circumstances in which nurses might prescribe, order or supply drugs, dressings, appliances and chemical reagents, taking account of such professional and ethical issues as responsibility and inter-professional communication;

ii. the categories of items which might properly be
prescribed, ordered or supplied by nurses and the
arrangements which would be needed for drawing up
and maintaining a list of such items;

iii. the methods by which drugs, dressings, appliances
and chemical reagents might be prescribed, ordered
or supplied by nurses, having regard to current
guidance on the safe and secure handling of
medicines' (Department of Health 1989, p. 3).

It is noteworthy that in the context of prescribing, the Crown Review
team's scope was not limited to any particular grouping of
community nurses – that is any notion that district nurses and health
visitors only should be considered for prescribing rights.

The remainder of the tasks set before Crown were again to consider points raised by the RCN in their initial arguments, particularly
in relation to the palliative care examples discussed above. That is
'to make recommendations on the circumstances in which a nurse
might properly vary the timing and dosage of drugs prescribed by a
doctor'. Finally, all of these deliberations needed to be set in the
context of cost, with the Review team being asked to consider implications for nurse training and resource implications in general
(Department of Health 1989, p. 3).

In spite of a 2-month delay causing some suspicion about a negative content and requiring an 'upbeat' intervention in the form of a
Virginia Bottomley press release (Department of Health 1989), the
Crown team was diligent in its work, and produced a report containing 32 recommendations only slightly adrift of its intended publication date. The so-called 'Crown Report' was warmly welcomed
by the nursing profession in general, and most definitely by the RCN
(RCN 1990). Essentially, all the RCN had asked for was contained
within the report. Crown recommended that nurses should be able
to prescribe from their own formulary of items needed for the delivery of nursing care, that doctors and nurses should collaborate in the
drawing up of 'group protocols' to facilitate the easy supply of medicines to groups of patients who had similar needs (e.g. immunizations) and in a similar system of protocols specific to individual
patients, to permit nurses to vary the time and dosage of medicines
prescribed. The report even gave a reasonable start date for all of
this to happen – April 1st 1992.

Practice Nurses Still Left Out

All was looking good then. However, it was the question of which
nurses should prescribe that came to taint the response to the Crown
recommendations. So far as the ability to write a prescription – what

Crown termed 'initial prescribing' – was concerned, the recommendation was that '... for the present, authority for the initial prescribing from the *Nurse's Formulary* should be introduced for nurses with a district nurse or health visitor qualification only' (Department of Health 1989, p. 25). The basic rationale given for this decision was that health visitors and district nurses could easily be identified on the register held by the UKCC as having completed further education since their initial registration. Crown also indicated that other specialist nurses were not likely to need to prescribe because they were mainly hospital based, were able to obtain supplies more easily and were in close proximity to prescribing doctors. The door was not closed to other nursing groups though, as Crown indicated that:

> 'Once initial prescribing by district nurses and health visitors has been introduced and evaluated, we recommend that consideration should be given to extending initial prescribing to other groups of specialist nurses' (Department of Health 1989, p. 27).

Practice nurses still did not get a 'look in' then, and as we will see subsequently, it is the Crown proviso to consider other specialist groups at a later date that will bring together the practice nursing professional quest for recognition through qualification, with the whole nurse prescribing debate. For its part though, the RCN was beginning to listen to its practice nursing membership, and discussion of the Crown recommendations by the governing Council led to a position statement whereby practice nurses were included within the group for whom the College would campaign for prescribing powers (RCN 1990). The RCN even went so far as to get one of its so called 'parliamentary panel' of supportive MPs – John Greenway – to ask the Secretary of State in the Commons whether practice nurses would feature in the Government's plans for nurse prescribing, with Virginia Bottomley replying positively that 'such an arrangement (introduction of nurse prescribing) would help not only practice nurses but health visitors and district nurses'.

It was not surprising the RCN began to champion the cause, because by 1990 the practice nurse membership base of the RCN was increasing exponentially (Jones 1996) and practice nursing proponents were beginning to demand that they should be extended the same right to prescribe as health visitors and district nurses (Carlisle 1990, Fullard 1990, Jeffree, Fry & Wagner 1990).

Moving back to the nurse prescribing mainstream, as was the case with much health care reform and report recommendations under the Conservative administration in the 1980s, the Crown Report was not to be implemented without further consideration, and the main questions were around cost. As was required of it, the Crown Report had made an attempt to consider the economic implications of its recommendations, but by its own admission 'providing detailed estimates of the costs and benefits of nurse prescribing has proved somewhat problematic' and largely because 'there is no such service in this existence in this country, nor any comparable service overseas which we could use as models, our costings would have to be based on a variety of assumptions, none of which can at present be tested' (Department of Health 1989, p. 58).

Cost or Benefit?

Clearly the Government was not going to implement a proposal as radical as nurse prescribing without having considered cost–benefit data rather more robust and detailed than that provided by Crown; it therefore commissioned the accountancy firm Touche Ross to undertake a more thorough analysis. Given that in order to meet the April 1st 1992 implementation date, Crown had set December 1991 as the deadline for bringing forward legislative change (Jones & Gough 1997), the announcement of the Touche Ross cost–benefit analysis brought about suspicion about the Government's true commitment to the initiative. Encouraged by the RCN, Virginia Bottomley was questioned by MPs in the Commons about whether the announcement of the analysis was in fact a delaying tactic. This resulted in the reply 'I hope to disabuse the hon. gentleman of such suspicions. The cost–benefit analysis is important and we hope to announce the details shortly' (Bottomley 1991). However, the rest of the Minister's response was a little more unsettling, because although she reiterated Government support, several points of potential delay were indicated:

> 'We will certainly make all the information available (from the analysis). However, there are other issues to be considered – such as deciding the precise formula, training, and the relationship between nurse and general practitioner prescribing. It is a complex matter, but has strong support and we shall carry forward that work.'

Touche Ross eventually began its analysis, but although it adopted a more rigorous approach than the Crown team were either equipped for or asked to do, they essentially faced the same difficulties. That is, there were no direct comparisons for a nurse prescribing model to be introduced in the UK, and most of the costs could only be the subject of conjecture. Touche Ross did manage to estimate that the cost of training the existing workforce of health visitors and district nurses to be around £8 million, yet they also anticipated savings in nurses' and GPs' time of around £12.5 million a year (Touche Ross 1991). This was not surprising given the original assertion in the case for nurse prescribing that district nurses were wasting time tracking down and badgering GPs to endorse their prescribing decisions. The problem here is that the nurse and doctor cash savings were not real, given that the sums quoted were already subsumed within the NHS budget and were unlikely to be released as true savings should nurse prescribing be introduced. This was certainly the case for the millions of pounds Touche Ross estimated as potential savings to patient and carer groups should nurse prescribing be introduced – the Government does not pay patients and carers anyway, so no real savings will be generated.

The Struggle for Legislation

Not particularly bolstered by the Touche Ross data, yet still having gone on record as supporting the principle, the then Conservative Government dragged its feet in moving forward on the issue of nurse prescribing. Parliamentary time was certainly not set aside to translate the Crown recommendations into the reality of practice through the necessary legislative change, and the all-pervading power of the Treasury and its influence on key Government decisions became evident. Virginia Bottomley may well have been seen to support nurse prescribing, but another agenda – the size of the NHS drugs bill – was beginning to cause concern. As Touche Ross was undertaking its analysis, the Department of Health published its document *Improving Prescribing* (Department of Health 1990), considering the implementation of an indicative prescribing scheme for GPs. The approach was to be a soft one, but the message was clear – spiralling drugs costs were to come under scrutiny and the Government would not consider the budget to be open-ended.

Practice nurses featured in this analysis, but unfortunately – as a result of their close relationship and direct employment by GPs – the adverse reaction was that any extension of prescribing rights to them would have an adverse effect on the GP drugs budget (Jeffree, Fry & Wagner 1990).

This theme of cost–benefit will continue to underlie our analysis of the introduction, or otherwise, of nurse prescribing, but we move again to consider the reaction of the RCN to the Government's attitude toward the whole issue.

The RCN was not prepared to see the Government's reticence to introduce the legislation required to undermine the principle of nurse prescribing. Without amendments to a whole range of Acts of Parliament, not least the regulations operationalizing the 1968 Medicines Act, nurses could never be recognized as prescribers. The RCN had one key weapon in its armoury – the existence of its

'Parliamentary Panel'. The RCN does not sponsor MPs and peers, but has a 'Parliamentary Panel' comprising about 12 members from all parties who support the RCN in Parliament, and who meet on a regular basis to discuss nursing issues. There were, until the 1997 general election, no nurses in the House of Commons, but other panel members were chosen for their interest in health, their ability to work on a cross-party basis, and their commitment to promote the interests of nurses and nursing. From late 1990 to early 1991 the RCN began a sustained lobbying activity of all MPs in the Commons, and in particular its own panel. In what could be considered to be both an ambitious and audacious move, the RCN was keen to capitalize on the 'private member's Bill' facility existing within the Commons. Through this facility, backbench MPs are able to introduce their own legislation, irrespective of the Government's own priorities. The chance of success is generally small, and it is usually the case that only uncontroversial bills with Government support are adopted, and even then only the top six have a real chance of being a success.

Nevertheless, given that the Government was not acting in 1990 to facilitate nurse prescribing through the appropriate legislation, the RCN decided – against the odds – to press ahead with its own four-clause Bill simply entitled *Nurse Prescribing Bill*. Those MPs entering the ballot were written to, including Parliamentary Panel members, suggesting that they support the issue of nurse prescribing if they were successful. When the ballot results were out, the 20 MPs selected were written to again with a draft copy of the Bill asking for their definite support. Unfortunately, the MPs selected high up the ballot order were already committed to other causes, but Dudley Fishburn MP who was drawn at position nine agreed to take the RCN Bill forward.

As had been predicted, Dudley Fishburn's Bill ran out of time in the Commons and came nowhere near reaching the statute books. However, the letter writing campaign increased awareness among MPs, and a subsequent opinion poll survey showed 69% supporting or strongly supporting nurse prescribing, with a further 28% in favour of the principle with some reservations (RCN 1991). Although the Fishburn Bill technically failed, the public relations campaign surrounding it was a great success. The RCN continued to pressurize the Government as a result, and enlisted the support of patient and carer groups to lobby William Waldegrave, the next Secretary of State to deal with the issue. Speaking at the 1991 RCN Congress in Harrogate Waldegrave told delegates '... we will do it (introduce legislation) unless the analysis turns up some unexpected serious problem' (Waldegrave 1991).

Again the Government rested back on the excuse of needing the Touche Ross cost–benefit analysis before moving forward, yet the report was ready in time for its contents to influence the parliamentary agenda as laid out in the Queen's speech of November 1991. Even though the results of the analysis were not totally conclusive, there certainly was not the 'unexpected serious problem' of which William Waldegrave was so wary. Nevertheless, nurse prescribing was absent from the speech, a clear indication that the Government had no intention of bringing forward the legislation required and the Crown recommendation of April 1992 as a start date for nurse prescribing was rendered unachievable. Faced with this legislative block the RCN went back to its same strategy – attempting to use a private member's Bill to circumvent governmental intransigence. This time around though, the outcome was more successful. The Conservative MP for Chislehurst – Roger Sims – came third place in the private member's ballot and decided to introduce a Bill to support nurse prescribing. Perhaps aware of the futility in putting off the inevitable, or more likely the chance of getting the issue over without being directly implicated, the Government eventually let it be known that they would support the Sims Bill. With tacit Governmental assistance the Bill was drafted and put before the Commons (House of Commons 1991).

In spite of Department of Health reluctance to act, and a lack of overt support in the past, the Sims Bill received widespread government support in its passage through both the lower and upper houses of Parliament (Jones & Gough 1997). Finally, 2 years after the publication of the Crown Report, the primary legislation permitting nurse prescribing – *The Medicinal Products: Prescription by Nurses, etc. Act* – was given Royal Assent in 1992. Although the Crown Report timetable was 1 year adrift, the nursing profession could rest assured that prescribing powers for nurses would at last be a reality – or would they?

More Delays

The Treasury influence had never gone away, even if forgotten by the RCN, and not openly acknowledged by the Department of Health. Given that Virginia Bottomley had assured Dudley Fishburn across the benches of the House of Commons in May, that nurse prescribing was on course for a revised implementation date of October 1993 (Hansard 1992), it was thought that there was nothing to fear from her forthcoming speech concerning NHS priorities for 1993. Perhaps it should not have come as such a surprise given the concern over NHS spending levels, but as Virginia Bottomley talked in November 1992 of a 2.5% increase in number of patients to be treated in 1993, she also dashed the hopes of all supporters of nurse prescribing:

'This increase in services is the result of the extra funds which have been announced today for the NHS next year and of the efficiency improvements which we expect the service to make ... We have had to take a number of hard decisions in drawing up these spending plans. We have had to focus on priorities so that there is more to spend on essential services, and I am therefore announcing today that further steps will be taken to reduce the rate of growth in the NHS drugs bill. I have also decided reluctantly to postpone the introduction of nurse prescribing' (Department of Health 1992).

In less than 8 months since the legislation was passed permitting its introduction, nurse prescribing was a victim to NHS spending priorities, and although unproven, a victim of Treasury association with the increasing cost of the drugs bill.

The link between the initiative and NHS spending – in particular the drugs budget – seemed too great to break. In March 1993 the Department of Health introduced the 'Prescribing Incentive Scheme' intended to encourage GPs through a series of costshifting financial incentives to minimize their prescribing bills (Department of Health 1993). The earlier soft approach envisaged in *Improving Prescribing* (Department of Health 1990) was clearly not working, and now the Department was forced to speak to GPs in the language they most understand – reduce your drugs costs and financial benefits for your practice will accrue elsewhere. Nurse prescribing was almost like a small boat drifting on this sea of drug cost containment. Speaking at the Medpharm '93 conference, Health Minister Brian Mawhinney followed through with this analogy as he put the whole issue in perspective when questioned by the author on the continual delays to nurse prescribing implementation:

'I would like to offer a personal opinion, if Ministers are allowed to have personal opinions that is. I would like to see nurse prescribing launched in a climate in which it could be properly assessed, a climate in which it would have a fair wind ... As I have said, the next twelve months are going to be tough for prescribing in general, and to launch nurse prescribing now would not do it justice' (Jones 1993).

The RCN was not, however, minded to give up the fight. The nursing and health care press in general were full of positive comments about nurse prescribing, and the 'lay-press' seemed to be very much in favour of the initiative. After more lobbying, a further concession was obtained from the Government – one that has quite an interesting background for practice nurses.

Given the problems with cost implications, the Department of Health devised a neat strategy of dealing with being condemned for not implementing nurse prescribing, plus their own agenda of convincing the Treasury that the scheme would not break the prescribing budget. The idea was a nurse prescribing 'pilot scheme'. Speaking at the 1994 national conference of practice nurses, Julia Cumberlege announced the criteria for the selection of pilot sites. There would be eight selected from applications from GP fundholding practices (thought to be the most financially reliable and having computer systems able to track the nurse prescribing budget) where there was a joint commitment toward the project with community trusts (Department of Health 1994). Of course the proposals were welcomed, but what of the practice nursing link?

What About Practice Nurses?

You will recall that Julia Cumberlege chaired the community nursing review that subsequently took her name. The Cumberlege Review suggested that qualified district nurses and health visitors should be allowed to develop their roles – including prescribing – and that the funding stream for practice nurses should be cut off. As discussed earlier, this did not appear to be in any way a vindictive move on the part of the Cumberlege team, but their proposals set other ideas in motion. First, practice nurses themselves were committed to survive, and began to consider their position in relation to health visitors and district nurses. At the same time, health visitors and district nurses began to consider their position in relation to practice nurses. Health visitor and district nurse numbers had remained static while those of practice nurses had increased exponentially (Jones 1996). In some areas conflicts arose about which group of nurses should be doing particular work – district nurses, health visitors or practice nurses (Butland 1991). In their defence, health visitors and district nurses were anxious to stress that they had years of training and a qualification mandatory to practice at their unique level of skill, whereas practice nurses were often employed with little experience and were not required to have any qualification other than basic registration (Andrews 1994).

This debate about whose experience and qualifications were best eventually spilled out into the area of nurse prescribing. Again, as discussed above, Crown had recommended that only community nurses who had a district nursing or health visiting qualification should be permitted to prescribe. Sarah Andrews, the Director of the Queen's Nursing Institute, summarized a prevailing rationale for this decision:

'I do not wish to imply that nurses other than health visitors or district nurses don't have the ability; clearly many have. At present, however, only those with mandatory recorded qualifications at a level beyond initial registration are those who we can be sure (or as humanly possible) are able to undertake this responsibility' (Andrews 1991, p. 1).

As director of an eminent body purporting to represent the interests of community nurses, Andrews clearly believed that the lack of a formal qualification for practice nurses rendered this group unsuitable for prescribing rights. Practice nurses were stunned by this kind of comment, the editor of the journal *Practice Nursing* particularly championing their cause:

'As every PN we have spoken to will agree, on a practical level it is ludicrous that they have been left out … It all comes back to the same old story. PNs are such a motley bunch that their qualifications and experience cannot be guaranteed in any straightforward way' (Crawford 1991b).

Crawford's further analysis of the situation no doubt struck a chord with practice nurses in general:

'PNs won't be allowed to prescribe, and they will continue to be left behind until they have parity with DN and HV colleagues in the form of a common core educational programme; without a qualification which says that all PNs are on an equal footing with DNs and HVs, they cannot be taken seriously by the legislators, who only have qualifications to go on. Until their profession recognises them, and they cease to be the poor relations of community nurses, they will continue to be left out in the cold by the rest of the world' (Crawford 1991b).

Even though these comments looked gloomy for practice nursing, there was evidence to show that practice nurses were influential so far as prescribing was concerned. A survey conducted by market researchers Martin Hamblin (1991) predated the findings of the survey undertaken by the RCN in 1995, but had similar results – practice nurses were proven to be instrumental in influencing the prescribing decisions of GPs. Again Crawford expounded on the theme:

'It seems that only the authors of the Crown Report on
nurse prescribing, and the upper echelons of the nursing
profession are either extremely naive or determined to
dismiss the facts. Including only district nurses and health
visitors in prescribing rights is to ignore a growing
number of nurses who are already prescribing (sic)'
(Crawford 1991b).

These assertions had a profound impact upon practice nursing, and
their professional project became one of seeking parity with other
community nursing colleagues. Such parity – it was hoped – would
lead to due recognition of practice nursing as a speciality in its own
right, with the potential to acquire associated rights and privileges,
such as the ability to prescribe.

So why did Julia Cumberlege – co-author and chair of a report that
sought to bring an end to practice nursing and prompted the Crown
Review to leave them out of initial prescribing rights – choose their
annual conference to announce the nurse prescribing pilot project in
1994? It would seem that Cumberlege had been badly briefed on the
one hand and practice nurses had become a victim of their own 'PR'
on the other. From the time that practice nursing was decried for
being anything but a homogeneous group of competent nurses, it
had campaigned against this image with resounding success. The
image of practice nursing in 1994 (and today for that matter) was
one of a highly competent and able workforce forming a group of
key providers of health care services. Cumberlege herself acknowledged this at the '94 conference, even admitting that the Review
team had been wrong in their assumptions back in 1986
(Cumberlege 1994b). Although this admission was greeted with
applause at the practice nurse conference, the silence that met the
announcement of the prescribing pilot sites acknowledged the fact
that at the time practice nurses had not gained recognition as specialists by the UKCC; they had not gained their own recordable qualification nor were they eligible to prescribe in pilot sites unless they
had a district nurse or health visiting qualification.

As we will discuss later, never to be outmanoeuvred, practice
nurses not only adopted a strategy for circumventing the need to be
initial prescribers, but also managed to achieve their goal of specialist status and qualification with the potential for them to be included as prescribers if they so wished. For now, we will consider the
pilot sites in more detail.

The Pilot Project

The nurse prescribing demonstration pilots were selected to represent roughly four fundholding practices in the north of England,

and four in the south. Following selection of the sites, secondary legislation was put before Parliament to come into effect on October 3rd 1994 (Sowerby 1994). This legislation actually made it legal for those nurses in the pilot sites who had a district nursing or health visiting qualification and who had completed the approved prescribing training, to prescribe from a limited formulary, in addition to allowing pharmacists to dispense from a nurse prescription (House of Commons 1994). The *Nurse Formulary* to be used was quite limited in content, essentially reflecting the draft prepared at the time the original legislation was passed (BMA, RPSoGB, RCN 1992), and representing those items highlighted as being useful by district nurses at the beginning of the campaign for prescribing rights in the early 1980s. It was only after the pilots had been in operation for 3 months that six prescription-only medicines (POMs) were added – bowel regulating, antifungal and wound care preparations (Department of Health 1997).

The pilot sites generally evaluated well, reinforcing the case made by advocates of nurse prescribing – time saving for nurses, doctors and patients, and a high degree of patient satisfaction (Department of Health 1997). Nurses were considered to have gained sufficient knowledge to prescribe items on the *Nurse Formulary* and were safe and competent in their practice (Department of Health 1997, pp 10–11). The real problem with the analysis of the pilots was the same as that faced by Crown and Touche Ross previously – the difficulty in obtaining an accurate economic evaluation. The pilot project was in reality too small to produce any realistic data and figures from the eight sites produced a variance of £83 000 net cost, to £159 000 net saving from the introduction of nurse prescribing. These figures included an initial 'set-up' cost ranging from £34 000 to £67 000 (Department of Health 1997). With a 'range of uncertainty' in the order of £240 000 these figures were unlikely to convince the Treasury that the introduction of nurse prescribing across the whole of the nation was a particularly good idea!

In an attempt to improve the data being gleaned from the pilot projects Julia Cumberlege announced that the original pilot site in Bolton would be extended to include a further 60 practices within the boundary of the community trust – nurse prescribing entered the second stage of piloting (Department of Health 1996a). The Bolton 'second wave' site has yet to be evaluated fully by the Department of Health, yet local analysis shows a similar result to that of the first wave pilots so far as nurse competence, time saving, and patient acceptability are concerned, although there may be a net cost saving across the trust area (Cropper 1998). Although the second wave of pilots (the original sites plus an expanded Bolton) were yet to be analysed, the Government further expanded the pilot project – now to be called 'demonstration sites' – to have sites in each English NHS region, and subsequently two sites in Scotland. By summer 1998, no further analysis had been made available from any of the demonstration sites.

The 1996 NHS white paper *Primary Care – Delivering the Future* (Department of Health 1996b) announced the 'third wave' of demonstration sites, adding a further seven trust-wide sites, so giving each English NHS region the opportunity to assess the benefits of nurse prescribing. Shortly after, two more sites were added in Scotland (Reed 1996). By summer 1998 none of the second or third wave sites had been formally evaluated by the Department of Health, nor had further analysis of the first wave sites occurred.

Practice Nurses Find a Way Round

As the call for nurse prescribing for district nurses and health visitors seemed to be stagnating, once again in our analysis we can return to consider practice nurses. Had they been sitting around awaiting the results of the pilots and demonstration sites? Of course not! As indicated earlier, while everyone else had pursued the ultimate 'holy grail' of initial prescribing, practice nurses latched onto one of the other recommendations of Crown that had been ignored by most others. This was the principle of the supply and administration of POMs through a group protocol agreed with a GP (Department of Health 1989).

As has been discussed (Hamblin 1991, RCN 1995) practice nurses have a proven ability to make decisions about the use of certain POMs – notably vaccines and items for the treatment of asthma and diabetes. These studies also acknowledge that GPs are willing for practice nurses to make drug administration choices at their own discretion and do not need to be routinely consulted before their administration. However, the vast majority of practice nurses do not have access to prescribing rights. What was needed was some form of system whereby doctors and nurses could agree a range of POMs that could be given by the latter, without the former having to provide a written instruction or prescription each time. The Crown Report provided the ideal solution in the form of group protocols (Department of Health 1989).

Protocols

A group protocol can take a number of forms. It basically consists of a simple proforma outlining the criteria against which certain medicines can be supplied or administered to individuals in specified situations. The protocol must name those nurses to which it applies, indicating their competence to undertake this activity. The protocol is signed by the doctor who would ordinarily have the responsibility of issuing a prescription or making a written request in the patient's notes (Jones & Gough 1997).

The Crown Report recommendation to use group protocols was not officially sanctioned by the 1992 Act, and no subsequent legislative change has been made to underpin their use. Rather the development of protocols for use by practice nurses (and indeed others) has been based on an interpretation of sections 58(2)(a) and 58(2)(b) of the Medicines Act (1968). In essence, this section of the Medicines Act provides that in addition to an individual prescription, POMs can be administered under the 'direction' of a doctor. The Act does not specify what form this direction should take – it could be verbal or written. For reasons of safety and clarity, written directions in the form of group protocols – as acknowledged by Crown (1997) – have become the norm.

The use of protocols has ensured that where it would be unfeasible for a doctor to issue individual prescriptions or written directions, nurses have been able to make appropriate choices of POMs to give to patients – for example the administration of childhood and travel vaccines, family planning and treatment in accident and emergency departments. The use of well-structured protocols has been welcomed by responsible bodies such as the UKCC (1997) and the RCN (Jones & Gough 1997). Over time, custom and practice have allowed a very wide interpretation of section 58 of the Medicines Act to develop, and in some instances this may be technically outside the law (Jones & Gough 1997, Williams 1998), and since 1996, when the legality of protocols was first called into question, the RCN has been trying to raise the Department of Health's awareness of the situation and to ask for clarification.

The Crown II Review – Making the Case

By early 1997, the Department of Health had become concerned about the ongoing debate around the use of protocols. Their concern was particularly aroused by emotive headlines in the nursing press emanating from a UNISON campaign to ask GPs to give a written undertaking to support nurses in their employ should there be legal action, together with increasing pressure from the RCN to properly evaluate the demonstration sites and extend prescribing rights to more nurses (Naish & Garbeth 1996). Once more the Department of Health turned to Dr June Crown to undertake a further review.

The Crown II Review was charged with performing a detailed examination of the use of group protocols and making recommendations about their legality and ongoing use, plus an assessment as to whether prescribing rights should be extended to professional groups not currently having those rights (Moores 1996). The Review team assembled in early 1997 and set out a series of questions, which were disseminated to all interested parties (Crown 1997). This gave the opportunity for bodies such as the RCN to present their agenda for the future of prescribing by nurses, and the need for clarification of the legal anomalies around group protocols.

Practice Nurses Included

In presenting its submission to the Crown II Review, the RCN recognized that the nursing profession had moved forward significantly since it first compiled evidence in support of nurse prescribing for the Cumberlege Review over a decade previously. Principally, aside from advances in practice skills and role expansion, the UKCC had determined a definition of 'specialist practice', describing the attributes of a nurse who had progressed above and beyond the level of practice noted as first level registration (UKCC 1990, 1994). Established examples of what could now be identified as 'specialist practitioners' were incorporated into the UKCC's recommendations for the future of nursing education and practice (UKCC 1994), including the development of a new educational programme for community nurses – the *Community Health Care Nursing (CHCN)* degree course (UKCC 1994). This development at last acknowledged that practice nurses were themselves an example of a specialist practitioner group with a 'general practice nursing' pathway being specified as an option in the CHCN programme. At last practice nurses had the ability to acquire a recordable qualification identifying them as specialist practitioners alongside their district nurse and health visitor colleagues.

Given that Cumberlege and Crown had identified the health visitor and district nurse qualifications (Department of Health 1989, Department of Health and Social Security 1986) as the only available markers of community nursing competence available and restricted their recommendation for extension of prescribing rights to these groups, it made sense to now consider extending those rights to other groups who could be similarly identified. The CHCN programme readily indicated that practice nurses could also be seen to be specialist practitioners. Practice nurses pointed out, however, that although many of them could demonstrate the qualities of a specialist practitioner, few had actually completed a CHCN programme. The UKCC and National Boards for Nursing acknowledged this point, making further concessions allowing practice nurses to credit their past experience and educational attainment against the recognized outcomes of existing courses meeting the Council's requirements for specialist practice preparation (e.g. the ENB A51 programme for practice nursing).

In recognition of these developments, when drafting its evidence to the Crown II Review, the RCN used the descriptor of specialist practice as a marker for the level of competency required to attain prescribing rights (RCN 1997), and suggested that practice nurses who can demonstrate specialist practitioner status should be included in the extension of prescribing rights.

The RCN evidence to Crown II linked specialist practice with the ability to prescribe any drugs or other items required for the delivery of nursing care. Its argument follows that specialist practitioners who have completed an additional nurse prescribing course (which would eventually be incorporated into specialist practitioner programmes) would prescribe within their specialist knowledge base and not exceed the boundaries of their competence. For example, a stoma care nurse could be expected to prescribe stoma and skin care products, but would not be prescribing insulin for diabetic patients. Similarly, a diabetic specialist nurse could prescribe insulins for patients, but would not prescribe pain control for a terminally ill patient (Jones 1997). The rationale behind these assumptions is that nurses are bound by an adherence to their professional *Code of Conduct* and the guidance within the *Scope of Professional Practice* (UKCC 1992a,b). Rather than restrict specialist nurses' prescribing powers by rigid regulation and specific formularies, the RCN argued that a concept of professional autonomy and competence, bound by an acceptance of individual accountability is the optimum means of ensuring that nurses are able to prescribe those products required for patient care (Jones 1997). This would mean that practice nurses who were able to define themselves as specialist practitioners and who had undertaken a nurse prescribing course would be able to prescribe POMs for their patients as their nursing care needs and competence range of the nurse dictated.

Review of Prescribing, Supply, and Administration of Medicines – Final Report

Having despatched the protocol issue, the Crown team turned their attention to the 'six million dollar question' – should health care professionals other than those who have them already be given prescribing rights?

The second week of March 1999 saw this question answered – basically yes. In its second and final report the Crown team accepted that the current restriction of prescribing to doctors (in the main) was out of step with a modern health service with increased responsibility on the part of all, better education and multidisciplinary working. Seeing the doctor as the person who makes the diagnosis and writes the prescription, and the nurse as the person who gives the medicine is an outdated concept (Department of Health 1999, para. 3.2), with recognition that 'In some instances, the decision about whether or not to prescribe a medicine is, for all practical purposes, taken by a team member who is not a doctor' (Department of Health 1999). Recognition of these principles – which the nursing profession has been emphasizing for the past 20 years – is easy; what Crown seeks to do is offer a framework whereby prescribing by a range of competent health care professionals can be made a reality.

The question of competence is key to the Review team recommendations, and having considered over 700 items of evidence presented to it, two distinct forms of future prescribing are proposed – 'independent prescribing' and 'dependent prescribing';

■ the act of 'prescribing for a patient presenting for the first time in an episode of care' is defined as 'independent prescribing' in that '... the prescriber takes responsibility for the clinical assessment of the patients (usually establishing a diagnosis) as well as for the appropriateness of any prescription which may be issued at that time' (Department of Health 1999, para. 6.14)
■ 'once a diagnosis has been established or a treatment plan prepared for an individual patient, the responsibility for clinical management may be transferred from the assessing clinician (an independent prescriber) to another health care professional' – to be known as a 'dependent prescriber' (Department of Health 1999, para. 6.16).

Independent prescribers are therefore seen to have the diagnostic and assessment ability to underpin an initial prescribing decision, whereas dependent prescribers not having this ability, still have sufficient knowledge and understanding to vary the dose of a drug or how and when it is given, and perhaps even prescribe an alternative within the same therapeutic category. These definitions of independent and dependent prescribing certainly resonate back to the Crown 1989 proposals – it's a shame they have taken another 10 years since its publication to be reconsidered. What Crown has done this time around though, is to give far more structure to how these prescribers might be defined and allowed to practice, and within the definitions provided, there is no reason why practice nurses will not be both independent and dependent prescribers.

Sadly, for all its innovative content, when it comes to independent prescribing Crown is still defensive of existing systems in that:

> 'The Team believes that doctors and dentists will continue to form the majority of independent prescribers for POMs. Any extensions, beyond district nurses and health visitors who are already legally entitled to prescribe from a limited list of medicines, are likely to be limited to specific therapeutic areas' (Department of Health 1999, para. 6.15).

For nursing, this proposal recognizes that some specialist groups possess the competence base when augmented by further education around prescribing practice to be independent prescribers. However, it amounts to setting up a myriad of formularies linked to specialist areas of practice, with only those having recognized qualifications being able to prescribe from their specific tightly regulated formulary. This goes against the recommendations of the RCN who suggested to Crown that individual accountability and determination of competence in a professional regulatory structure should be sufficient to govern prescribing habits rather than a legally enforced formulary system. Drawing up specialist formularies, policing and updating their content, and pharmacists being able to identify which nurses can prescribe what as they are presented with prescriptions will cause logistical problems.

So, at the end of the day, how does the Crown Review team see nurses becoming prescribers?

The first step is to establish an independent body – the New Prescribers Advisory Committee (NPAC) – to consider proposals from professional groups wishing to have prescribing rights extended to their members. It will be NPAC's job to provide the recipe for these rights to be granted as they set criteria (Box 9.1)

The membership of NPAC has yet to be agreed, but it will include people who are there for their own expertise rather than representing any particular organizational interest. Crown does see the need to have input from a patient group, professional body, regulatory body and existing prescriber point of view. Regardless of how NPAC is made up it is obvious that this committee will be instrumental in determining nurse prescribing over the next few years.

Box 9.1

Criteria to be Set by the NPAC for Granting Prescribing Rights (Department of Health 1999, para 6.28)

- The clinical need for the proposed extension of prescribing
- The definition and registration arrangements for the professional group concerned, ensuring that there are clear criteria for determining which individuals may be included in the group. They may include consideration of the education and training requirements of the group
- The need for additional prescribing to be 'independent' or 'dependent' in the senses defined above
- The broad category(ies) of the medicines that might be prescribed
- The need for prescribing by the new group to be funded by the NHS

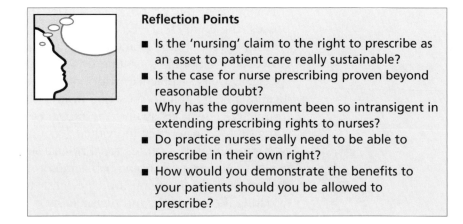

Reflection Points

- Is the 'nursing' claim to the right to prescribe as an asset to patient care really sustainable?
- Is the case for nurse prescribing proven beyond reasonable doubt?
- Why has the government been so intransigent in extending prescribing rights to nurses?
- Do practice nurses really need to be able to prescribe in their own right?
- How would you demonstrate the benefits to your patients should you be allowed to prescribe?

Conclusion

The Crown recommendations have yet to be fully accepted by the Secretary of State – the period for consultation ended on June 7th 1999, and we do not know whether the Department of Health, the Treasury and the Government will be willing to accept them. Time will tell, but suffice to say, the case for nurse prescribing has existed for almost two decades, and there is little evidence to suggest that it is not a valid case. Specialist nurses – those working in general practice included – must continue to articulate the benefits to patient care should they be permitted to prescribe. The arguments are sound, but the battle has yet to be won.

References

Allen M 1991 Practice nursing profile: Meradin Peachey. Practice Nursing January p. 5

Andrews S 1991 Nurse prescribing: post-basic education, the key to expansion. Practice Nursing January p. 434

Andrews S 1994 Desperately seeking recognition. Practice Nursing February pp. 132–133

Atkin K, Hirst M, Lunt N, Parker G 1993 Nurses count. A national census of practice nurses. Social Policy Research Unit, University of York

BMA, RCN 1988 Nurse prescribing: a discussion paper. RCN-BMA2 CNAEXMEET. Unpublished paper held in RCN archives, London

BMA, RPSoGB, RCN 1992 Draft nurse prescribers' formulary. British Medical Association, Royal Pharmaceutical Society of Great Britain, Royal College of Nursing, London

Bottomley V 1991 Oral answer to questions on nurse prescribing. Hansard February 5

Butland G 1991 Practices who don't release staff for training should be hit in the pocket. Practice Nurse January p. 432

Carlisle D 1990 Who prescribes? Nursing Standard 86(9):16, 17

Crawford M 1991a Practice nursing profile: Ruth Cherry. Practice Nursing October p. 4

Crawford M 1991b PN diploma courses get the go-ahead. Practice Nursing July/August p. 1

Cropper M 1998 The progress of the nurse prescribing scheme. Personal communication – paper presented to the Association of Nurse Prescribing conference. March 18, Manchester

Crown J 1997 Review of prescribing, supply and administration of medicines. Letter inviting submission of evidence to the review. Dr June Crown/NHS Executive, Leeds

Cumberlege J 1994a Message to Practice Nurse journal readers. Practice Nurse March p. 263

Cumberlege J 1994b Nurse prescribing – one step nearer. Baroness Cumberlege announces criteria at practice nurse conference. Department of Health press release 94/147. March 24. Department of Health, London

Department of Health and Social Security 1986
Nursing: a focus for care. Report of the community
neighbourhood nursing review. (The Cumberlege
Report). HMSO, London

Department of Health 1989 Report of the advisory
group on nurse prescribing (Chair Dr June Crown).
HMSO, London

Department of Health 1990 Improving prescribing.
HMSO, London

Department of Health 1992 NHS to treat record
numbers of patients as spending rises to highest
levels ever. From fax transmission of press release
sent by Parliamentary News Service on 13.11.92 to
RCN Press Office

Department of Health 1993 Prescribing incentive
scheme 'will benefit patients' says Dr Brian
Mawhinney. Department of Health press release
H93/620. 11 March 1993. Department of Health,
London

Department of Health 1994 Nurse prescribing – one
step nearer. Press release 94/147. 24 March.
Department of Health, London

Department of Health 1996a Lady Cumberlege
announces extension to nurse prescribing. Press
release 96/13. Department of Health, London

Department of Health 1996b Primary care – delivering
the future. HMSO, London

Department of Health 1997 Evaluation of the nurse
prescribing pilot sites. HMSO, London

Department of Health 1999 Review of prescribing,
supply and administration of medicines. Final
report (Chair Dr June Crown). The Stationary
Office, London

Evans J 1992 PNs – A picture. Practice Nursing
September p. 9

Fry J 1988 General practice and primary health
care 1940–1980s. Nuffield Provincial Trust,
London

Fullard E 1990 Report of the advisory group on nurse
prescribing – December 1989. Memorandum to
Terry Brown, Associate General Manager,
Kensington, Chelsea and Westminster FPC. cc to
Mark Jones, RCN 16 March 1990. Unpublished, held
in RCN archives, London

Hamblin M 1991 Practice nurses research summary.
Mark Allen Publications, London

Hansard 1992 Entry for 03 May 1992. In: Royal
College of Nursing 1992 Nurse prescribing – the
case for implementation. Parliamentary briefing.
RCN, London

House of Commons 1991 The medicinal products:
prescription by nurses etc. act 1992
(commencement no. 1) order 1994. Statutory
instrument 2408 (C.48). HMSO, London

Jeffree P, Fry J, Wagner V 1990 Prescribing and
the practice nurse. Practice Nurse March pp.
443–446

Jones M 1993 Brian Mawhinney and nurse
prescribing. Unpublished memorandum to Derek
Dean, Director of Nursing Policy and Practice,
describing comments made by the Health Minister
at Medpharm '93. Held in RCN archives, London

Jones M 1996 Accountability in practice. Quay Books,
Dinton

Jones M 1997 Fighting for the freedom to prescribe.
Nursing Standard 11(48):13–14

Jones M, Gough P 1997 Nurse prescribing – why has
it taken so long? Nursing Standard 11(20):39–42

Lane K 1969 The longest art. Allen & Unwin, London

Medicines Act (The) 1968 HMSO, London

Naish J, Garbett R 1996 'Don't administer drugs says
union'. Nursing Times 92(47):5

RCN 1990 Comments on the report of the advisory
group on nurse prescribing – report to RCN
Council March 1990. Paper RCN/90/38. Royal
College of Nursing, London

RCN 1991 MPs opinion poll – nurse prescribing.
Royal College of Nursing, London

RCN 1995 Whose prescription? Royal College of
Nursing, London

RCN 1997 Evidence submitted to Crown II. Royal
College of Nursing, London

Reed M 1996 Nurse prescribing. Letter from Margaret
Reed, Nursing Officer. Directorate of Primary Care,
Scottish Office, Edinburgh

RPSoGB 1988 Report of a meeting between
representatives of the Pharmaceutical Society and
the Royal College of Nursing. Pharmaceutical
Society of Great Britain. WBR/VG 30.03.88.
Unpublished minutes held in RCN archives, London

Sowerby M 1994 Nurse prescribing. Unpublished
letter from Mike Sowerby, Project Manager, Nurse
Prescribing NHS Executive, to Mark Jones,
Community Health Adviser, Royal College of
Nursing. 21 September 1994. Held in RCN archives,
London

Stilwell B 1991 Practice nurses role needs further
definition. Practice Nurse January p. 466

Touche Ross 1991 Touche Ross, Department of
Health 1991 Nurse prescribing - Final report: a
cost-benefit study. HMSO, London

UKCC 1990 The Report of the post registration
education and practice project. United Kingdom
Central Council for Nursing, Midwifery and Health
Visiting, London

UKCC 1992a Code of professional conduct. United
Kingdom Central Council for Nursing, Midwifery
and Health Visiting, London

UKCC 1992b Scope of professional practice. United Kingdom Central Council for Nursing, Midwifery and Health Visiting, London

UKCC 1994 The future of professional practice – the council's standards for education and practice following registration. United Kingdom Central Council for Nursing, Midwifery and Health Visiting, London

UKCC 1997 UKCC response compiled by Maureen Williams, Professional Officer, Health Visiting and Community Nursing to the review of prescribing, supply and administration of medicines. UKCC Council Paper. Annexe 1 to CC/97/29. United Kingdom Central Council for Nursing, Midwifery, and Health Visiting, London

Waldegrave 1991 Speech addressing RCN congress, Harrogate

Williams M 1998 Public protection and the nurse prescribing scheme. Abstract and paper presented at the Association of Nurse Prescribing conference. March 18. EMAP Healthcare, London

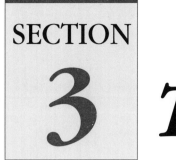

SECTION 3

The Future

10 *Achieving Practice Nurse Potential through Specialist Practice*

Patsy Dodd

Introduction

The achievement of practice nurses in their development since the mid 1980s is unparalleled in any other sphere of nursing as practice nurses have moved from the treatment room nurse to that of a valued and respected member of the primary health care team. Yet has the full potential of the practice nurse been realized by both the nurses themselves or the other members of the primary health care team? The aim of this chapter is to explore the real meaning of specialist practitioner and the effect it will have on general practice nursing.

   The chapter will argue that the opportunity afforded through the changes in nurse education will facilitate practice nursing to raise its level of practice to a higher level, and in doing so will demonstrate quality nursing care directly related to population needs. The chapter will reflect upon both the experiences of the author and other nurses in challenging and moving the boundaries of nursing practice forward.

Key Issues

- Defining the title Specialist Practitioner
- UKCC's definition of specialist practice
- Care and programme management

- Clinical practice
- Clinical development
- Clinical leadership

Specialist Practitioner – What Does it Mean?

The definitions of a specialist practitioner highlighted in Box 10.1 provided by a variety of professionals highlight the confusion surrounding the title. The introduction of numerous titles in nursing has led to a state of confusion in the profession, which is exacerbated

> **Box 10.1**
>
> **Defining the Title**
>
> 'A practice nurse thinks whereas a specialist practitioner knows'
> (General Practitioner)
> 'A nurse who has undergone specialized training and is now able
> to provide that little bit extra of specialized skills in the
> community' (Hospital Consultant)
> 'Unsure' (District Nurse)
> 'A nurse who has undergone further training in a particular topic'
> (Health Visitor)
> 'A nurse who concentrates on one field of nursing' (Nursery
> Nurse)
> 'A person who has undergone further training concentrating on
> a particular area of expertise' (Project 2000 Student)
> 'A person who has training in a specific area to allow them to
> practice and give care in that area' (Midwife)
> 'A practitioner involved in providing specialist care' (Student
> Midwife)

> **Box 10.2**
>
> **Definitions (Thompson 1996)**
>
> **Specialist Nurse**
> Usually a senior nurse who has specialist experience and training in a
> particular field of nursing, who cares for a group of patients within
> that field (e.g. diabetes).
>
> **Nurse Practitioner**
> More of a generalist who has a broad spectrum of patients to care for
> and a high level of responsibility, which includes controlling her own
> caseload, manning minor illness clinics and prescribing treatment
> (though still not signing the FP10)
>
> **Community Specialist Practitioner**
> Has undergone statutory standards of education to degree level and
> is the only recordable qualification of the three with the specialism
> being practice nursing not just asthma or diabetes

by the UKCC's reluctance to acknowledge all but a few. Thompson
(1996), however, attempts to clarify the issue defining the terms as
outlined in Box 10.2.

Although offering a welcome degree of clarity to defining titles,
Thompson (1996) has not dealt with the issue of the 'nurse clinician'.
This is particularly relevant to our current debate because nurses
working in general practice who have undertaken a master degree
are renaming themselves nurse clinicians. In separating the role of
the nurse clinician from that of specialist practitioner, it would
appear the role is often dependent on how nurses are permitted to

develop their roles in their own practice setting. One nurse clinician described her role as an acute clinical assessment role and a manager of chronic disease. This compares evenly with that of specialist practitioner, but the educational background of each role is entirely different. Confused? Read on.

What then is the real definition of a specialist practitioner and how can the role be defined? What are the advantages or disadvantages of practice nurses undertaking such programmes?

Specialist Community Practitioner Qualification

The UKCC's recommendations for nurse education in April 1995 highlighted not only the need for nurses to continually update practice, but also laid the blueprint for new programmes of education leading to the qualification of specialist practitioner. The UKCC defined the specialist practitioner as:

> 'exercising higher levels of judgement, discretion and decision-making in clinical care. They will be able to monitor and improve standards of care through supervision of practice, clinical audit, the provision of skilled professional leadership and the development of practice through research, teaching and the support of professional colleagues' (UKCC 1996).

Within the community setting, the UKCC identified eight areas of specialist community health care nursing as listed in Box 10.3.

Initially, the new specialist community nurse qualification caused both anger and anxiety to practice nurses, given the lack of consideration given to nonrecordable courses they had undertaken over the preceding years. The educational opportunities during the transitional period and practice nurses' responses are examined in detail in Chapter 1; however, it is important to consider the examination of

---

Box 10.3

The Eight Areas of Specialist Community Health Care Nursing (UKCC 1996)

- General practice nursing
- Community mental health nursing
- Community mental handicap nursing
- Community children's nursing
- Public health nursing – health visiting
- Occupational health nursing
- Community nursing in the home – district nursing
- School nursing

specialist practice as the use of the transitional arrangements has impacted upon others' perceptions of practice nurses as functioning at specialist level. This may become ever more important as nurses increase their role within primary care.

From October 1998 the academic level of study for all modules of education leading to the specialist qualification had to be no lower than first degree level, with 50% of any programme containing theory and 50% practice. The learning outcomes concentrated on four main areas:

- care and programme management
- clinical practice
- clinical practice development
- clinical practice leadership

These areas will be discussed in detail, but you might be asking yourself why bother to become a specialist practitioner at all? This was a question I asked myself before undertaking the course. I had been a practice nurse for 14 years and had extended my role appreciably so what more could be achieved? Yet the need for practice nurses to undergo further training to gain equal status with other community nurses remained constant, with practice nurses often being seen as the least trained member of the primary health care team.

Similarly, the shift from secondary care to primary care has witnessed an increase in membership of primary care teams in response to political, organizational and clinical pressures (Pringle 1992). Lowry (1996) defines the future primary health care team as 'a team of equals rather than a group of professionals within a medically dominated hierarchy' and suggests developing nurse-led general practice as an alternative to the medically dominated general practice. In 1996 this might have been scoffed at, but since 1998 there is every opportunity for nurses to lead in developing primary health care services and to move away from working within a structure dominated by a medical or general management ethos.

Are nurses capable of achieving this? This development of clinical leadership will be discussed later in the chapter, but it should be noted at this point that the opportunities for practice nursing to move specialist practice forward are crucial to taking advantage of opportunities that have now arisen. Perate (1997) argues that as general practice responds to the myriad of changes within the NHS there is the opportunity to offer a broader and more varied range of services. The extension of services has resulted in new roles for practice nurses, and with new initiatives associated with increasing the public's health there has been a marked increase in activity in primary health care. Often it is found that the practice nurse is central to the success of new initiatives, so the need for postregistration education and continual updating of knowledge and skills is imperative. Practice nurses are seen at the heart of the Government's plans to develop a primary care-led NHS with the increasing role of delivering that care being recognized by the NHS Management Executive (1993)

So, can practice nurses ignore the implications of a primary care-led NHS or will they move with it and extend their role accordingly? Moving practice can be and often is uncomfortable and difficult; the easier option is all too often to become the victims of ritualistic practice. Yet an examination of the learning outcomes in the four areas highlighted by the UKCC for the specialist practitioner will enable practice nurses to realize that the targets set are achievable if there is enough enthusiasm to move forward. It is definitely not a time to sit idle.

So what are the learning outcomes and how can they be achieved? The following sections will highlight the UKCC's specific learning outcomes. Each area of practice development will be discussed, with exemplars from practice evidencing how practice nurses have moved their practice forward.

Care and Programme Management

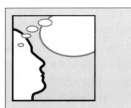

Reflection Points

- How is care planned in your practice?
- Who organizes the care provided?
- How is the care delivered?

The UKCC clearly defines what is expected of a specialist practitioner within this area with the nurse on completion being able to:

- supervize and manage clinical practice to ensure safe and effective holistic research-based care
- initiate and contribute to strategies designed to promote and improve health and prevent disease in individuals and groups by identifying and selecting from a range of health and social agencies, those that will assist and improve care
- recognize ethical and legal issues that have implications for nursing practice and take appropriate action

The expected learning outcomes might appear reasonably straightforward to some, but are they actually achievable at your practice? Are there any structures to identify what services should be offered?

Care management is defined as 'the process of tailoring services to individual needs and a method of organising care' (Ovretveit 1992). Yet, given the diversity of the population it is impossible to exam-ine specific care to be offered by each individual practice without determining the practice population needs.

How are needs defined? What is need and whose need is it? The organization's, patients' or professionals'? Need and demand are difficult to separate, with health economists acknowledging that the needs of the individual are not always of benefit to the wider public. This can allow for a situation that produces inequality and would subsequently fail to allow the needs of minority groups to be met. The complexity of defining need often inhibits planning services based on need and difficulties then arise in determining the health needs of the practice population. However, once needs are identified the planning services require a close link between methods of resource allocation and planning models. Problems might then arise with GPs following a medical model of care that is often different from the nursing model.

Community health profiles can be used to support a nurse in two ways:

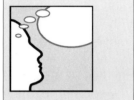

Reflection Points

- Will the GPs you work alongside be receptive to new ideas?
- How will you convince them what services are needed?

- first the change of emphasis to a more community-based health service has meant we must now be both effective and efficient practitioners
- second, the changes in the organization and delivery of care have meant nurses are increasingly required to act as advocates for their patients

Profiling is a means of providing relevant data. Public health departments use epidemiological and census material to provide annual reports, regions and localities identify community needs and community nursing staff produce profiles examining their caseload. These profiles provide broad qualitative data, but lack individuality. Some health authorities are now producing practice profiles built from computerized records, disease registers and the public health annual report. Using profiles already in existence is obviously a less arduous task than to produce your own practice profile, and will facilitate the nurse to concentrate on analysis. An analysis of the data collected in a profile will empower nurses to examine their own practice in relation to the areas they are currently involved in and identify areas that might have been ignored, but the data highlight as previously unmet needs.

Are profiles effective? It is not always major changes that make you become a more effective practitioner. On attempting to produce a profile within my own practice it was clearly identified that there was a particularly high incidence of asthma, and on further investigation, insufficient appointments to accommodate the need. This had been a constant complaint voiced by the receptionist and had fallen on deaf ears – those ears being mine! You might see this information gained as quantitative data where we as nurses often look at qualitative issues, but surely the quality of care these asthmatics were receiving should be questioned due to overbooked clinics or even delays in getting an appointment at all. Once the need for more appointments was identified, reorganization of clinics had to be considered.

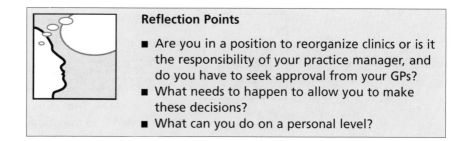

Reflection Points

■ Are you in a position to reorganize clinics or is it the responsibility of your practice manager, and do you have to seek approval from your GPs?
■ What needs to happen to allow you to make these decisions?
■ What can you do on a personal level?

Practice nurses have a professional responsibility to ensure that patients receive quality care, and as such are instrumental in working collaboratively with GPs and practice managers in the organization of care. Indeed, many practice nurses are now seen to take an active lead in the organization of clinics, and in doing so challenging the tradition of waiting to be told what clinics to run (Rink et al 1996). Reorganization of clinics might appear a daunting task, with many practice nurses underestimating their own skills as managers. Too often nurses devalue themselves as 'management material', but on examination of their role, management is evident in every working practice.

An example of reorganizing overbooked clinics is shown here in a study by Joan Woodman from Colne (Woodman 1997). The practice she worked in was the largest of three in Colne with five GPs, three practice nurses and associated staff serving a population of 11 500 patients. There was no hospital in town and the nearest minor injuries unit was 5 miles away in the community hospital. Joan explored the possibility of many of the patients being seen by the practice nurse instead of the GP. A 6-month trial was initiated with three main issues examined in running a nurse triage scheme in general practice:

■ competency and training needs
■ legal issues
■ time management

A nurse formulary was developed with the GPs for minor illnesses and it was acknowledged the reception staff would be the key to the success of this scheme.

The results of the trial were as follows: 190 patients were seen, with an equal split between adults and children, 65% were female, 16% had to be referred to a GP. Only three patients seen by a nurse returned within the week to see a GP. However, there were some reservations noted by the nurses:

■ did providing a triage service dilute or enhance the practice nurse role
■ is nursing enhanced by providing a rescue service for the overworked under-resourced medical profession
■ with a possible shortage of qualified nurses in the future can we really afford to take on any more 'medical activities'

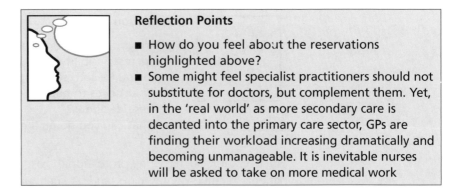

Reflection Points

■ How do you feel about the reservations highlighted above?
■ Some might feel specialist practitioners should not substitute for doctors, but complement them. Yet, in the 'real world' as more secondary care is decanted into the primary care sector, GPs are finding their workload increasing dramatically and becoming unmanageable. It is inevitable nurses will be asked to take on more medical work

The Colne pilot study concluded by confirming 'if nurses are to achieve high standards of care for all patients the profession should work towards qualifications for particularly specialised roles' (Woodman 1997). This confirms the need for practice nurses to gain further qualifications relevant to their role, and specialist practitioner fits this definition well, but could the specialist practitioner eventually become the one with the unmanageable workload? To prevent this happening it is essential to examine the roles of all members of the primary health care team and also the practice team.

To allow care to be organized both efficiently and effectively, individual expertise needs to be acknowledged (Wiles & Robinson 1994), and the value of skill mix within the primary health care team be appreciated. As team work evolves from the initial assessment of needs to the delivery of effective care (Lowry 1996), all team members are expected to share common health goals and objectives relating to patient care. The resultant management of care cannot become the sole responsibility of any one professional, but by using individual practitioner's skills and expertise quality care will be established.

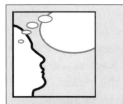

Reflection Point

How often within your own practice are all roles and expertise of other members acknowledged?

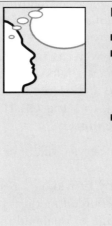

Reflection Points

■ How do you communicate as a team?
■ Do you within your own practice hold regular primary health care and practice team meetings? If not perhaps now is the time for you to organize them
■ Returning to the original questions at the beginning of this chapter – look at them again and explore ways of managing change within your practice – a daunting task for some as changes are not always readily accepted. This should be seen as yet another challenge and my experience of practice nurses in the past is that they find it difficult to resist a challenge

A key factor to consider in the establishment of primary care teams is to set up regular meetings. This facilitates the opportunity for team members to openly discuss any issues impacting on care provision. This is critical if care is to be effective and meet patients' and the community's needs.

Clinical Practice

Through the development of specialist practice nurses are able to challenge both themselves and others in the move towards evidenced-based care delivery. Indeed, it may be worth considering how much of our practice is ritualistic rather than evidenced based. When clinics are running apparently well and have done so for a long time do we ever examine how they can be improved or do we sit back and continue to run our cosy trouble-free clinics?

In the move towards evidenced-based practice the UKCC's expectations of a specialist practitioner are listed in Box 10.4.

This list seems to be exhaustive, but by taking time to look at each item, much of what is advocated may already be practised, but still needs to move forward. How do you move from ritualistic practice into innovative practice?

The UKCC's *Scope of Professional Practice* (1992a) provided practice nurses with the opportunity of developing their own nursing role in new directions. This suggests working more autonomously – an

---

Box 10.4

UKCC's Expectations of a Specialist Practitioner (UKCC 1994)

- Ability to assess health, health-related and nursing needs of patients and clients, their families and other carers by identifying and initiating appropriate steps for effective care for individuals and groups
- Set, implement and evaluate standards and criteria of nursing intervention by planning, providing and evaluating specialist clinical nursing care across a range of care provision to meet the health needs of individuals and groups requiring specialist nursing
- Assess and manage critical and clinical events to ensure safe and effective care
- Support and empower patients and clients, their families and other carers to influence and participate in decisions concerning their care by providing information on a range of specialized nursing care and services
- Facilitate learning in relation to identified health need for patients, clients and carers
- Provide counselling and psychological support for individuals and their carers

argument that is well debated. Practice nurses often describe them-selves as autonomous practitioners (Paniagua 1995a), but why when opportunities have arisen for practice nurses to develop services and use innovative skills is it only with permission from and by negotia-tion with the GP (Mitchinson 1996)? The debate will continue, but practice nurses have demonstrated innovative and creative methods of nursing, showing they do respond flexibly and sensitively to the indi-vidual needs of the practice population (Paniagua 1995b). The devel-opment of innovative practice, however, should not be undertaken without considering the quality of care provided. But what skills do we use as nurses to ensure clinical practice is of the highest quality?

One tool used in the evaluation of the nurse's own levels of prac-tice is that of critical incident analysis. Critical incident analysis, through the adoption of reflective practice, can be effective in improving care given. Palmer, Burns & Bulman (1994) argue that the best possible environment for innovative practice is one where col-leagues are not only committed to professional practice, but also to becoming reflective practitioners. Some might think reflecting on an incident highlights where things have gone wrong, but it actually prevents the practitioner from becoming complacent with everyday aspects of work and allowing their practice to become habitualized (Palmer et al 1994).

An example of reflection is given by a practice nurse in Merseyside:

> 'I was busy providing support to a lady who was distraught and distressed. During this consultation I received a phone call from one of the receptionists saying they had a mother on the phone. The mother was concerned as her asthmatic daughter was very breathless. There were no doctors present at the surgery at this time. I made a quick decision that assessment of her asthma was required and instructed the receptionist to ask her to bring her daughter to the surgery. As my consultation drew to a close, I began to reflect on my decision of requesting the child be brought to the surgery.'

With more time to analyse the situation would the decision be dif-ferent? How many times are we caught up in a busy clinic to be inter-rupted by receptionists requesting decisions from patients' requests? Often receptionists feel the nurse to be more approachable (Paxton, Heaney & Porter 1996), and decisions are almost expected of us, but the dangers of rash decisions are identified in the incident:

> 'On reflection, I realized that the child was older and taller than I initially thought and her peak flow rate was extremely low. I then realized I should have instructed

the mother to take her immediately to the accident and emergency department. I tried to contact them by telephone but they had already left. I become extremely concerned about what state of health she would be in when she arrived at the surgery ...'

Was the nurse at risk of contravening clause 2 of the UKCC's *Code of Professional Conduct* which states:

'No action or omission on your part, or within your sphere of responsibility is detrimental to the interests, condition or safety of patients and clients' (UKCC 1992b).

Realizing the rapid decision made might not have been the most appropriate the nurse rang the GP on his mobile phone and explained the situation. The child attended the surgery and was given the appropriate treatment by the GP, and returned home.

This reflection showed how vulnerable the nurse felt working alone in the surgery when GPs are out on home visits; she also learnt not to make decisions without knowing and understanding the full facts, not only to protect herself from litigation, but more importantly to protect the patient from any possible harm.

The critical incident highlights the problems around decision making and the importance of reflecting. Decision making is perhaps the difference between a practice nurse and a specialist practitioner. How is decision making defined? Jenkins (1995) describes it as 'a skill that can be learned with the individual's potential to become an effective decision maker being enhanced by education and practice' – surely this is what the specialist practitioner programme provides. Nurse education has a long history of providing practical experience that has not always been directly related to the theory being taught (Kenworthy & Nicklin 1989). The specialist practitioner programme has moved forward from this with specified theoretical elements being complemented by relevant practical skills. All learning experiences are centred upon your own practice and the needs of your practice population. Reflective practice is an essential part of learning because experiences are discussed in the appropriate context, and decisions can then be made to enhance the quality of care delivered.

Specialist practice requires nurses to be both accountable and take ownership for clinical decisions. This is a difficult concept for some nurses in general practice, who maintain that clinical decisions are the sole responsibility of the GP. Perhaps this is best explained by Hammond (1966):

'Clinical decisions are the result of a unique process which begins with a problem or a state of discrepancy requiring a decision. One's own value system provides the framework and must be examined and understood as it affects the decision. Each decision is heavily influenced by certain assumptions one might take, and the environment in which the decision is made. Generally alternatives or options are considered as the decision maker looks for courses of action which might be followed.'

The next part of the process is the determination of the probable outcomes that each course of action might result in, considering both the risks and benefits to be gained. At times this process occurs at the same time as alternatives are examined. While mentally considering courses of action, one or more options become most viable as the ones to be chosen. The decision-making process is completed when the best alternative is selected and implemented (Jenkins 1995).

Decision making is practised each time the nurse consults with a patient; it might not be the final decision, but do not underestimate skills you already have. How can we become total decision makers when legal or external factors prevent us? This is perhaps best described through the example concerning changing patient treatment. For example, if you consider that there is a need to alter an asthmatic's medication, do you make a decision, but still seek the qualification and signature of the GP? This example implies that the GP really makes the decision, but because of the impact of external factors, are GPs always able to make a decision, or is it often forced upon them? The complexity of decision making is highlighted through the example of an elderly patient who needed a nursing home placement (the GP's decision) – resources were not available and a representative from social services following their assessment made a decision to place the patient in residential care. So who really decides?

However, with decision making comes responsibility and the ability to substantiate any decision made should be only when the practitioner has an in-depth knowledge of the issues. Specialist practitioners gaining both theoretical knowledge and practical skills should justify the decisions they make, but this alone is not enough; it is also the ability to examine existing practice and determine how this can be improved. An example is given by Christine Ellaby of Cheshire when she looked at respiratory care in her practice; she writes:

'As a result of the 1990 contract practice nurses were becoming more involved with the care of patients with asthma. This led to many nurses undergoing diploma level courses and establishing nurse-led asthma clinics. Within a total fundholding pilot site consisting of three general practices (approximately 22 000 patient

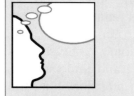

Reflection Points

- Are you aware of clinical decision making in your practice?
- Are you following the process outlined by Hammond?

population) it was decided to review clinical practice within this area of chronic disease management. This involved looking at certain clinical activities carried out by both GPs and practice nurses with the intention of identifying good practice and also to ascertain if patients were receiving adequate managed care. The survey enabled three different groups of practice nurses to come together to discuss individual practices dealing with asthma care. The survey identified many aspects of care both by the GPs and the practice nurses, which indicated different levels of clinical input; for example, there was a significant variation in levels of prescribing prophylactic therapy. This correlated with the amount of nurse involvement, in that the more the nurses were involved, the more prophylactic therapy was prescribed and fewer acute exacerbations. As a result of this finding all three practices have invested more nurse time to asthma care.'

Alongside this the survey identified that respiratory problems took a high percentage of the GPs' appointments. Many of these patients had minimal contact with the practice nurse. It was therefore decided to introduce spirometric testing to all the practices. The nurses took responsibility for setting up a pilot group of patients who may or may not have had a diagnosis of asthma or chronic obstructive pulmonary disease (COPD), but they had to be over 40 years of age, have a smoking history, and be receiving bronchodilator therapy. The nurses established strict guidelines for the use of spirometric testing and reversibility testing and adhered to specified treatment changes based on the objective testing. The results of this pilot have been to identify more accurately COPD and/or mixed respiratory disease and asthma. There has been improved patient compliance and knowledge, improvements seen in patients' symptoms and patients have been able to increase their physical activities.

'More importantly the nurses have been able to build on their original asthma-related clinical skills to develop and manage an area of chronic disease management that was previously the domain of GPs. Subsequent to the project, the nurses have developed closer networking skills and utilised their expertise to enable them to develop clinical practice at a time when there appears to be little professional support or medical guidelines available. On a final note, a positive organized management strategy was established for that client group with evidence-based practice to support their interventions' (Ellaby 1998, unpublished).

This nurse-led project clearly demonstrates how ritualistic practice can move onto innovative practice, as well as collaborative working between neighbouring practices in the examination of how care is delivered. The expertise of others was valued and good networking can reduce the isolation felt by many practice nurses.

Evaluation of the project was undertaken through a comprehensive audit process. Clinical audit is a process involving systematic and critical analysis of practice and identification of change resulting in improvement in quality of care (Malby 1995). Here, the problems of unnecessary GP appointments and level of care were previously unrecorded; by means of audit, problems were identified and resolved. However, audit is not always welcomed because some see it as highlighting deficiencies within practice without offering strategies for improving care provision. For audit to be successful within your own practice setting it needs to be patient-centred, show evidence of improved care, involve all members of the primary health care team and be relevant to your own practice (Fox 1997). Nursing audit can only aspire towards improving the quality of care by measuring the performance of those providing that care in relation to desired standards (Lenci 1995).

The nurses in the project involving patients who had respiratory problems aimed at improving the standard of care patients received. However once standards are set are there any legal implications if those standards are not met? Nurses working autonomously can be at risk if documented standards set are not met (Tingle 1992), so care must be taken to ensure that the standards set are achievable and realistic. Once standards are set protocols can be drawn up to clearly define where the nurse's role ends and the GP's begins. This is increasingly important as primary care realizes the impact of *Clinical Governance* upon care delivery (Crinson 1999). Evidence shows that nurses are more likely to use protocols than GPs (Cotton 1997), seeing them as a means of sharing care effectively, but still working within the law. Clinical protocols can be used in litigation, but it is argued that practice nurses involved in their design and implementation demonstrate that they have been proactive, thoughtful and careful in addressing the provision of quality nursing care (Tingle 1995).

As nurses become more autonomous they must be involved in the development of protocols because they have been shown to change clinical practice and improve patient outcome, with local adaptation providing the best likelihood of successful implementation (Grimshaw & Russell 1993). Evidence-based practice will demonstrate the viability of any project and assist to move any clinical practice forward, but it can also provide valuable information to examine new areas of practice, which leads on to the next area to discuss – clinical practice development.

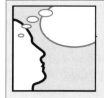

Reflection Points

Sue Richards (1997), the nurse representative in the medical defence union looked at the litigation issues around protocols and asks you to ask yourselves:

- Are protocols written out?
- Are they negotiated with the GPs and the primary health care team?
- Do protocols name the nurses to whom the particular care is delegated?
- Have you and the GPs signed and dated them?
- Do you regularly review protocols to update them in line with accepted clinical and nursing practice?

Box 10.5

Role of the Specialist Practitioner in Clinical Development (UKCC 1996)

- To create an environment in which clinical practice development is fostered, evaluated and disseminated
- To identify specialist learning activities in a clinical setting that contribute to clinical teaching and assessment of learning in a multidisciplinary environment with scope of expertise and knowledge base
- To initiate and lead practice developments to enhance the nursing contribution and quality of care
- To identify, apply and disseminate research findings relating to specialist nursing practice
- To explore and implement strategies for quality assurance and quality audit and determine criteria against which they should be judged, how success might be measured and who measures success

Clinical Practice Development

Clinical practice, as discussed allows practitioners to expand exising practice, whereas clinical development is exploring the possibility of introducing new areas depending upon the practice population needs. In considering the clinical development function of the specialist practitioner the UKCC outline the role as shown in Box 10.5.

The expansion of the role of the practice nurse based upon evidence-based practice is explicitly identified in the UKCC's definition of clinical development. Yet, there is a limited research base available to inform practice nursing. In addressing this nurses must become research aware and research active to contribute to the research base that underpins their clinical practice (While 1998). Yet the development of the role as identified above is dependent upon the relationship the nurse has with other members of the primary health care team, and in particular, the GP.

The development and expansion of the nurse's role is fundamental if nurses are to offer realistic nurse-led primary care. In striving towards this goal, practice nurses must consider the issues of professional competence and the nature and quality of patient professional relationships, because these are key predictors of overall consumer satisfaction (Williams & Calman 1991). Brooks & Phillips' (1996) study of consumer satisfaction clearly highlighted that women patients in general valued the work of practice nurses in undertaking routine procedures previously undertaken by the GP. Indeed, nurse–patient consultations in general practice are seen to have a great psychosocial component (Peter 1993) because the practice nurse is perceived as both approachable and accessible (Brooks & Phillips 1996). Although nurses may diagnose and make appropriate referrals, there remains strong opposition to nursing acting independently and autonomously (Georgian Research Society 1991). The greatest opposition to the development of nursing diagnosis has come from the GPs. Undoubtedly, the diagnostic and monitoring function of the nurse has expanded dramatically over the past decade, with the emphasis on practice nurses to be accountable for their actions as diagnosticians, decision makers and clinical judgement makers. These are a fundamental component in developing new areas of nursing practice.

If innovative nurse-led care is to be introduced, an examination of population needs and support for the development of the project from other team members is essential. Roles of all members need to be examined and developed accordingly. The identified need for change has to be explored taking into consideration the effects of new initiatives on the whole team. Successful implementation will often depend upon collaboration. How can this be achieved? McGregor (1960) defines collaboration as:

> 'The limits on human collaboration in the organisational setting are not the limits of human nature but of management's ingenuity in discovering how to realise the potential represented by its human resources.'

The development of practice should not be restricted to the nurses, but consider other members of the primary health care team, such as the receptionists. As practice nursing expands, it is appropriate to consider skill mix, and who shares their workload. Many receptionists have skills that are not used or would welcome opportunities to extend their role. In exploring this issue, Jenny Brown, a practice nurse in Liverpool, examined the role of health care assistants, and its subsequent impact upon the practice nurse role.

The project aimed to identify whether support workers did have a role to play and how National Vocational Qualifications (NVQs) could be used to expand existing roles and introduce skill mix into general practice. A receptionist was trained and assessed to NVQ level 2 and the project ran for 12 months. The evaluation revealed that the practice nurse had more time to spend with patients, more patients were seen and the patients themselves appreciated the wider service. The health care assistant was accountable to the practice nurse and worked strictly to protocols devised and agreed by the practice nurse and the GP. The findings from the project were positive, with a successful evaluation leading to its expansion at two further practices, with the range of duties incorporating those identified by NVQ level 3. Practice nurses should not view support workers as a threat, fearing that their posts may be lost, but as an asset to allow highly trained professionals to use their time more effectively (Brown 1995). Here it is not just accountability for the nurse, but for support workers as well. Inappropriate delegation of some tasks could well have legal implications, although 'the statute law does not prescribe who is to perform certain health tasks, but standards must be set, protocols introduced and set criteria met' (Hunt & Wainwright 1994). Providing any delegation follows this law, the implementation of health care assistants will enable the practice nurse to lead new developments within the practice and explore new areas of practice.

The challenge for primary care is the development of innovative structures and processes that will meet the cumulative effect of changing demographic profiles and service demands. The key to successful development is the effectiveness of interprofessional working based on a collaborative approach (Livesey 1997). The implications are that nurses are now in a position to develop their own programme of care for clients, assess needs, provide appropriate treatment, investigate, advise, educate, counsel and follow up referrals. They are capable of development free from medical control and are unchallenged by a nursing hierarchy with the traditional bureaucratic control (Paniagua 1995a).

Clinical development of all nurses working within primary care emphasizes the need to continue to draw on public health work and community development approaches to promote a vision of primary care that allows a response to both health and health care need (Gough 1997). However, the success in developing practice will depend upon the particular ingenuity and determination of each individual to prove his or her worth (Paniagua 1995b). Examples of nurse-led initiatives to meet the public health agenda are not yet commonplace, yet as Ann Ryan shows they are achievable. Ann

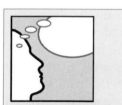

Reflection Points

■ Are practice nurses really unchallenged by a nursing hierarchy with the traditional bureaucratic control?

■ How many practice nurses are free from medical control?

works in a busy surgery situated in an area of high social deprivation. The health profile of the practice identified a high unemployment rate and high deprivation, particularly among the teenager population. There were many young single mothers. This information led her to addressing the issue of how teenagers acquired information about sexual health. Her intention was to implement a new service in her practice by providing sexual health education to teenagers. This would also attempt to meet the specific *Health of the Nation* (Department of Health 1992) target to reduce teenage pregnancies. The question raised was 'Do young people in Britain have adequate access to education and information regarding their health and sexuality?'.

There appeared to be three main ways to acquire information:

- in school
- from parents
- from the media

Ann found difficulties in all three areas. Her intention was not to purely enhance her own role, but to complement the service provided by others to enhance care for a particularly vulnerable group.

Looking firstly at sex education in the local schools she identified that the teachers themselves feared they may be committing a criminal offence by providing contraception advice to pupils under 16 years of age. This led to reluctance on their part to give advice beyond that laid down in the curriculum; also classes of 20 or more at a time did not allow individual problems to be addressed. Ann identified that the limitations of education often led young adults to seek information elsewhere, namely through the media. However, she found the media often portrayed sex as fun and was not always responsible in its attitude. The third area providing information was parents; she found that the parents were at times authoritative and judgemental in accepting their offspring's sexual relationships.

Having explored the mechanisms already in place she determined that there was a need for implementing a new service in general practice. Ann examined her own role and felt she needed to facilitate the opportunity for young people to discuss any problems. This necessitated the need to work more closely with the school nurse. Ann noted it was not important where the teenager acquired information from, but that it was adequate and met the individual's needs. How then did she introduce the service?

Ann found most teenagers reluctant to consult the general practice for advice on personal matters due to confidentiality, embarrassment, approachability and availability of appointments. As most teenagers would not attend formally structured clinics Ann targeted teenagers already attending clinics, for example, those attending the asthma clinic. She had previously taken the opportunity to discuss with the parent the service for the teenagers who needed to discuss any personal issues. The knowledge of some families allowed Ann to inform parents of her availability in the hope they would tell their teenage children. The development of this service will be slow and it will be extremely difficult to evaluate its effectiveness. Ann sees its success being measured in terms of increasing self-esteem and awareness, greater knowledge and empowering decision making about personal feeling, not in reducing the number of pregnancies and abortions, which is the usual tool for measuring success. This highlights the importance of quality care yet the difficulty in measuring outcomes. Ann concludes:

> 'The provision of sexual health education in general
> practice may not have a significant impact on government
> targets but providing education will promote sexual
> health by increasing knowledge and awareness enabling
> the development of interpersonal skills and
> responsibilities, exploration of attitudes and the greater
> dissemination of appropriate biological information' (Ryan
> 1997, unpublished).

This exemplar of good practice stresses the need to identify what the practice population really needs, and not government-identified normative needs. Targets are set, but with practice populations being so different, it is far more useful to profile your own practice needs and implement services to meet those needs.

As practice nurses we are often 'bogged down' with disease management clinics, with more and more care moving from the secondary care sector to general practice. It is enlightening to witness nurse-led collaborative preventative care in the primary care setting. Nevertheless, disease management clinics and secondary prevention services are becoming more and more the responsibility of the practice nurse. In the following exemplar of nurse-led care Pauline McHew of Widnes explores the possibility of initiating a clinic for patients who have rheumatoid arthritis in general practice. She explains:

> 'Following several discussions with various members of
> the primary health care team, rheumatoid arthritis was
> identified as being an area of chronic disease that had
> been neglected and could be managed more effectively.
> It was agreed that the practice nurse was in an ideal
> position to facilitate the management and care of patients
> with rheumatoid arthritis. The training needs of the
> practice nurse were identified jointly with the local
> university-based school of health.'

Through the university, an association was formed with the rheumatology specialist nurse at the local hospital who agreed to provide the practical training. Funding for this training was provided by the health authority. The time scale of the course was flexible because this was a new initiative, but the practical training was estimated to be completed after 12 weeks. This allowed time to be spent with all members of the rheumatology team, including the consultant, rheumatology specialist nurse, physiotherapist and occupational therapist.

An assignment was undertaken that included management of a patient who had rheumatoid arthritis. A protocol of care and guidelines for drug management were devised collaboratively. The role of the nurse emphasized education in all aspects of care for patients and their families, monitoring of blood for drug side effects, and acting on any abnormal results by appropriate referral to other members of the rheumatology team. The provision of regular follow-up and open access will reveal early problems if they should develop. The clinic is continually audited and is proving to be successful. Regular updates in training will continue to be undertaken' (McHugh 1997, unpublished).

This initiative shows a planned approach to care delivery; having identified a need, training was undertaken both academically and practically, and by working collaboratively with a specialist in that field patients receive quality care. As Sharp (1997) identifies, the move of services to primary care will facilitate nurses to have the opportunity to expand practice. It is therefore inevitable that if nurses seize the opportunities, practice development will progress.

Clinical Practice Leadership

The two initiatives identified above acknowledge the potential of developing nursing roles within the general practice setting. Indeed, some may describe them as leaders in their field – but what makes a leader? Do practice nurses have leadership qualities? Who are seen as leaders in general practice? The final area to discuss in relation to specialist practitioner is leadership, which is perhaps the most difficult to clearly define. The UKCC's definition of leadership within the role of the specialist practitioner is given in Box 10.6.

Practitioners who have advanced their knowledge and enhanced their skills through experiential education and experience can exercise increasing clinical discretion and accept greater professional

Box 10.6

UKCC's Definition of Leadership within the Role of Specialist Practitioner (UKCC 1994)

- The ability to lead and clinically direct the professional team to ensure the implementation and monitoring of quality-assured standards of care by effective and efficient management of finite resources
- Identification of individual potential in registered nurses and specialist practitioners through effective appraisal systems. As a clinical expert advise on educational opportunities that will facilitate the development and support of their specialist knowledge and skills to ensure they develop their clinical practice
- Ensure effective learning experiences and opportunity to achieve learning outcomes for students through preceptorship, mentorship, counselling, clinical supervision and provision of an educational environment

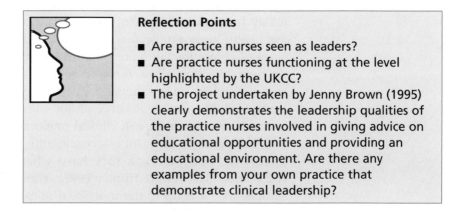

Reflection Points

- Are practice nurses seen as leaders?
- Are practice nurses functioning at the level highlighted by the UKCC?
- The project undertaken by Jenny Brown (1995) clearly demonstrates the leadership qualities of the practice nurses involved in giving advice on educational opportunities and providing an educational environment. Are there any examples from your own practice that demonstrate clinical leadership?

responsibility through advanced practice (UKCC 1991). If practice nurses are to become leaders they must have a clear understanding of the needs of the practice team and the practice. Yet, there is still an assumption that GPs should always be seen as leaders. The discussion surrounding primary care groups has accepted GPs as leaders of these groups. Doctors have always held a more powerful position in the health care hierarchy than nurses, but is this our own doing? Nursing history originated during the Crimean war with unquestioning obedience to superiors and strict adherence to routines, and when formal nursing education was introduced it was mainly structured and dominated by doctors (Baird 1997).

The change from the medical model of care to a primary health care model has raised the profile of practice nurses. It is now recognized that a practice nurse's contribution in the development of a primary care-led NHS is a key element (Department of Health 1996). However, the opportunity for nurses to lead will only become a reality if the value of nursing practice, in terms of its effect on patients, is demonstrated, and once the nursing claim for greater independence and professionalism gains momentum (Baird 1997). For this to become reality, nursing needs leadership at all levels (Lowry 1996). Leaders must identify the route ahead, encouraging and inspiring others to follow and allowing change to become positive, exciting and challenging, rather than discouraging and threatening (Steward 1989).

Leadership in any setting could entail evidence of appropriate qualifications, with specialist practitioner becoming a requisite for seniority posts. Practice nurses have won a significant battle in achieving equal status with other community nurses, but the real victory will be when the specialist community practitioner qualifications are recognized as demonstrating leadership and expertise within practice nursing. Carey (1997) pinpoints what nurses can do, emphasizing the unique contribution of nursing to health care provision.

The government has recognized the value of practice nursing, identifying that we should be considered for lead nurse posts, but in reality how often do practice nurses hear of career opportunities in the health authority or management vacancies in your local trusts? Lines of communication are poor and there is a great need to develop networks that allow news to reach us (Richards 1997). This is confounded by nurses themselves, and a general lack of confidence in their abilities to deal successfully with management tasks. The contradiction lies in that in clinical practice nurses often feel able to assert themselves and discuss confidently key issues affecting their profession, but few think they have what it takes in management and leadership (Kent & Hunter 1997). There is no secret formula for leadership – it is up to the individual nurse to determine what skills are required and the probability is you already have them. An interesting study was undertaken by Weeks (personal communication 1997). She selected 16 practice nurse leaders to analyse leadership qualities identified in those leaders. A theory was generated from what were believed to be the 12 characteristics required for future practice nurse leaders (Box 10.7).

The study highlighted the amount of personal time that was given by these practice nurse leaders. Eight said it would be impossible to carry out their roles without support.

Weeks highlights the support needs as coming from a variety of people, namely colleagues who cover clinics to allow you to attend meetings, the GPs you work for, peers who can be 'sounding boards' for new innovative ideas and health authority staff. However, support from families is essential for free time to be given up for the additional unpaid role. It was also found that 12 of the leaders had other leadership roles (i.e. parent teacher association, school governor or chairing other groups). This might suggest some

Box 10.7

The Characteristics Identified by Weeks (1997) as required for Practice Nurse Leaders

- Communication with others
- Integrity and self awareness
- Assertiveness
- Commitment to practice nursing
- Ability to drive policies forward
- Enthusiasm
- Ability to influence people
- Representative of practice nursing
- Leadership attributes
- Ability to predict the future (have a vision)
- Decision making ability

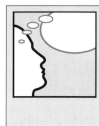

Reflection Points

- Is a lack of support the stumbling block that prevents practice nurses taking on leadership roles?
- All too often leadership is expected to be done in your own time but with increased workloads who can afford the time?

are 'born leaders' – an expression frequently used. Some had initially begun their leadership role in local practice nurse groups, being founder members and then went on to regional or countrywide associations. They have become peer reviewers of practice nurse magazines, and now recognized conference speakers.

This study indicates that leadership qualities can be developed slowly, but many do have the ability to become leaders. How can practice nurses be encouraged to become leaders and how can leadership qualities be developed? Weeks (1997) suggests prospective leaders need to be identified, with peers supporting their attendance at committee meetings, educational seminars, conferences and policy discussions. An examination of academic ways of achieving the qualities needed should be explored. The development of the specialist practitioner will determine the need for clinical leadership skills to meet new challenges and opportunities.

This study also highlights the need for the financial and support aspects to be addressed. Many leadership roles were self-funded in the post, but this should not remain an option. Suggested sources of support were:

- practice nurse groups
- health authorities

> **Box 10.8**
>
> **Three Examples of Ways Practice Nurses Can Lead (Bagnall 1997)**
>
> ■ A nurse-led provider organization could be set up to meet the primary health care needs of school children offering a range of services including school health visiting, GPs, community psychiatry, social work, community paediatrics, physiotherapy and educational psychology
> ■ Head an integrated service for people who have neurological disorders, such as Parkinson's disease or epilepsy. The team could include neurological consultants and nurses, GPs, physiotherapists and voluntary organizations (e.g. Parkinson's Disease Society). This model could work for services for other disease groups such as locomotor, respiratory and digestive disorders
> ■ Lead a nursing team providing a service that bridges acute and community settings, providing a seamless service between hospital and the community

■ Universities
■ Royal College Nursing
■ GPs

The conclusion of this study showed there is a need to develop new leaders for the future. Could this be you?

Bagnall (1997) suggests three examples of ways practice nurses can lead (Box 10.8).

The primary care pilot projects allow nurse-led projects to be implemented, but financial and organizational barriers appear to be restricting the number of nurse-led proposals being submitted (Gupta 1997).

The introduction of primary care groups has facilitated community nurses to be involved in commissioning health care as well as providing it. Opportunities are there and, as specialist practitioners, practice nurses justifiably merit the possibility of being considered to become members of such groups and so become leaders of community nursing practice.

Conclusion

Perhaps to conclude it would be useful to look at the definition of a specialist practitioner and what skills are needed to fulfil that role from someone who has completed the specialist practitioner programme. Yvonne Salisbury of Wirral writes:

> 'A specialist practitioner is a nurse who has demonstrated via a structured learning programme that he/she is

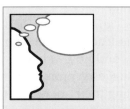

Reflection Points

■ What opportunities do you identify to develop your leadership skills?
■ Are there any barriers or constraints to developing your leadership skills?

confident and competent to practise autonomously within their particular sphere of nursing. In general practice you should empower individuals, families and the community to identify their health needs and plan, implement and evaluate action to meet those needs. Resource implication often affects the quality of service patients receive, but the ability to identify, implement, manage and work within resources available will demonstrate the skills of a specialist practitioner.

Also by using analytical, political and social skills, being aware of current trends, health implications, public health risks and having an involvement in practice and local policies you can act as a facilitator and educator to empower both patients and other staff. Collaboration with all members of the primary health care team and other community teams (e.g. social services, voluntary and secondary services), will produce the quality of service desired' (Salisbury 1998, unpublished).

This definition shows the specialist practitioner role extending into political and management areas by confirming the need to be both academically and clinically knowledgeable. The specialist practitioner will assist to demonstrate educational and professional equality with other members of the community nursing service.

On a final note, having completed the specialist practitioner programme I find GPs, other members of the primary health care team and health authority representatives valuing my opinion on various topics, which is a welcome experience. The respect I receive shows I am now seen as a professional in my own right, not as historically know as the 'doctor's handmaiden'. The threat of a GP recruitment crisis will result in more opportunities arising for specialist practitioners to undertake even more tasks that have been traditionally carried out by GPs, supported through collaboration with health authorities, educational institutions and other members of the primary health care team and our own professional and regulatory bodies. It is our chance to grasp these opportunities and fulfil our potential as specialist community practitioners who make a unique and valued contribution to practice.

Acknowledgements
I would like to thank the following for their contributions towards this chapter: Christine Ellaby, Sheila Fairclough, Pauline McHew, Ann Ryan, Yvonne Salisbury and Sandra Weeks.

References

Bagnall P 1997 Reasons to be cheerful. Nursing Times 93(5):34–35

Baird A 1997 Nursing and healthcare culture. Practice Nursing 8(10):42–44

Brooks F, Phillips D 1996 Do women want women health workers? Women's views of the primary health care service. Journal of Advanced Nursing 23(6):1207–1211

Brown J 1995 The handmaiden's tale. Practice Nurse

Carey L 1997 Practice nursing: has it served its purpose? Practice Nurse National Conference, Practice Nurse, London

Cotton P 1997 Protocol development: attitudes among GPs and practice nurses. Practice Nursing 8(6):27–29

Crinson I 1999 Clinical governance: the new NHS, new responsibilities. British Journal of Nursing, 8(7):449–453

Department of Health 1992 Health of the nation. HMSO, London

Department of Health 1996 Primary care: delivering the future. HMSO, London

Fox J 1997 Clinical audit and the practice nurse. Practice Nursing 8(6)

Georgian Research Society 1991 The attitude of GPs towards practice nurses – a pilot study. British Journal of General Practice 41:19–22

Gough P 1997 Primary care nurses must resist GP model. Primary Health Care 7(10)

Grimshaw JM, Russell IT 1993 The effect of clinical guidelines on medical practice: a systematic review of rigorous evaluations. Lancet 342:1317–1322

Gupta K 1997 Concerns grow over nurse pilot bid numbers as final deadline passes. Practice Nurse 14(9):32

Hammond KR 1966 Clinical inference in nursing: a psychologist's viewpoint. Nursing Research 15(1):9–14

Hunt G, Wainwright P 1994 Expanding the role of the nurse. Blackwell Scientific Publications, Oxford

Jenkins H 1995 Improving clinical decision making in nursing. Journal of Nursing Education 24(6):242–243

Kent C, Hunter D 1997 Management material. Nursing Times 93(5):36–37

Kenworthy N, Nicklin P 1989 Teaching and assessing in nursing practice. Soutain Press, London

Lenci B 1995 Nursing audit. Practice Nursing 6(15):128

Livesey H 1997 Integrating the nurse practitioner role in primary care settings. Primary Health Care 7(10):26

Lowry M 1996 Developing nurse-led primary healthcare. Professional Nurse 11(12):821–822

Malby R 1995 Clinical audit for nurses and therapists. Scutari Press, London

McGregor D 1960 The human side of enterprise: theory x and y. McGraw-Hill, New York

Mitchinson S 1996 Are nurses independent and autonomous practitioners? Nursing Standard 10(34):34–38

NHS Management Executive 1993 New world, new opportunities. HMSO, London

Ovretveit 1992 Health service quality: an introduction to quality methods for health services. Blackwell Scientific Publications, Oxford

Palmer A, Burns S, Bulman C 1994 Pushing back the boundaries of personal experience: reflective practice in nursing. Blackwell Scientific Publications, Oxford

Paniagua H 1995a The scope of advanced practice: action potential for practice nurses. British Journal of Nursing 4(5):269–274

Paniagua H 1995b Practice nursing: will it survive? British Journal of Nursing 4(20):1173–1174

Paxton F, Heaney JG, Porter AM 1996 A study of interruption rates for practice nurses and GPs. Nursing Standard 10(43):33–36

Perate I 1997 Taking a sexual health history: the role of the practice nurse. British Journal of Nursing 6(17):978–983

Peter A 1993 Practice nursing in Glasgow after the new GP contract. British Journal of General Practice 43:97–100

Pringle M 1992 Partners in practice: the developing primary care partnership. British Medical Journal 305:624–626

Richards S 1997 Get yourself connected. Practice Nursing 8(20):172

Rink E, Ross F, Godfrey E, Roberts G 1996 The changing use of nursing skills in general practice. British Journal of Community Health Nursing 1(6):201–203

Sharp J 1997 A nurse-led service in the community. Primary Health Care 7(9):12

Steward R 1989 Leading in the NHS: a practical guide. Macmillan, London

Thompson S 1996 Defining specialism in asthma. Practice Nursing 7(20):301

Tingle J 1992 Legal implications of standard setting in nursing. British Journal of Nursing 1(14):728–731

Tingle J 1995 Clinical protocols and the law. Nursing Times 91(29):27–28

UKCC 1991 Report of proposals for the future of community education and practice. United

Kingdom Central Council for Nursing, Midwifey and Health Visiting, London

UKCC 1992a Scope of professional practice. United Kingdom Central Council for Nursing, Midwifery and Health Visiting, London

UKCC 1992b Code of professional conduct. United Kingdom Central Council for Nursing, Midwifery and Health Visiting, London

UKCC 1994 The future of professional practice: the Council's standards for education and practice following registration (PREP). United Kingdom Central Council for Nursing, Midwifery and Health Visiting, London

UKCC 1996 The Council's standards for education and practice following registration (PREP). Transitional arrangements – specialist practitioner

title/specialist qualification. Registrar's Letter 15/1996. United Kingdom Central Council for Nursing, Midwifery and Health Visiting, London

While A 1998 First steps towards ethical research. Practice Nurse 15(3)

Wiles R, Robinson J 1994 Teamwork in primary care: the views and experiences of nurses, midwives and health visitors. Journal of Advanced Nursing 20:324–330

Williams S, Calman M 1991 Convergence and divergence: assessing criteria of consumer satisfaction across general practice, dental and hospital care settings. Social Service Medicine 33:601

Woodman J 1997 Nurse triage: easing the workload. Practice Nurse 14(9):554–558

11 *Autonomy in Practice – Is It a Reality?*

Lynda Carey   Mark Jones

'Women should be treated as autonomous decision makers'
Mary Wollenstonecraft
(1792)

INTRODUCTION

In their consideration of the position of women as providers of health care on behalf of the World Health Organization, Helena Pizurki and colleagues reach the conclusion that:

> 'of all the professions subject to sex-role stereotyping, nursing seems to be the most severely handicapped in that nurses are doubly conditioned into playing a subservient role: first by society generally, and secondly by the medical establishment' (Pizurki et al 1987, p. 58).

This chapter will assess the reality of this statement as it applies to nurses working within contemporary UK general practice, asking whether their role is one of de facto subservience with consequent elimination of any notion of autonomous practice.

This is a fundamental issue given that practice nurses have in the past cited the autonomous nature of their practice as a key factor in their choice of career (Mitchinson 1996). Indeed, historically, for many nurses the initial attraction of general practice was the opportunity to work independently away from the traditional hierarchy that dominated nursing up until the 1980s (Atkin et al 1994). Yet, it is questionable whether the move away from traditional nursing hierarchy towards general practice has enabled nurses to become empowered or merely replaced nursing hierarchy with the controlling power of the GP. Fundamental to this discussion is the concept of autonomy, and whether it can be a reality for nurses working within general practice. Central to this is an analysis of the relationship between GP and practice nurse with reference to gender and power dynamics, perhaps illustrating all is not what it might seem between apparently status rich curing doctor and caring focused devoted nurse.

Given the material highlighted, the chapter is not intended to be an easy read. Instead it is included within this text as an opportunity to re-examine a number of the wider concepts that underpin practice. Readers are not encouraged to accept the ideas wholeheartedly, but to consider them with intent and allow them to provide a greater understanding of the manner in which they work. It is intended to be inspirational and as such offer an opportunity for nurses to explore the wider issues.

Key Issues

- Defining autonomy
- Feminist analysis
- Analysing the practice nurse and GP relationship

- Autonomy and power – where does the power base lie
- Autonomy – the impact upon care provision

Defining Autonomy

Defining autonomy and autonomous practice within nursing is not an easy task; even though the concept is widely heralded and discussed, little real attention has been paid to defining the concept. This is evidenced by both Ross & Mackenzie (1996) and Haggard (1997) who discuss factors influencing nurse autonomy without attempting to define its meaning to nursing practice. It is therefore unsurprising to find that nurses describe themselves as autonomous practitioners without any discussion of their practice. The Oxford English dictionary (Fowler & Fowler 1989) defines autonomy as 'the right of self government'. Similarly, Morris (1998, p. 247) defines autonomy as 'the freedom to make choices'. These definitions identify autonomy as part of a wider philosophical debate that recognizes that freedom and rights are crucial factors in the decision making process. Gillon (1986) defines autonomy more comprehensively as 'the capacity to think, decide and act on the basis of such thought and decision freely and without let or hindrance'.

This is an important definition to consider within the general practice setting, because are practice nurses in a position to act without consideration to the relationship of the GP?

On a wider scale, it is questionable whether nursing can achieve autonomous practice unless it achieves recognition for its contribution to health care delivery; without such identification nurses will never achieve equality and so become independent decision makers. In contrast to the above perspective Jenson & Mooney (1990) maintain that autonomy cannot be examined within an individualistic perspective, because individuals must always consider the implications of their actions upon others. They argue that in examining the concept of autonomy it is important to recognize that individuals are 'embedded in relationships of interdependence and power'. It is the relationship of interdependence and subsequent balance of power that is important for practice nurses to consider in determining whether autonomous practice is a reality or a fantasy. Nevertheless, before considering the potential of practice nursing it is worth reflecting on the degree to which nursing is recognized in the provision of health care.

Recognizing the Contribution of Nursing to Care Provision – a Feminist Analysis

Advocation of a feminist approach to examine the subject of nurse power and nurse autonomy is not well developed; indeed nursing, in the main, has failed to adopt this perspective within its analysis. This is not to dismiss nurse theorists and educationalists – as Morse (1995) states, feminism has failed to impact upon many spheres of women's lives. The reluctance of women to acknowledge and engage with this group of sociological theories is in part highlighted as a failure to identify feminism as a means of understanding women's roles in society, instead labelling it only as a political movement, that is stereotypically described as anti-men in its nature (Morse 1995). McLoughlin (1997) believes the failure to value the contribution of a feminist perspective has resulted from a lack of common understanding of what the perspective can offer, with an overemphasis on stereotypical images of feminist activists. However, Morse (1995) maintains that the issue is more fundamental, with women yet to recognize the discrimination that they experience every day of their lives.

In advocating a feminist analysis there is a need to challenge the assumption, held by many nurses, that feminism does not have a place within a discussion of nursing and its role development. Feminist theory is important in any examination of nursing because nursing is essentially defined as women's work (Smith 1994), and never more so than in practice nursing, where 99.9% of the workforce are women (Atkin et al 1993). It is important in both recognizing that society has defined the caring nature of nursing as intrinsically linked to the perceived role of women in society, but also in challenging this concept and recognizing the difference of women and the contribution they can make to society.

In its broadest sense, feminism allows for an examination of the systems of dominance and women's role in their maintenance. It does not concern the exclusion of men, but aims to offer a counterculture. Berg (1979) defines feminism as 'the acceptance of individual conscience and judgement', arguing that '... a woman's worth stems from her common humanity'. This definition is important to understanding the concept of nursing as it addresses the humanistic approaches epitomized within the newer philosophy of nursing.

The universal belief underpinning all feminist theory is the view that there is inherent inequality within society based upon gender. Gender is a socially constructed issue, with the roles of men and women not determined biologically, but dependent upon the roles placed upon them within society. Feminists have long argued that the gender inequality is grounded in the patriarchal structure of society. Patriarchy being defined as the dominance of male culture in society has led to the exploitation and oppression of women (Tong 1992). Mackinnon (1997) identifies the central problem as the organization of the structure of society; she therefore reasons that before it is possible to examine other concepts, such as autonomy, it is necessary for feminist theory to examine the justification for patriarchal dominance within society.

Patriarchy is central to the continued dominance of medicine over nursing. Within the United Kingdom structure of health care, patriarchal dominance has always existed, with the medical provision exerting control over other groups of health care providers. This well-documented structure has yet to be effectively challenged by nursing, but as French (cited in Tong 1992) highlights, without a challenge to a hierarchy there can be little real cooperation in the efforts of society as a whole. Specifically, Witz (1990) argues that in examining the position and status afforded to nurses within the health care system, it is critical to recognize that nursing is women's work and intrinsically linked with caring and women's more informal role in society. She holds that before nursing can become autonomous there is a need to challenge women's role in society; this may be an increasingly daunting task given that the issues raised by the women's movement are becoming less valued within our society (Witz 1990).

Yet, if nursing is fundamentally based upon caring, then the value placed upon it will be based on the value given to women's work within our society because caring is associated with women (Smith 1994). This is important for the future development of both nursing and practice nursing because we work in a system that places greater emphasis on curative models of health care provision. As nursing's foundation is built upon a philosophy of caring it will always be undervalued within our society in comparison to the curative nature of medicine. This is best demonstrated by Tong (1992) who highlights that even though in an objective assessment of a profession's worth, nursing is of equal worth to medicine, subjectively it is still considered a subordinate profession. According to Witz (1990), this is because professionalism and professional status is not objectively defined, but instead is an historically bound event, with one group determining their boundaries to the exclusion of other groups. This she cites is most apparent in medicine with its initial crude tactics used in the exclusion of women into the profession and its subsequent control and influence over nursing. Indeed, even Nightingale, in her promotion of the role of the nurse, described nursing as subordinate to the doctor (Nightingale 1978). Similarly the power of medicine is increasing, as the overriding philosophy of a market for health care places more and more emphasis upon the outcomes of care provision over the contextual nature of caring.

However, acknowledging the barriers to development, the system is being challenged; indeed Barker, Reynolds & Stevenson (1997) cite the example of mental health nurses as the first group to challenge the paternalistic nature of medicine. Witz (1990) disputes this approach, identifying that nurses have still failed to overrule the power of the medical profession. This, she argues, is due to the underlying culture of the organization that maintains the ultimate power decisions with those of the medics. In support of this, Snowball (1996) argues that the ability to make autonomous decisions can only be achieved within a culture that facilitates the process of decision making.

Importance of Decision Making

It is doubtful that autonomous decision making within general practice is realistically achievable unless issues such as the cultural expectations of nurses are addressed. This is evidenced in the study by Carey (1994), which highlighted the reluctance of nurses to become involved in wider practice decision making. Of the 10 nurses surveyed only two participated in practice decision making, the rest identifying issues such as lack of time as the reasons for non-involvement. Whether this is in part due to the socialization of nurses to what Friere (1989) highlights as the consensus of the oppressed, that maintains the power with the oppressing group, is uncertain. It may in reality be a reluctance by doctors to relinquish the necessary power to facilitate nurses to become autonomous practitioners.

Challenging this perspective, Porter (1991) argues that nurses do impact on the decision making process, but only through suggestion rather than more explicit means. This covert approach is highlighted by Carter (1994), who identifies the historical context of deference, arguing that this reinforcement of decision making reinforces the power relationship between the nurse and medicine. Similarly, Witz (1994) argues that autonomy is not to be claimed, but instead must be examined within the context of the environmental factors that impact upon autonomous decision making. If this is valid then it is important to question whether the exclusion of nurses from explicit decision making is indeed hindering the development of nurses as autonomous practitioners (Witz 1994). In the context of practice nursing, it is therefore important to examine the factors that explain why practice nurses are in a relationship within general practice that is ultimately one of subordination.

In contrast, Ross & Mackenzie (1996) dispute the concept of autonomy as an absolute state, instead arguing that the recent move towards acknowledging nurse decision making such as the *Scope of Professional Practice* (UKCC 1992) has increased nurse autonomy. The move towards a 'knowledgeable doer' is central to decision making and the adoption of a problem solving approach to care that focuses on the individual rather than the disease process. All of the nurse practitioners within Carey's study (1994) reported clinical decision making and an awareness of the subsequent accountability that resulted in the decision making. Even though the practice nurses made decisions, they identified the need for reassurance concerning decisions, and described how they would seek reassurance from the GP. This emphasizes the potential reluctance of nurses to take responsibility for autonomous decision making.

Maintaining Patriarchal Dominance: Analysing the Practice Nurse and GP Relationship

The role of nurse in general practice could be identified 50 years before Florence Nightingale conceived of the concept of formal training for nurses. The doctor engaged in community practice – the general medical practitioner (GP) – has been described as one of the oldest providers of medical care, dating back to the Apothecaries Act of 1815 (Fry 1988) and with it the contribution of the GP's wife to the work of the practice was recognized. The 'doctor's lady' (as she was often known) took on the work of secretary, accountant and nurse. She was seen as the linchpin of the practice – the ultimate ancillary assistant (Lane 1969). Haug (1976) believes this all fitted in rather well with the attitudes and values of these early day GPs, who tended to exude an air of paternalism towards their patients, with their wives and nurses being suited to the mothering role, offering care and compassion to the patient and running the occasional errand, for example delivering medicines (Loudon 1985).

Today, the role of practice nurse is rather more clearly defined, all being registered nurses, and many possessing specialist qualifications specifically designed to underpin their role in general practice. But does the family model still fit? In spite of leaping the best part of two centuries into the future, 99.9% of practice nurses are still female (Atkin et al 1993), and the majority of senior GP partners are men. Indeed, Greenfield et al (1987) highlighted that in employing practice nurses GPs were keen to employ older women who had young children, namely the very characteristics that blur the boundary between the private and public domain of caring within the context of UK nursing. The perception held by GPs that the 'good' nurses exhibit the same qualities as a mother, offers a unique insight into how they distinguish the professional status of nursing. Nevertheless, there clearly are women working in medicine; however, when found in general practice they are generally relegated to the position of junior partner with little influence over the running of the practice. Ironically, it is generally their commitments as carers in the context of their own families that entails part-time working for the female GP and condemns them to such an inferior position within the practice family. Even when female GPs and male practice nurses do exist, it is theorized that the assignment of the male gender to medicine (in terms of patriarchal dominance) and feminine to nursing (in relation to female subordination) outweighs these 'aberrations' – female doctors and male nurses cannot escape the gender assignment of their professional grouping (Porter 1991).

As most practice nurses are direct employees of the GPs they work with, their contract often identifying the senior partner as the person to whom they are accountable, it is relatively easy to see the GP as head of the practice family. Incidentally, although some practice nurses have been shrewd enough to negotiate profit and decision sharing relationships with GPs, current rules and regulations actually prevent nurses becoming true partners, and most significantly the practice only receives a range of cash incentives if existing partners are replaced by a medical practitioner. It would seem then that men run general practice, with GPs being credited with valued skills of diagnosis and cure or the power to refer elsewhere for cure; nurses (and others) are employed by the practice, meeting the requirements for caring, administration and generally supporting the medical function of the practice and its income generation capacity. GP = dad, practice nurse = mum, patients = the kids?!

What Does Everyone Want for Christmas?

Simplistic as the above family analysis of general practice may be, it serves the purpose of acting as springboard for more detailed discussion as this chapter progresses. At this point it is useful to consider the aims and objectives – the 'wish list' of those involved in the practice, and how the 'family' dynamics come into play to achieve them. After all, can any father really be in charge – even when he thinks he is, and doesn't mother always have a strategy for getting her own way and keeping the children happy?

The GP

Without wishing to sound too cynical, if we set aside the idea of providing a good health care service to a local community, the prime motivator to a GP must be to attract sufficient income to enjoy a satisfactory lifestyle while maintaining the business that is his general practice – including the overheads for such things as wages and utility charges. General practitioners generate income in a variety of ways, the most significant being or having been a per capita allowance respective to their total patient list, 'item of service' payments for a range of activities, a commitment to health promotion work and various ad hoc fees, for example for insurance medicals, signing passports, etc. A significant factor is that aside from having to have patients registered with them, GPs can delegate a great deal of the work they are paid for to their employees – notably practice nurses – and up until 1990 it was the effort put in by the doctor and his nurse that enhanced the income stream.

The 1990 date is significant because at this time the government imposed a new contract upon GPs (Department of Health and Welsh Office 1990), which for the first time set targets for immunization and cervical cytology uptake, in addition to requiring an annual review of elderly patients, new-patient health checks and the introduction of health promotion sessions into their practices. The hitherto rather open-ended funding system was now replaced with one that (per capita payments aside) rewarded GPs for the amount of work carried out or withheld payment if targets were not met. The 1990 contract gave many GPs a bit of a jolt as they realized that they might not reach these new targets and their income would be threatened. So what was the answer? Practice nurses of course!

Why the new GP contract caused such a flurry in practice nurse recruitment is summed up neatly by Pyne when he suggests that:

'General practice has become more sophisticated. It has become clear that even the best organised doctors cannot provide all the services which patients expect without help' (Pyne 1993, p. 15).

There was therefore a double-edged incentive for GPs to take on practice nurses: first to minimize their workload, and second to maximize profit (Mungall 1992) – both pretty good motivators!

Practice nurses suddenly became the number one item for the average GP's Christmas list. For example, Evans (1992) finds in her survey of practice nurses for Walsall Family Health Services Authority (FHSA), that there was a 300% increase in employment since the introduction of the contract. Davies (1994) indicates that before the new contract GPs in the South Wales valleys were actively seeking to employ new practice nurses, with a 60% increase in number occurring in the months before its introduction. Similarly, Robinson, Beaton & White (1993) found that over 50% of GPs they surveyed indicated that they had taken on practice nurses, 83% had expanded the role of existing nurses to cope with the increased workload from the new contract, and 99.2% of the GPs sampled believed that nurses should be taking on all of the health promotion work. The most comprehensive survey of practice nurses, *Nurses Count* (Atkin et al 1993) would seem to confirm that these local trends are indicative of a national picture, with the results of this survey indicating that most nurses (74% of the 12 437 sample) had been in their present post for less than 5 years, and over half for less than 3 years. The GPs knew that although they might have survived without practice nurses, they would struggle and would not be able to maximize income. Practice nurses were willing to come and work for them, and with the ability to generate an 'on average' income of £17 000 for their GP employer everyone was happy. But what did the nurses want from the deal?

The Practice Nurse

Even though we identified practice nurses of a kind being around in the early 19th century, they are really a recent phenomenon, with numbers only becoming significant in the early 1980s. From that time, practice nursing began to appeal to those nurses who had family commitments and required part-time work (the average nurse working 18 hours a week in 1985 [Bowling 1988] and maintaining this average in the early 1990s [Atkin et al 1993]) and to those nurses who felt general practice offered more freedom and less restriction in the form of nurse managers (Jones 1996). Yet, up until the time of the new GP contract, the gradual increase in practice nurse numbers had really gone unnoticed. Their exponential increase in number thereafter certainly grabbed the attention of colleagues in other fields of primary care nursing as district nurses and health visitors, respectively, saw their monopoly on the care of sick people in the community and health promotion at risk of being eroded.

The clash of who sticks in the needle, does the smear or promotes health, was almost inevitable as GPs wanted to ensure that their nurses undertook this work so that they would receive payment and reach the new contract targets. Almost overnight, newly employed practice nurses were expected to become experts in childhood immunizations and health promotion (activities previously dominated by health visitors) and the assessment of elderly people (a patient group catered for largely by district nurses). As indicated by Gardener (1994) these events led to a 'dark period' in nursing history. During 1990 and 1991, the nursing press was full of articles and editorials denigrating practice nurses as 'untrained' and 'professionally naive' (Gardener 1994, p. 12). There were so many expressions of concern to the RCN and the UKCC that practice nurses may not be competent to do this work, that both organizations considered it necessary to issue impromptu guidance on these issues (RCN 1990, UKCC 1990).

Although health visitors and district nurses were seemingly on the defensive about practice nurses, practice nurses themselves felt that they had something to prove in relation to these colleagues. Practice nursing had grown ad hoc, and unlike the other groups did not have a recognized post-basic qualification. Studying the literature relating to practice nurse development, the arguments seem to have been between practice nurses and their district nurse and health visitor colleagues about who should do what, the latter groups expressing their importance by virtue of possessing post-basic qualifications, whereas practice nurses did not. Practice nurses were adamant that this had to change and that their contribution had to be fully recognized. This quest for equality by qualification had begun some years before the introduction of the new GP contract, the key event bringing it to a head being the publication in 1986 of the report *Neighbourhood Nursing – A Focus for Care*, otherwise known as the 'Cumberlege Report' (after the chair Julia Cumberlege) (Department of Health and Social Security 1986).

The Cumberlege Report produced many good ideas about the future of community nursing; however, these went largely unheeded by practice nurses, for whom the suggestion that if the roles of health visitors and district nurses were augmented and made more flexible, then there would be no need for their employment by GPs, was almost too much to bear. Significantly, Cumberlege argued that direct reimbursement of nurses' wages would be inappropriate and would hinder the development of the nurse's role. On reflection it is perhaps worth considering whether the widespread public rejection of Cumberlege's 1986 Report has had a significant impact upon obstructing practice nurses as autonomous practitioners. Nevertheless, rather than give up at the prospect of their evolution coming to a rapid end, the Cumberlege Report seemed to galvanize practice nurses into action. As an eminent practice nurse of the time pointed out:

> 'Cumberlege did us a great favour. To be told we were bottom of the bucket by people who had fewer qualifications than many of us was starting to annoy us' (Ruth Cherry, nurse member Hereford & Worcester FHSA, first practice nurse to serve on an FHSA Committee – reported by Crawford 1991, p. 4).

It is particularly interesting to note that whereas the Cumberlege Report was an England-only report, the backlash against it and what it stood for became a UK-wide phenomenon. Practice nurses sensed as one the need to protect their role and claim recognition alongside their community nursing colleagues. At this point the practice nurses embarked upon an interesting alliance with their GP employers, one perhaps that was to jeopardize their ability to become truly autonomous practitioners for all time – or at least until the bargain they were to strike fell apart.

Presents for Everyone!

We already know that GPs wanted practice nurses to work for them to generate income and help fulfil the terms of their 1990 contract. As representatives of the dominant force in our patriarchal health service – the doctors – and practice/family status as boss/father – they were a force to be reckoned with. Consciously or not, practice nurses realized they were also a force and could use it to meet their own objective – recognition as equals by other community nurses and as specialists in their own right by the UKCC.

Rather than see it as any form of weakness, unlike others, practice nurses were keen to show that they had managed to educate themselves adequately without any national recognition, and that such recognition was long overdue. Many practice nurses felt that they were discriminated against simply because they had not undergone a similar post-basic training as their health visitor and district nurse peers. The nursing profession reinforced this by denying practice nurses access to certain advanced practice roles (a case in point was the debate surrounding the possible introduction of prescribing rights for nurses).

Charting the recent history of practice nursing, we can see a parallel track of GPs rallying to the defence of their nurses in their professional quest. The Cumberlege Report was met by a barrage of criticism by GPs at national level, threatening as it did their ability to retain practice nurses on a profitable basis. Before Cumberlege GPs received reimbursement from their Family Practitioner Committee for 70% of the practice nurse's salary and as they were able to retain the profit from all the work they were steadfastly opposed to the recommendation that such a scheme should cease in favour of the expansion of health visitor and district nursing roles (Department of Health 1993, p. 49). As a combined entity, GPs and practice nurses fought off this threat; although history does not record who was the dominant force in the battle it goes without saying the voice of the GP was significant. Furthermore, as practice nurses approached, negotiated with and campaigned against the UKCC, demanding equitable status via a recognized qualification and education programme, GPs pitched in alongside them arguing that their nurses were as good as any other and certainly deserved this recognition. When it looked as if practice nurses would be excluded from the new specialist definitions being determined for community nurses as part of the PREP proposals, GPs came to their defence chastizing the UKCC as 'empire builders' (Dewdney 1992). Unfortunately, it was the realization of what practice nurses were really seeking through this credentialist strategy and its potential cost that began to upset the strategic GP/nurse alliance.

Practice Nursing: The Fight for Recognition

Throughout the history of nursing there has been a dichotomy of opinion about whether a solid educational base earns the title 'nurse' or experience and innate ability are more fitting. Florence Nightingale opposed state registration, fighting instead for nursing to be recognized by virtue of a skill base controlled by a strong management function, while Mrs Bedford-Fenwick fought long and hard to have the claim to the title of 'nurse' protected by law and official registration. Practice nurses, who by and large have no 'formal' education into the role (Atkin et al 1994) have been keen to suggest that their comprehensive nursing background and acquisition of skills in an ad hoc manner ideally prepare them for the job. In seeking recognition, practice nursing's strong point appears to be the wealth of experience and aptitude among its members, and the freedom obtained from GP employment. Porter (1991) indicates these conditions are right for a strategy of clinical professionalism as a means of role advancement, whereby they free themselves from the hierarchical management structure and claim recognition for their specific expertise. Ultimately though, the realization is that the only way of achieving recognition is by gaining their own qualification. The social closure enacted upon practice nurses by the rest of nursing, even down to legalistic tactics such as denial of prescribing rights, forces them into adopting a credentialist strategy.

'Listening' to practice nurses discussing education and qualifications as part of a focus group analysis into the subject illustrates the significance of the issue. One nurse contends:

> 'Until we have training that is recognized …
> we can talk around this table until tomorrow, but until
> they (the UKCC) actually recognize that there is also a
> need for a practice nurse training, with a qualification …
> we're not going to get anywhere.'

Her colleague added a useful summary of the point in question:

> 'It's alright having all the courses but as long as we aren't
> recognized what's the point? You don't get recognized for
> doing a good job if you haven't done a proper course,
> like health visitors and district nurses I mean. We have all
> got loads of experience, and we know it, but we all get
> left behind because we don't need a qualification for our
> jobs. I mean – alright – we need to know what we are

doing and that, but there's no need to have a piece of paper or anything saying we can do it. It works against us all the time, in grading and everything. The others see us as amateurs.'

The previous speaker then went on to add:

'Unless we have a qualification we are going to be replaced by D and E grades that are going to be practice nurses and we are going right back to 20 years ago when we are going to be just treatment room nurses' (Jones 1996, pp. 54–55).

Practice nurses then have an innate desire to prove themselves through a credentialist strategy. The conflict with GPs arises when to obtain a qualification practice nurses require:

- courses to be established that are convenient for them to follow
- time out of the practice
- funding for a course
- to feel 'safe' to articulate their educational needs

All of these points raise problems in the nurse/doctor alliance.

I Just Need You to Do the Job – OK?

'Yeah, you see education is, is, eh luck, if you're in a practice where you've got a good doctor he will say oh yeah I support that, great, but another one who says, oh anyone could do your job. Basically, er, if your GPs aren't with you, you're stuffed.' This practice nurse being interviewed by Jones (1994) was typical of colleagues who told of the influence GP employers had over access to education. The fundamental driver for the reluctance of GPs to let practice nurses attend courses – either at their own expense or that of the practice – seems to be a philosophical mismatch between the GP view of the practice nurse as an employee who works, and the practice nurse view of themselves as practitioners who practise. As we discussed earlier, GPs have a series of tasks and services that they are required to provide to their patients, and these can be broken down into jobs that their employees – the nurses – need to do. The practice nurse perception of the need for comprehensive nursing care underpinned by appropriate education can be lost on GPs who have little concept of nursing values and merely want the job done. As one practice nurse commentator puts it:

'They've got the contract haven't they? We do the work, we get paid for it, OK? But if you want to get out

for a course, you are not doing the work are you now?
And who's going to do it for you when you aren't
there – they aren't – I mean, they can't!' (Jones 1994,
p. 55).

Her opinion was unfortunately a reflection of GP opinion, as the GP
adviser to East Sussex Health Authority's consensus conference on
practice nurse educational needs commented:

'Many aspects of practice nursing are repetitive, routine
and technical in nature. Some of these skills are akin to
riding a bike – once learnt never forgotten' (Dewdney
1992, p. 79–80).

What Power does the Practice Nurse Possess?

Given the development of the practice nurse's role, it is pertinent to
examine the concept of power and whether practice nurses are
really able to make a fundamental difference at a practice level. Hart
(1996) states that for equality to be achieved within a practice setting it is crucial to establish a flattened structure to the organization.
This then requires greater communication and a release of control
by the GP. For this to happen there needs to be an open system of
communication between all groups; yet the reality for many general
practices is a system where the practice meetings are exclusively
held by or are led by the doctors, to the exclusion of other groups.
The issue of communication is critical for autonomous practice and
practice nurse development. Yet, the dichotomy arises in that practice nurses are likely to describe the relationship with the employing GP as a social relationship, and often describe it as positive if
the GP does not interfere with their everyday work (Carey 1994). It
is questionable whether this social communication empowers or
reinforces the hierarchy.

The reality of the relationship between GPs and practice nurses is
that they have, and still do, engage in a relationship of mutual
exchange. The GP has represented the nurse's interest – nurses have
capitalized upon their patriarchal dominance in the health care system almost as a surrogate in their own credentialist strategy. The
nurse has helped GPs do their job and maximize their profit margin,
but if the relationship has contributed towards practice nurses feeling unable to complete their strategy as restrictions are placed on
their access to education, has the price been too high to pay?
Practice nurses have bound themselves closely to the doctor's own
professional project, yet the closeness of that bond, ultimately represented by an employment contract, means that as soon as the GPs
are made to feel uncomfortable, as nurses articulate learning needs,

refuse to undertake certain activities, etc., the alliance breaks down. At the same time, however, practice nurses have been keen to free themselves from the constraints of employment in the mainstream NHS (e.g. nurse management, inflexible practice) and have gone so far as to attack their natural 'sisters' in mainstream nursing, either directly or through conflict with nursing's governing body – the UKCC.

Should the Practice Nurse Leave Home?

Doctors are still keen that practice nursing remains within their control; indeed several authors suggest that the only real way forward for practice nurse education is within schemes similar to GP vocational training, using GP mentors alongside experienced practice nurses (Mungall 1992, Robinson, Beaton & White 1993, Styles 1994, Fisher 1995). However, if as Witz suggests 'The key element of any professional project is to gain control over education, training, and practice of an occupational group by members of that occupation themselves' (Witz 1992, p. 138), then surely practice nurses must free themselves from the ties with GPs they have been at least partly responsible for so that they may become truly autonomous practitioners?

Practice nurses have won major concessions from the UKCC as a result of their lobbying efforts and are now recognized as specialist practitioners in their own right. Perhaps the time is right for them to investigate the possibility of realigning themselves with mainstream nursing and drawing their power from this – their first family – rather than the surrogate version existing within general practice? General practitioners will continue to fight for their own existence and dominance in the health care system – witness their success in monopolizing the organization of primary care groups – with or without practice nurses. As the likes of the RCN argue for nurse representation to primary care groups, GPs are more than happy to say they are able to represent the practice nurse's interest, and it is likely that those nurse members who are elected will be drawn from community trust nursing sectors rather than general practice. Again their ties with GPs and disassociation with nursing militate against any sense of autonomy or self-direction on the part of the practice nurse.

So what are the possibilities for practice nurse autonomy in this melee of gender, power and identity? Considering GP employment first, and without getting into a major health policy discussion, there is an unintended consequence of health care 'reform', such as the introduction of the new GP contract in 1990: at least some representatives of one group of professionals are driven into a cycle of target hitting and profit maximization, at the expense of another group of professionals who feel unable to speak out about their potential lack of education and training to do the work that is expected of them. The nursing and medical professions need to combine forces to address these issues and tackle the root of the problem, whether this is professional arrogance, professional pride or an effect of a market economy imposed on our health care system.

As for the relationships of practice nurses with the rest of nursing, the UKCC has now seen fit to recognize practice nurses as specialists in their own right, and research shows practice nurses to be the most satisfied among those working in the community – at least on the face of it (Wade 1993). Maybe practice nurses now need to be encouraged to forget their struggles of the past, and begin to work within the new frameworks of nursing practice on offer and realize that their credentialist struggle has paid off – almost!

Challenging Medical Domination

No nurse is truly autonomous, in that they have a job description and contract of employment governing their working practices, yet practice nurses currently face unique constraints in their relationship with GP employers. Autonomy in the truest sense is about mutual recognition of the value of each other's role, competence and ability. The question is will practice nurses as a national group – not just ardent individuals and local groups – find this recognition while employed directly by GPs working to a totally different model and theoretical approach to health care provision?

Witz (1994) identifies that nurses will only be able to achieve autonomous status when they challenge medicine; this she argues is achievable through the adoption of a nursing philosophy for care provision. It is therefore important to consider the work of Salvage (1992) in relation to a 'new nursing' philosophy. In the move towards nurse autonomy Witz (1994) identifies the need for nurses to support the development of nursing into a new contextual framework, which redefines nursing away from a medically orientated handmaiden approach. This approach focuses upon a patient-centred care-driven model of care underpinned by holistic practice. She cites the move towards the 'knowledgeable doer' alongside the introduction of the nursing process as a significant drive towards the development of new nursing. She argues that the increased knowledge and organization of care away from medically driven tasks has the potential to define the core skills of nursing and thereby impact upon the professional status of nursing.

However, given that GPs have tended to employ older nurses (Atkin et al 1993), many practice nurses may not have been exposed to this philosophy. In particular, this cohort of nurses has not undergone the same socialization process as more recently qualified nurses. It is perhaps, unsurprising that practice nursing has failed to successfully incorporate this 'new' philosophy, given the dominant culture of nursing itself, based upon a hierarchical disciplined profession, grounded upon the traditions of a medical model that rewarded a deference towards medicine (Hart 1996). McLoughlin (1997) believes that as nurses we have been socialized to such an extent that nurses exhibit what Friere (1989, cited in Rhead & Strange 1996) describes as the characteristics of an oppressed group, namely horizontal attacks and a belief in the myths of the oppressors. This is a powerful analogy for practice nursing, in its continued debate concerning what exactly is its present and future role, couched as it often is in terms of its perceived higher value in comparison to other groups within community nursing. This continued infighting by nurses sustains and strengthens the medical profession's ideological control of nurses. The unanswered question therefore remains, that if as nurses we worked collaboratively would there be a real opportunity to challenge the dominance of medicine?

If this is to become a reality then it is possibly time to challenge the myth of medicine as a driving force in the shape and structure of practice nurses' work. The impact on the management of chronic disease by the practice nurse is now widely accepted (Department of Health 1993), yet as nurses we have accepted the validity of the medical model in the treatment of disease without examining alternatives or even questioning whether we are impacting on the lives of the individuals we care for. Bryar (1994) argues that the adoption of the medical model reduces the nurses' ability to work within a nursing framework and therefore reinforces the dominance by the medical profession over nursing.

This is not to say that nursing is not challenging the medical dominance, but it is questionable whether this challenge will impact on practice nursing or be successful in the wider arena. The failure to adopt this philosophy can in part be explained by the isolation of nursing within general practice. The insular nature of practice nursing from the wider nursing body has in part been caused by practice nurses themselves, but is exacerbated by the employment status of nurses.

What is the Consequence of Autonomous Practice for Patient Care Delivery?

Although the chapter has argued that practice nurses are not autonomous practitioners, and indeed it is questionable whether absolute autonomy is even achievable in the near future, it is worth exploring the potential impact of autonomous practice on patient care delivery. An exploration of the wider issues focuses discussion away from the purely professional issues, and may therefore offer an opportunity for nurses to argue strongly for greater independence. Fundamental to this discussion is an examination of power and the impact of empowerment on care provision.

The benefits of adopting feminist philosophy are in challenging the power base and the structure of health care provision, which can ultimately assist with the transfer of power from the professional, and thereby move towards a goal by which the clients are themselves empowered (McLoughlin 1997). The concept of empowerment is well documented (Sines 1994, Skelton 1994) as is the need for the nurse to adopt the philosophy in assisting individuals to adopt healthy life choices: a fundamental role of the nurse within the general practice setting. However, the problem in challenging the present system is recognized by Webb (1986), who highlights the difficulty given that the health system continues to reward a self-perpetuating inequality and sexism.

Nurses, as stated earlier, are not truly autonomous, but neither are they entirely powerless. As professionals, practice nurses hold a large degree of power in an individual consultation with a patient, yet given the organizational structures and the socialization process, nurses are not always ready to take responsibility for their decisions. The failure to take responsibility for clinical issues serves to reinforce the unequal balance of power that exists between nurses and doctors, and must at least in part be the responsibility of practice nurses themselves. The failure to accept responsibility is identified by Hugman (1991) as a component of the empowerment process, with power being released and taken. It is therefore important for practice nurses to take greater responsibility for clinical decisions. The impact of such an approach on care provision can be potentially immense in considering the importance of power empowerment and advocacy in patient care delivery.

Much has been written about the importance of empowerment in the process of promoting health, and as such this concept has a fundamental impact upon the role of the practice nurse in promoting health. However, it is doubtful if practice nurses will be in a position to empower patients to make positive health choices if as nurses we have not taken the opportunity to take responsibility for decision making. Wuerst & Stein (1991) argue that nurse autonomy is a central factor in empowering patients in making health choices, although this is disputed by Hugman (1991), who recognizes that as professionals nurses are not always willing to allow patients to make decisions.

Nevertheless, Hancock (1997), states that autonomy is fundamental to the development of practice, citing that without autonomy practice is fragmented and ritualistic in its approach. Ritualistic practice does not give the opportunity for patients to challenge and make their own decisions, and for this reason may be a comfortable framework for practice; however, it may also be fundamentally ineffective. Therefore, in aiming to become autonomous practitioners, practice nurses must not only challenge the power of the GP, but also change their own practice to empower the patients they work with. This may be a difficult concept for a number of nurses given that it will require nurses to change their practice away from the medically dominated management of chronic disease towards a social model of health.

Similarly, the concept of advocacy is well cited, although much disputed within nursing practice (Gastrell & Coles 1996). In discussing whether practice nurses can act as advocates to patients it is necessary to examine the impact of autonomous practice of the nurse. As already identified practice nurses have a direct commitment to the GP as their employer; Gastrell & Coles (1996) argue that this causes a divided loyalty for nurses who feel that they cannot act against their employers. This then raises a significant issue about whether practice nurses should either accept that they cannot act as an advocate or challenge the medical domination. In challenging the power of the GP, the nurse is increasingly in a position to act as a patient advocate. This, therefore, is potentially one of the greatest motivators in rising to the challenge, and impact upon patient care.

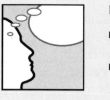

Reflection Points

- Reflect upon your own practice – how much autonomy do you have?
- How do you strive to empower patients to make their own decisions? Do patients have freedom of choice?

Achieving Autonomous Practice – the Politicization of Practice Nursing

This chapter has argued that autonomy is a fundamental issue for the progression of practice nursing, yet as discussed there are a number of issues to be addressed before nurses can truly describe themselves as autonomous. In striving towards autonomy as a goal and aid to professionalism nurses must claim the situation for themselves; indeed it would be naive to believe that GPs are willing to devolve power to nurses without a challenge. In addressing this issue, Witz (1994) recognizes that localized power is vital in shaping the future of nursing, but how are practice nurses working to come together to address these issues? In claiming power from medicine, nurses must become politicized and challenge the medical dominance. This is particularly difficult for practice nursing because to date there is little evidence of taking political action outside the domain of nursing itself. The need to raise awareness of nursing issues in the political arena is ever more necessary as the health care structure changes and there are increasing opportunities for nurses to contribute to the redevelopment of primary care. The question remains whether practice nurses as a group will take this opportunity and challenge the dominance of medicine in primary care?

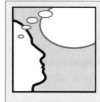

Reflection Points

■ Consider the mechanisms by which practice nurses can become politicized
■ What contribution do you feel that you could make?

Conclusion

Practitioner autonomy is a central issue for nursing and can only be achieved through the redefinition of nursing roles that are centred upon nursing values (Witz 1990). This supposition is supported by Trnobranski (1997) who stresses that the key impact for nurses within primary care, and perhaps even more so for practice nurses, is that the role is not defined by themselves, but instead by others, most notably by GPs and central government. This is not to argue that practice nurses have not structured and developed their roles, but has the fundamental issue of control and development been maintained? Without the adoption of a feminist perspective it may not be possible to achieve autonomous practice, for without the basic understanding of the constant struggle held by the dominant male culture impacting on the nursing profession, it is not feasible for nurses to achieve their true potential (Grams & Christ 1992). This is perhaps even more apparent within practice nursing, given the gendered relationship between the GP and the nurse.

An examination of a counterculture offered by a feminist analysis is critical to the examination of nurse autonomy within general practice. This perspective offers an explanation of how nurses have become disempowered, if indeed they ever had any power, and mechanisms for ending the subordination of nurses by doctors. These are strong words, which some practice nurses may reject, feeling that they are not living in an oppressive system, but a system built upon personal relationships with the GP. Nevertheless, nursing has been oppressed by a system that favours the medical provision since its very instigation in the 19th century. The challenge for the nurse working within the general practice setting is to examine the system of hierarchy within health care and the structures by which we are suppressed. It is through the examination of these structures at both a national and local level that nurses will realize the opportunity to deliver holistic care provision as autonomous practitioners.

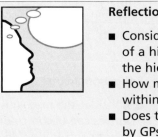

Reflection Points

- Consider the issue that practice nurses opted out of a hierarchy of practice, precisely at the time the hierarchy was disappearing. Do you agree?
- How much decision making occurs in reality within practice?
- Does the direct employment of practice nurses by GPs liberate or inhibit autonomous practice?

References

Atkin K, Hirst M, Lunt N, Parker G 1993 Nurses count: a national census of practice nurses. Social Policy Research Unit, The University of York

Atkin K, Hirst M, Lunt N, Parker G 1994 The role and perceived training needs of nurses employed in general practice: observations from a national census of practice nurses in England and Wales. Journal of Advanced Nursing 20:46–52

Barker PJ, Reynolds W, Stevenson C 1997 The human science of pyschiatric nursing: theory and practice. Journal of Advanced Nursing 25:660–667

Berg B 1979 The remembered gate: origins of American feminism. Oxford University Press, New York

Bowling A 1988 The changing role of the nurse in the UK – from doctor's assistant to collaborative practitioner. In: Bowling A, Stilwell B (eds) The nurse in family practice. Scutari Press, London

Bryar R 1994 An examination of the need for new nursing roles in the primary health care team. Journal of Interprofessional Care 8(1):73–75

Carey L 1994 The role of the nurse in general practice: a comparative study of the role of the practice nurse and nurse practitioner. Unpublished MSc dissertation, University of Liverpool, Liverpool

Carter H 1994 Confronting patriarchal attitudes in the fight for professional recognition. Journal of Advanced Nursing 19:367–372

Coles L 1996 Clinical care at home. In: Gastrell P, Edwards J (eds) Community health nursing, frameworks for practice. Ballière Tindall, London

Crawford M 1991 PN Diploma courses get the go-head. Practice Nursing. July/August p. 1

Davies G 1994 Meeting needs. Practice Nursing 22 March p. 19

Department of Health 1993 The challenges for nursing and midwifery in the 21st century. HMSO, London

Department of Health and Social Security 1986 Neighbourhood nursing – a focus for care. Report of the community nursing review (the Cumberlege Report). HMSO, London

Department of Health & Welsh Office 1990 Terms and conditions for doctors in general practice. The NHS (general medical and pharmaceutical services). Regulations 1974 Schedules 1–3 Amended. HMSO, London

Dewdney E 1992 The search for consensus. Practice Nurse June pp. 79–80

Evans J 1992 PNs – a picture. Practice Nursing September p. 9

Fisher H 1995 Training support for practice nurses. Professional Update 3(10):75–77

Fowler FG, Fowler HW 1989 The Oxford english dictionary of current English. Clarendon Press, Oxford

Friere P 1989 The politics of education. In: Murray P, Moon B (eds) 1989 Developments in learning and assessment. Hodder & Stoughton, London

Gardener L 1994 In search of unity. Practice Nursing 8 March p. 12

Gastrell P, Coles L 1996 Ethics in practice. In: Gastrell P, Edwards J (eds) Community health nursing: frameworks for practice. Ballière Tindall, London

Gillon R 1986 Philosophical medical ethics. John Wiley, Chichester

Grams K, Christ M 1992 Faculty workload formation in nurse education: a critical theory. Journal of Professional Nursing 8(2):96–104

Greenfield S, Stilwell B, Drury M 1987 Practice nurses: social and occupational characteristics. Journal of the Royal College of General Practitioners 37:341–345

Haggard L 1997 Commissioning services to meet identified needs. In: Hennessey D (ed) Community health care development. Macmillan, London.

Hancock HC 1997 Professional responsibility: implications for nursing practice within the realms of cardiothoracics. Journal of Advanced Nursing 25:1054–1060

Hart E 1996 Action research as a professionalizing strategy: issues and dilemmas. Journal of Advanced Nursing 23(3):454–461

Haug MR 1976 Issues in general practitioner authority in the national health service. In: Stacey M (ed) The sociology of the NHS. University of Keele, Keele, pp. 23–42

Hugman R 1991 Power in caring professions. Macmillan, London

Jensen UJ, Mooney G 1990 Changing values in medical and health care decision making. John Wiley, Chichester

Jones M 1996 Accountability in practice. Quay Books, Dinton

Lane K 1969 The longest art. Allen & Unwin, London

Loudon ISL 1985 Medical care and the general practitioner 1750–1850. Clarendon Press, Oxford

Mackinnon C 1997 Feminism, marxism, method and the state: an agenda for theory. In: Tietjens Meyers D (ed) 1997 Feminist social thought: a reader. Routledge, London

McLoughlin A 1997 The 'F' factor: feminism forsaken? Nurse Education Today 17:111–114

Mitchinson S 1996 Are nurses independent and autonomous practitioners? Nursing Standard 10(34):34–38

Morris Y 1998 Ethics. In: Blackie C (ed) Community health care nursing. Churchill Livingstone, London

Morse GG 1995 Reframing women's health in nursing education: a feminist approach presented at 'teaching women's health': a multi-disciplinary conference for teachers of medicine and nursing. Nursing Outlook 43(6):273–277

Mungall I 1992 The road to better training. Practice Nurse May pp. 56–61

Nightingale F 1978 Notes on nursing: what it is and what it is not. Duckworth, London

Pizurki H 1987 Women as providers of health care. WHO, Geneva

Porter S 1991 A participant observation study of power relations between nurses and doctors in a general hospital. Journal of Advanced Nursing 16:728–735

Pyne R 1993 Frameworks. Practice Nursing 21 September pp. 14–15

RCN 1990 Practice nursing – your questions answered. Royal College of Nursing, London

Rhead M, Strange F 1996 Nursing lecturer/practitioners: can lecturer/practitioners be music to our ears? Journal of Advanced Nursing 24:1265–1272

Robinson G, Beaton S, White P 1993 Attitudes towards practice nurses – survey of a sample of general practitioners in England and Wales. British Journal of General Practice 43(366):25–28

Ross F, Mackenzie A 1996 Nursing in primary health care: policy into practice. Routledge, London

Salvage J 1985 The politics of nursing. Heinemann Nursing, London

Salvage J 1992 The new nursing: empowering patients or empowering nursing. In: Robinson J, Gray A, Elkan R (eds) Policy issues in nursing. Open University Press, Milton Keynes

Sines D 1994 The arrogance of power; a reflection on contemporary mental health nursing in practice. Journal of Advanced Nursing 20(5):894–903

Skelton R 1994 Nursing and empowerment: concepts and strategies. Journal of Advanced Nursing 19:415–423

Smith JP 1994 Nursing, women's history and the politics of welfare. Journal of Advanced Nursing 19(3):609–612

Snowball J 1996 Asking nurses about advocating for patients: 'reactive' and 'proactive' accounts. Journal of Advanced Nursing 24:67–75

Styles 1994 Empowerment: a vision for nursing. International Nursing Review 41:77–80

Tong R 1992 Feminist thought: a comprehensive introduction. Routledge, London

Trnobranski P 1997 Power and vested interests – tacit influences on the construction of nursing curricula? Journal of Advanced Nursing 25:1084–1088

UKCC 1990 Statement on practice nurses and aspects of the new GP contract 1990. United Kingdom Central Council for Nursing, Midwifery and Health Visiting, London

UKCC 1992 Scope of professional practice. United Kingdom Central Council for Nursing, Midwifery and Health Visiting, London

Wade BE 1993 The job satisfaction of health visitors, district nurses and practice nurses in areas served by four trusts: year 1. Journal of Advanced Nursing 18: 992–1004

Webb C 1986 Feminist practice in women's health care. Wiley, Chicester

Witz A 1990 Patriarchiarchy and professions: the gendered politics of occupational closure. Sociology 24(4):675–690

Witz A 1992 Professions and patriarchy. Routledge, London

Witz A 1994 The challenge of nursing, In: Gabe J, Kelleher D, Williams G (eds) Challenging medicine. Routledge, London

Wuerst J, Stern P 1991 Empowerment in primary health care: the challenges for nurses. Qualitative Health Research 1(1):80–99

12 *The Future of Practice Nursing*

Lynda Carey

Introduction

In recent years health care provision has changed dramatically, and it is with a degree of certainty that we can assume it will continue to change again as society evolves. It is the rapid transformation that we have witnessed as a society that have and will continue to directly impact upon the role and function of the nurse, including the practice nurse. The need for nursing practice to change was clearly identified by the UKCC as early as 1990, as they state:

> 'If nurses are to rise above the turmoil of uncertainty in health care, they must challenge traditional attitudes in practice and shape a future for the lasting benefit of patients and clients' (UKCC 1990).

Given that the recent development of the role of the practice nurse was as a direct response to the changing needs of health care delivery, it is critical for practice nurses to continue to challenge practice and develop new approaches to care. Indeed, a continued theme throughout this text has been the developing characteristics of practice nursing work from its inception as assistant to the GP, to that of a recognized valued contributor to primary care provision. The development over the past century has, as one would expect, been immense; however, it is the specific, dramatic and rapid development since the late 1970s that differentiates practice nursing from other community nurses. As previous chapters highlight, practice nurses have grown and proved themselves to be highly motivated, competent and, at times, creative practitioners; but what next? Where does the future of the practice nurse lie?

In addressing the questions facing practice nursing, this chapter will not presume to predict the future of practice nursing, except perhaps to state that it will be different from existing practice. Instead, it will critically examine the existing strengths of practice nursing that may facilitate the change process, while discussing and raising the issues that may ultimately lead to undermining of the role of the practice nurse. An examination of the threats facing practice nursing may raise difficult issues for nurses in practice, yet it is only through an open discussion of these concerns that practice nursing will be able to move forward and achieve its potential as a key health care provider. Having examined the issues, the chapter will conclude with an analysis of the potential of practice nursing in future care delivery.

Key Issues

- Threats to practice nurse development
- Underlying strengths of practice nursing

- Opportunities for development
- Potential for practice nurses in health care delivery

Threats to Practice Nurse Development

A discussion surrounding the insecurity of the role of the practice nurse is perhaps strange in a text devoted to practice nursing, and perhaps even more obtuse within a chapter that aspires to examine the future potential of the role of the practice nurse. Yet, it is in examining the threats to practice development and assessing their impact on nursing that practice nursing can find its true potential to move forward. In exploring the challenges to practice, it may be necessary to reflect not only upon traditional nursing practice, but also the need to contest the medical domination that has isolated practice nursing from mainstream nursing.

Medical Domination

Dent & Burtney (1997), in their examination of the role of the practice nurse, identify how practice nursing has developed, not as a response to the nurse or patient needs, but rather as a response to the needs of the medical profession. This, they argue, is evidenced by the example of health education and promotion, a core role and function of the practice nurse, quoting the work of Williams & Calnan (1994), who highlight that the GPs were happy to delegate this 'dull and boring' role. Within this context, the role of the practice nurse has ultimately been controlled by the medical profession. This is in contrast to other nurses who are enhancing their role, adopting new skills through an explicit new nursing framework.

The domination by the medical profession is explored in greater depth in Carey & Jones' earlier chapter, where we argue that practice nurses have fundamentally failed in challenging the power of the medical profession, opting to work closely for them, rather than aiming to identify a distinct power base within the general practice setting. Practice nursing grew up as a direct response to the needs of GPs enforced by government legislation, with the sole aim to increase the emphasis of health care from a disease orientated approach towards a health focused delivery of care (Dent & Burtney 1997). This led to a situation of GPs employing nurses with little consideration of the potential role. Left in this position, practice nurses grasped their opportunities and positively responded in developing a role to meet the needs of patients. However, as GPs, expectations of nursing were awakened, the drive for nurses to move and extend their role into the traditional sphere of medical practice grew (Reveley 1998). It is therefore unsurprising to find that the role developed by practice nurses was not what was originally intended; this has led to a small but growing frustration by a number of GPs, who have once again turned to nursing to meet their increasing health care demands, but this time the new role of the nurse practitioner – a role that like practice nursing has so far failed to clearly define its boundaries of practice.

It is perhaps simplistic to consider the control by medical practitioners over practice nursing as solely an issue of role transference, because it is undoubtedly influenced by the problem of employment. The nature of practice nurse employment has the greatest potential to inhibit practice nurse development. A relationship based on employment is unequal, and although there are examples of nurses acting as independent practitioners within the primary care setting, it is unclear if practice nurses will be able to move practice forward until this issue is addressed. It is therefore important for practice nurses to challenge the tradition of GP employment. This may not be as difficult as one may first anticipate as GPs increasingly identify a reluctance to employ nurses. If nurses are faced with this opportunity, then it is perhaps time to grasp it.

The domination by the medical profession highlights a fundamental flaw in the development of nursing as a whole, but is particularly significant for nurses within general practice. This places practice nurses in a potentially vulnerable situation. Although on an individual level practice nurses may be powerful as a distinct nursing discipline, they are distinguished by the characteristics of the powerless (Friere 1989). Reasons for this powerless state must include the relatively short existence of practice nursing as a recognized discipline as well as the characteristics of the nurses themselves.

Practice Nursing

Without doubt a significant factor that will influence practice nurses and enable them to achieve their true potential is practice nurses themselves! Historically, the move into practice nursing was identified as an option for nurses who had family commitments – this was very much as a direct response to the part time nature of the work

(Atkin et al 1993). The original practice nurses were not drawn from a historically challenging group of nurses, although as Gupta and Jones separately highlight in their earlier chapters, they were a powerful force in demanding recognition of their rights with other nurses.

This is not to deny that practice nurses have been effective in setting up a nursing service in general practice; they obviously have been! However, the employment of almost exclusively female nurses into the role on a part time basis ensured that GPs were in the first instance unlikely to attract nurses who wanted an explicit career pathway. As Atkin et al (1993) identify, many of these initial recruits to practice nursing were attracted by the nature of work, which fitted around family commitments, rather than the desire for a new career.

The characteristics of the initial recruits to practice nursing distinguished the discipline as a group who were unlikely to challenge the power of GPs in developing care. Indeed, the nature of the part time GP employment only served to alienate practice nurses from mainstream nursing. This, at times, self exile distanced the nurses from both nurse education and contemporary nursing issues. Furthermore, the continued failure of practice nurses to embrace potentially empowering processes, such as clinical supervision, as a means of gaining support in an otherwise isolated work environment, has only served to add to their vulnerability.

Adoption of a Separatist Approach to Role Development

The growth of the role, function and number of practice nurses in the early 1990s unequivocally impacted upon other community nurses. Indeed, there was much initial resentment towards practice nurses as other community nurses were wary of the expanding role and function undertaken by this group (Jeffree 1998). Yet community nurses, although initially threatened, adapted practice and increasingly undertook wider roles, which demonstrated their flexible approach to care provision. The most striking example of this has been the changing practice offered by the District Nursing Service, who have enhanced their role both within the home environment and the general practice setting. The early intimidation by the emerging practice nurse role has been replaced by a greater emphasis on a multidisciplinary approach to care, and the realization of the need for a partnership in care.

Yet, it is debatable whether practice nursing has continued to grow and forge new roles, as other nurses have over the past decade. This is witnessed within the recent history of practice nursing. Having won a degree of recognition from the UKCC practice nurses have to a lesser degree sat back and enabled other community nurses to gain a significant move forward, sometimes at the expense of themselves. Indeed, practice nurses at times, continue to

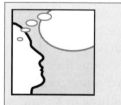

Reflection Point

Consider the suggestion that the biggest threat to practice nursing is practice nurses themselves. Reflecting on your own experiences is there any evidence to support this view?

identify other community nurses as a threat to their existence and can be reluctant to work together to resolve care issues, fearing eradication of their own role. The failure of practice nurses to positively engage with other community-based nurses has led to a position where nurses, rather than working together, are in some instances actively competing. This highlights the view of Rhead & Strange (1996) that nursing is too often intent upon internal fighting rather than challenging the hegemonistic control held by the medical profession. For example, practice nursing has continued to at times publicly compete with nurse practitioners in addressing where each is placed within the hierarchical structure defined within nursing. In examining this issue it is worth debating whether this has been to the benefit of either group or simply served to highlight the fragmented nature of nursing.

The lack of a unifying voice and the heavy reliance upon individual relationships with GPs, coupled with the isolating nature of the role, places practice nurses in a precarious position. This is potentially further jeopardized by practice nurses themselves, who have not adopted the wider opportunities to engage with other practice nurses or indeed other community nurses. With hindsight, this may have been a dangerous strategy for practice nurses to adopt, for as central government begins to invest power in community nurses, the separatist nature of the discipline may mean practice nurses are once again excluded from the decision making process. This is best illustrated within the example of the development of primary care groups, where practice nurses are disadvantaged, given the still comparatively small number of nurses in general practice, and the, in certain instances, tribalistic pattern of voting nurses on to the boards.

Indeed, as a national group, practice nurses have relied too heavily on their personal relationships with GPs, without adopting a cohesive national structure that allows them to address issues at a national level. In her earlier chapter, Karen Gupta highlights the initial strength of the practice nurse associations at a local level in developing the discipline, but has the time for the local association been and gone? Is it not time for a stronger national association that can impact on health policy rather than act as a link for the local organizations? For this to occur there is a need for practice nurses to become politically aware, in terms of national politics, and within the discussion of nurse politics.

Lack of a Clearly Defined Role

The isolated nature of practice nursing, both on a day-to-day basis and a political level, has been hindered by the overriding failure to explicitly define the role of the practice nurse. It is this lack of clarity surrounding the role that has resulted in practice nursing being defined as task orientated in its approach (Quinney, Pearson & Pursey

1997). The perception of a task-orientated approach not only maintains medical dominance, but as Raatikainen (1994) demonstrates, is characteristic of nurses who are powerless in their ability to move practice forward. In direct contrast to the situation practice nurses are faced with, other community nurses have developed a nursing-led power base that protects and offers a future for their role in the development of primary care-based nursing. Perhaps the most pertinent example of this approach is the development of the health visiting service at a national level. It is indisputable that health visiting has in recent history been under threat (Dolan & Kitson 1997) with the introduction of general practice fundholding in the early 1990s. Given that GPs were then in a position to buy community nursing services, increasing questions were raised about the outcomes and effectiveness of the health visiting service. Faced with this explicit challenge, health visiting fought back. Through the campaigning of the professional body, the status and contribution to health care delivery of health visiting have been raised, a mighty feat given that they have successfully managed not to fall into the trap of measuring their contribution within explicit medically driven outcomes of care.

This is in contrast with practice nurses who have too often focused upon their contribution to the achievement of medical outcomes rather than the holistic nature of care, thereby undermining the relationship they have with patients and service users. The failure to define the practice nurse's role is evidenced within the UKCC specialist practitioner document (UKCC 1996). This long awaited document, which set out core competencies of the role, only significantly differentiated the role from that of the district nurse through the clinical environment for care provision, namely in the general practice surgery rather than within the patient's home. This signalled a significant neglect on both the part of the UKCC and practice nursing itself to identify a distinct area of specialist practice. Given this lack of vision it is unsurprising that practice nursing is defined by the employing GPs, yet its potential strength lies in identifying its unique contribution to primary health care provision.

Knowledge and Education

The failure by the UKCC to define the role of the practice nurse may in part be understandable given that as a governing body it consulted the providers of practice nurse education along with other groups about what they perceived the role to be. This was potentially difficult for nurse education, because the majority of nurse educators responsible for practice nurse education in the early 1990s did not come from a practice nurse background; more often than not they held a health visitor or district nurse qualification. This is not to say that these nurse educators were not committed to practice nurse education, but nevertheless their understanding of the nuisances of the role was gained secondhand, and for a number of practice nurses this resulted in a lack of credibility.

This perceived lack of credibility in nurse education has been particularly threatening for practice nursing, for nursing can only gain the power to change when it challenges medicine in general practice from a nursing perspective (Witz 1994). It is the nursing perspective that enables the nurse/patient interaction to be holistic in nature. The adoption of such an approach will complement medicine and move practice nursing out of its present position. For this to occur, nurses need knowledge. Yet, as identified earlier in the text, practice nursing has at times only adopted an informal approach to education and knowledge for practice, rejecting a mainstream nurse education approach to professional development. It would be wrong, however, to suggest that practice nurses are alone in their perceptions of what education can offer them. Indeed, UK nursing has only in its relatively recent history adopted and recognized the importance of theoretical underpinning of practice. The perception of nursing as a vocational purely practical skill is still being reinforced within the widest context of society and central government.

Nevertheless, the failure to engage with mainstream education has potentially grave implications for practice nurses. This has undoubtedly led to an unrealistic perception of the role and value of education. At one end of the continuum, there is the naive belief that nurse education holds all the knowledge to solve all the problems and developments of practice, whereas at the other end of the continuum there is the equally naive though sceptical belief that nurse education does not meet the needs of practice nurses. Nurses who have this latter belief have instead attempted to legitimize the practice of learning from their employing GPs. This is perhaps, a dangerous option because GPs are not nurses, and therefore do not understand the nursing approach to care. Similarly, it is questionable whether GPs are in a position to identify competence in nursing. This situation was tragically identified in the 1990s when a very small number of nurses endangered patients' lives through incorrect practice taught by the GP. Given this scenario, it is surely unsafe for practice nurses to rely on knowledge from GPs only and recognize that nurse education has a place in meeting the educational needs of the practice nurse community.

It would be wrong to say that this situation, within which practice nursing potentially finds itself, is solely the responsibility of GPs. Indeed, a degree if not the majority of responsibility must lie with nurses themselves, who have often been reluctant to enter mainstream education, instead undertaking education that followed a medical disease-orientated approach. If practice nursing is to continue down this route it will never compete with medicine and as such will always be perceived as a subservient role, waiting for the medical profession to discard the aspects of health care it no longer deems necessary.

Yet, the reality is that nurse education has not always acknowledged practice nursing, thus leading some practice nurses to feel unvalued by the nurse educational establishment. This has led to a situation where even though nurse education has incorporated practice nurses into core activity, the failure to engage with education has continued, with some practice nurses showing a reluctance to share knowledge and skills with nurses both at a pre- and post-registration level. Accepting, that the process of education requires commitment and motivation, it is disturbing that a significant number of practice nurses demonstrate this reluctance. Justification for this action is often laid at the door of the GP in terms of the demands for financial recompense for education. This is not as simple as one may at first identify; rather it can be argued that it is nurses themselves who are reluctant to take on this wider role, and as such are not eager to push the issues with the employing GPs. Similarly, even when nurses are willing to participate in the process of education either at the recipient or facilitator level, the reluctance of the nurse to challenge the GP's position must be considered. This is a important issue for nurses because it continues to allow nurses to be restricted from knowledge by another profession. If practice nurses are to gain recognition they must challenge this position and actively engage in education.

Why are practice nurses reluctant to engage in the education? Education is undoubtedly a challenging experience, both for the student and the educator. Acting in the role of practice educator, nurses are open to an examination of their existing practice from students, who will require evidence-based rationale for methods and approaches to working. This is difficult for all nurses, but perhaps more so for practice nurses, who given the isolating nature of their work, have not participated in the wider debate of evidence-based nursing practice. This is apparent in the initial heavy reliance upon pharmaceutical companies for information for nursing practice in the early days of practice nursing.

The lack of formal education opportunities for practice nurses and recognition of their informal learning was in part appeased by the UKCC's transitional arrangements for community nurses. However, the question about whether the transitional arrangements really offered practice nurses an opportunity for recognition or have further marginalized them from other community nurses must be addressed. This is an area of much debate, particularly as the employment of practice nurses still does not require nurses to hold either the specialist practitioner qualification or title.

It can be argued that instead of disadvantaging practice nurses, the transitional arrangements favoured them, and that this is testament to their strength of lobbying. But was it really the need for recognition of the contribution of the practice nurse to care delivery, or perhaps the realization that the cost of enabling practice nurses to engage in mainstream higher education on a national level was too expensive, that persuaded the argument? It is evident that a number of GPs are still unaware of practice nurse educational opportunities, seeing them as unnecessary to fulfil the task-orientated approach of care delivery. Similarly, the widespread education of practice nurses is potentially a dangerous option at both a political and GP level. Raatikainen (1994) identifies the most important factor in establishing power as knowledge; by restricting the vast majority of practice nurses from higher education, GPs are restricting their opportunity to gain knowledge, to challenge and thereby to move nursing forward.

Evidence-Based Practice

Evidence-based practice is a relatively new phenomenon to practice nursing and given the overriding dominance of the medical profession, it is unsurprising that practice nurses have failed to examine the wider research evidence in the application of care provision. This is particularly evident in the failure to examine and apply nursing research within the clinical setting. Although one could argue that this is potentially a damning reflection on practice nursing, practice nurses are not alone. Indeed, Kitson et al (1996) highlight that the number of health care interventions that are based upon evidence is small. Why then have practice nurses failed to adopt research-based practice? Kitson et al (1996) argue that the failure to implement research findings has resulted from the imposition of guidelines that are not meaningful to the practitioner, failure to understand standard-setting methodologies and failure to examine the implementation from a contextual perspective. They argue that practice is best developed through an inductive approach. This facilitates creativity, innovation and reflective practice in conjunction with a systematic review of the literature. The reflective approach to practice is reinforced as a positive aspect of nursing practice.

Participation in the research process for many practice nurses has been marginal, and at times limited only to the collection of data for drug company-sponsored clinical trials. This failure to actively engage in the research process has disadvantaged the position of practice nurses. In realising their future potential practice nurses must examine and recognize the opportunities for research in practice (Davies 1999). The value of evidence-based practice is increasingly important as nurses are required to measure the effectiveness of nursing interventions as the clinical governance agenda becomes an increasingly explicit element of health care provision. This may not be as achievable as the Government perceives unless the issue

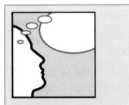

Reflection Points

- How does research-based evidence impact upon your daily practice?
- What mechanisms are available to you to ensure that your practice is evidence based?

of access to resources, both journals and information technology, is addressed. The exclusion of access to many practice nurses inhibits their ability to examine research and analyse its impact on practice.

The move towards evidence-based practice requires not only access to resources, but a fundamental willingness by nurses to examine and analyse their own practice. Reflective practice aids this process (Freshwater 1998), yet as a group practice nurses have not widely engaged in the move towards reflective practice. Reflective practice is an important tool in facilitating individuals to explore their own practice and examine the clinical decision making process. It requires individuals to question their practice and is therefore important in enabling nurses to move away from ritualistic practice towards an evidence-based approach.

Opportunities for Practice Nursing

Having explored the threats to practice nursing, it is crucial at this point to redress the balance in examining the existing strengths and future opportunities for practice nursing. It is worth recognizing that you may feel somewhat despondent about the future of practice nursing, yet it is important to reiterate that there are a number of key assets that will ensure a role for the practice nurse in the new emerging health care service. Fundamental to the discussion within this section, is the realization that in moving into the practice nurse's role, many nurses took an unprecedented risk, stepping into an area of practice previously unknown to nurses. These nurses were obviously risk takers, a key strength to draw upon in shaping the future development of the practice nurse's role. In exploring the future of practice nursing it will be necessary for practice nurses to take similar risks.

Achieving Recognition – The Nurse–Patient Relationship

The relationship between the practice nurse and patient has grown substantially over the past decade as the nurse has become recognized as a source of support and knowledge to the practice population. The acceptability of the nurse to the patient arguably offers the greatest potential strength to practice nursing. The perception of the nurse as a valued health care professional within easy access to the majority of the population can, now that it has been accepted, no longer be withdrawn. It is therefore, worth re-examining the nature of the nurse–patient relationship, and its impact upon the future role of the practice nurse.

Nursing undoubtedly serves a different function to medicine in the delivery of effective health care. The philosophy of nursing care, as discussed in earlier chapters, is significantly different from that of medicine. In recognizing this Henderson (1994) cites Foucault in identifying that nurses perceive the human body differently from the medical profession. This different perception he argues enables nurses to identify different knowledge – it is this different knowledge that is instrumental in forming the nurse–patient relationship. The value of the nurse–patient relationship cannot, Thomas & Bond (1996) argue, be underestimated within the financially driven health care service. They argue that as health care delivery has moved towards a consumerist perspective, the values of the consumers (or patients) is becoming increasingly important.

Given that nursing is an expensive resource, it is therefore important for nurses to be aware of consumers' perceptions of care. From a naive perspective, practice nurses can claim that they are valued, citing the often high demand for their services and patient informal feedback, although as a professional group we have failed to critically examine the consumer-identified needs and deliver the appropriate care. Practice nurses are not alone in this area, but given that practice is changing it is important to draw on existing strengths to examine how we can meet patient needs for improved health care delivery. Thomas & Bond (1996) argue that in addressing this issue it is vital to look beyond the patient satisfaction survey to more creative approaches. As knowledge is often said to equate to power (Raatikainen 1994), the knowledge that patients value the service is a strong bargaining position for practice nurses to use in the development of health care that meets the practice population needs.

The importance of responding to patient needs at both an individual and population level, building upon the key issue of relationships, is critical, with practice nurses identifying the building of relationships over a substantial period of time as an important issue in their care delivery. The concept of relationship building can lead the nurse to adopt the role of advocate; this is an area of much contention (Mallik 1998), and it is questionable whether the nurse can act within an advocacy role. The issue is complicated for practice nursing given that it is questionable whether practice nurses can act as advocates for patients if their position is compromised by their direct employment by GPs. Nevertheless, they are valued by patients and therefore have the potential to raise both their profile and the standard of health care delivery.

The Changing Nature of Health Care Provision – The Importance of Promoting Health

As nursing enters the new millennium, the structure and function of health care delivery is evolving, moving increasingly away from a service dominated by illness to an ever intensifying emphasis on health and the factors contributing to an individual's health status.

This explicit component of health care delivery requires a re-examination of professional roles as a greater emphasis is placed on health promotion. This has for a long time been perceived as the domain of nursing, with practice nursing demonstrating a strong commitment to this area of practice since the introduction of the GP contract in 1990. Although initially an area of practice delegated by the GP, practice nursing has established itself to such an extent that health education within chronic disease management is a firmly established constituent of the role (Quinney et al 1997).

Health education within the disease management model offers the opportunity for practice nursing to establish a solid position within the GP setting and thereby further develop nursing practice. The contribution of the practice nurse in the management of chronic disease management has been long articulated (Department of Health 1993), although not always without criticism (OXCHECK 1994). Piper (1997) highlights that even though nursing input has been shown to be valued by patients, there is little evidence of a reduction in both drug interventions and mortality rate figures. This is undoubtedly a dilemma for practice nurses, given that nursing interventions are not solely aimed at morbidity and mortality indices, but rather the therapeutic interaction between the nurse and the individual.

The significance of effective chronic disease management from a nursing perspective is important in not relying solely upon drug interventions, but increased success in emphasizing a holistic approach to care delivery. This was evidenced as early as the mid 1980s through the work of Stilwell, Restall & Burke-Masters (1988), who identified the benefit of a holistic assessment of health care. A holistic approach to disease management is important in assessing individual needs and identifying appropriate health education strategies. On a cautionary note, the importance of a holistic assessment and management of chronic disease requires practice nurses to work in a different manner to their present role. The current situation of short consultation times does not allow nurses to practise in a holistic manner or use effective health promotion strategies. Nevertheless, the potential to further raise the status of health promotion within the general practice setting remains.

The different approach that nurses offer may itself raise tension within the provision of health care, given that the emphasis on health rather than illness is not solely based upon an altruistic belief, but stems as Gastrell highlights in Chapter 4, predominantly from an economic stance. Health care delivery must increasingly demonstrate its effectiveness, both clinically and economically. This is best achieved through the identification of local health care needs. The move towards an increased awareness itself offers an important opportunity for practice nursing, not only because this group has through the audit process been constantly asked to demonstrate its effectiveness, but also because of the relevant skills developed during this process over the past two decades. The emphasis on cost-effectiveness and achievement of nationally set targets is not new to general practice or practice nurses, who were often set the task of achieving targets on a local level. The examination of targets and the undertaking of audit has enabled practice nurses to gain experience, which can be used as the first building block in identifying and examining issues surrounding clinical effectiveness. Additionally, the process of audit should have enabled practitioners to examine their practice. The only concern within this scenario centres upon whether nurses have recognized the opportunities previously offered by audit, and now clinical effectiveness in the delivery of care, or whether nurses have viewed these tools as oppressive elements of the NHS rather than real opportunities to develop their practice.

Generalist Role

The structure of health care changes to meet the new demands of society, as already stated, will inevitably be shaped predominantly by economic considerations, with the increasing demand for services not matched by a substantial increase in revenue for health care delivery. This grim yet realistic scenario will require all professions to re-examine their roles in meeting health care demands. As community nurses explore their roles, it is anticipated that there will be increasing debate surrounding the need for specialist versus a more generalist approach to care delivery. The strength of the practice nurse situation lies in the unenviable position that the generalist role is often an economically more viable alternative than the specialist role of other community nurses.

Indeed, the dominance of the medical profession in the development of practice nursing has led to a situation where the role of the practice nurse mirrors that of the GP. This is advantageous as it offers direct access to medical services via the GP system, itself heralded as a model of good practice in ensuring equity of access to health care. The adoption of a similar model for nursing care opens up new opportunities for the development of practice nursing. The pitfall, however, is that practice nursing is in grave danger – in adopting a generalists role it will be perceived to only take on others' roles rather than defining its sphere of practice. The challenge is to maintain a generalist approach, yet still develop a distinctiveness in practice.

Relationship with the GP

The development of the practice nurse's role as mirroring that of the GP has the potential to be beneficial, not only in its generalist approach, but also in facilitating the maturing of a framework for closer working. Setting aside individual relationships, practice nurses do have a strong personal relationship with GPs, and it is this relationship that has the potential to promote practice nurses into new arenas. General practitioners are potentially the most powerful health professionals in the newly configured health service, holding powerful positions on the primary care groups, as well as controlling access to secondary care service. The close working relationship that practice nurses in particular have with GPs undoubtedly places them in a strong position to influence the emerging health care agenda.

The most influential factor in enabling practice nurses to have a positive relationship with the GP, with the possible exception of employment, has been the flexibility by which practice nurses have demonstrated they can work. The flexibility and ability to adapt to the nursing needs of the population are key strengths for practice nurses. However, as identified earlier in the text, there is a need to recognize that the demands of the changing health service will require them to continually view their role as a dynamic one and not static. Within this perspective the lack of role clarity has liberated nurses to forge positive working relationships with individual GPs. The flexibility of practice nurses' working patterns is partly, as Karen Gupta identifies in Chapter 1, due to the lack of managerial control that other community nurses experienced in the late 1980s and 1990s, but also indicative of the characteristics of early practice nurses who took the risk of working in a new environment. The lack of a nursing management structure has enabled practice nurses to adapt their service to meet health needs without the constraint of a large bureaucratic organization. This, for the most part, has proved a very positive experience, but it has also placed a number of nurses in a precarious position, as they have been encouraged to develop practice.

In recognizing this strength practice nurses need to consider how they can best use their relationship with the GP. This may appear as a Machiavelian approach to accessing power, but it is potentially a powerful tool in the development of practice if nurses use it to develop nursing practice.

Expanding the Boundaries of Practice – Realizing Nurse-led Care

The flexibility of the practice nurse and the willingness to adapt has enabled the role to move into new areas of nursing practice. To date the development of practice has predominantly centred upon a disease-orientated approach; for the most part, this has failed to incorporate a nursing perspective, instead adopting a medical philosophy of care provision. Although adopting a medical model of practice,

practice nurses have nevertheless developed and acquired a new set of skills, and thereby extended their area and scope of practice. Jenkins-Clarke, Carr-Hill & Dixon (1998) highlight the significance of delegation in the development of primary health care, this primarily being the delegation of advice and reassurance from the doctor towards a nursing role. The significance of advice giving and reassurance in the context of general practice, is at present unmet in terms of minor illnesses, and Jenkins-Clarke et al (1998) therefore suggest that the role of the nurse needs to expand towards a triage role. This demonstrates that along with the expansion of the boundaries of nursing has come the realization that nursing differs from medical practice. The challenge for nurses is to articulate the difference and therefore truly adopt an expanded role.

One of the greatest opportunities that exists for nurses in primary care is the development of nurse-led care. This affords nurses the opportunity to articulate the contribution of nursing within a framework that is nurse- rather than medicine-led. This approach has been adopted by the nurse practitioner movement and although this chapter is not advocating a wholesale move towards the adoption of the nurse practitioner model, it does form a useful framework for the future of practice nursing.

What is Nurse-led Care?

Nurse-led care is an important consideration for practice nurses in particular, because of, as Jenkins-Clarke et al (1998) highlight, the growth in primary care-based health care, with an increasing move towards the United States surgery-based care. The growth in surgery-based care is significant in securing a future for practice nurses (Jenkins-Clarke et al 1998). The move in conjunction with an increase in both the content and scope of practice nursing (Atkin & Lunt 1996) can only lead one to suggest that the future of practice nursing will be in an area that increasingly allows the GPs to delegate more of their workload to nurses.

Jenkins-Clarke et al (1998) highlight that although the extension of the nurse's role is often perceived negatively, for practice nurses it is a positive opportunity for role development. This is indicated by the shifting of workload among practitioners from medicine towards a nursing focus. The shift in workload that results from the changing structure of health care raises the issue of whether nursing is still reacting as a handmaiden to general practice or is positively controlling and developing the situation. The situation can be nurse led if nurses adopt the core elements highlighted in Box 12.1.

These factors are fundamental in developing nurse-led care that can then in turn be used in the expansion of nursing care to new areas of practice: for practice nursing mostly notably in the management of acute minor illness (Rees 1996). The drive towards

> **Box 12.1**
>
> **Core Elements for Nurse-Led Care**
>
> - Philosophy of nursing care provision
>   — it is important in actualizing the potential of nurse-led care that the fundamental driving force is not that the nurse delivers care, but that the care that the nurse delivers adopts a nursing philosophy; this is best described by Salvage (1989) as 'new nursing' and centres on a holistic approach to care provision
> - Autonomy
>   — although a debatable concept, it is important for practice nurses to consider autonomy as it relates to their sphere of nursing practice; nurses must increasingly participate in decision making, taking responsibility for care delivery within a nursing framework

> **Box 12.2**
>
> **Areas for Practice Nurse Development (RCN 1997)**
>
> - Assessment of individuals' physical and physiological health status using a full history taking and physical examination
> - Discrimination between normal and abnormal
> - Evaluation to decide upon treatment (sometimes in consultation with GP) – problem-solving approach
> - Management of care through protocols
> - Setting of long-term health goals

a focus of practice nursing care within this arena is inevitably driven by the need for a reduction of the GP's workload, a reduction in the number of prescriptions issued and the need to raise patient education about the management of acute minor illness. Given this remit, it is unsurprising that the practice nurse will develop within this arena.

Indeed, it can be argued that there is a need for the practice nurse role to develop to incorporate the nurse practitioner mode of working, characterized by the features listed in Box 12.2.

Within this remit GPs may be eager for nurses to develop (Jenkins-Clarke et al 1998). In identifying the positive aspects of such an approach, Stilwell (1988) argues that it facilitates the opportunity for nurses to work in a holistic manner, and is therefore a natural move forward from the pure health promotion and disease management perspective that has framed practice nursing practice for the past decade. In the delivery of effective health care provision practice nursing can offer the benefits listed in Box 12.3.

Box 12.3

Benefits Offered by Practice Nursing

- Time
  - Stilwell (1988) and Jewell (1994) highlight that nurses have significantly longer consultations than GPs, averaging 15 minutes in length. This is important because nursing is predominantly based upon therapeutic communication, yet it is still very limited and as such its management requires great skill
- Communication skills (Trnobranski 1994)
- Quality of care
  - quality is difficult to measure in nursing given that quantitative measures of care outcomes frequently fail to capture the essence of the nursing care provided (Mason 1997). Nevertheless, as nursing roles expand nursing care must be perceived to be at least equal to that given by the GP (Jones 1997). Without this demonstration of quality, nurse-led care will be seen only as a substitute for medicine

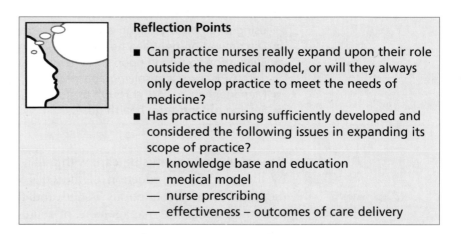

Reflection Points

- Can practice nurses really expand upon their role outside the medical model, or will they always only develop practice to meet the needs of medicine?
- Has practice nursing sufficiently developed and considered the following issues in expanding its scope of practice?
  - knowledge base and education
  - medical model
  - nurse prescribing
  - effectiveness – outcomes of care delivery

Realizing the Potential – The Future of Practice Nursing

Having examined the threats and strengths of practice nursing, the discussion now moves towards how the profession can achieve its full potential as a significant contributor to primary health in this new millennium. In discussing this it is perhaps worth reflecting upon the words of Alison Kitson:

> 'Nurses who are in control of their own systems of care, that is who are professionally accountable, responsible and engaged in continuous evaluation of their work are better equipped to deal with the rapid changes in the health care agenda' (Kitson 1997, p. 33).

Practice nurses have this potential, the threats to their development are not insurmountable, there exist a number of factors that strengthen the position of practice nurses, and such opportunities for development are obtainable. These most notably are around the issues of integrated nursing teams, professional development and clinical leadership.

Integrated Nursing Teams

The future of practice nursing lies with all community-based nursing, in the increasing recognition of the contribution of all nurses to care delivery and this is best met within the adoption of integrated nursing teams. The concept of an integrated nursing team is not new, as Bull (1998) highlights; however, as an organizational structure for care provision its development has been patchy. This is despite the move towards general practice attachment of health visitors and district nurses that was clearly identified as a consequence of the introduction of the 1990 GP contract and fundholding (Department of Health 1990). The concept of integrated nursing teams is, however, not solely concerned with the attachment of a number of practice staff, but requires nurses to work collaboratively in the setting of nursing objectives for the population (Rowe et al 1998).

The move towards the development of successful integrated nursing teams is seen as an important move in developing nursing within a primary care focus that can competently meet both population and organizational needs (Rowe et al 1998). It perhaps may appear sceptical to say that the move towards closer integration of community nursing practice is as a result of economic issues; however, it will facilitate the increase and greater potential of all community nurses, including practice nurses. The integration of community nursing is in part as a response to the realization that community-based nurses, especially health visitors, district nurses and practice nurses do have common issues in the delivery and management of their role. As the debate has continued within many areas of nursing concerning skill mix and best use of resources, community nurses, with the exception of district nurses, have avoided this issue. Within this context of greater integration of nursing teams it is important to separate the concerns surrounding grade mix with the wider issue of skill mix.

Integrated nursing teams are important in enabling practitioners to work closely to agree the core issues for practice and in doing so to re-examine the areas of overlap in working practices, so that practitioners can realise their potential (Rowe et al 1998). The process of integration does not necessitate the offloading of previously unwanted tasks or parts of the role, but requires the nursing team to work closely to identify the key skills to deliver care. Such an approach undoubtedly enables practitioners to work to their full potential in meeting the population's health care needs. The integration of nursing into team working will require all nurses to examine their own professional development needs depending upon their contribution to care delivery.

Professional Development

The development of new approaches to working by community nurses, and in particular practice nurses, is an important consideration in the development of practice. However, the professional standing and individual recognition have not been influenced by practice nurses, but by the professional bodies. Indeed, the lack of clarity surrounding the development of the professional is hindered by the present drive towards the concept of 'higher advanced practice', currently being debated by the UKCC. The concept of higher advanced practice has emerged from the long debate over the past years concerning advanced practice (UKCC 1998), and serves to offer nurses the chance to define their practice in terms of practice that demonstrates innovation, development of skills and increased evidence of outcomes.

However, it would be wholly wrong to assume that practice nurses will be significantly different from other groups within nursing in achieving recognition of their practice at a higher level, although for the first time it will allow a small number of nurses to achieve this recognition. The development of higher practice will recognize exceptional nursing practice – there are practice nurses who are presently ready to demonstrate this (UKCC 1998). This is an important development concerning nursing practice because for the first time it allows nurses from different disciplines to be recognized at the same level. It does not restrict the practitioner to a prescribed academically based educational programme; this will allow nurses the opportunity to identify their educational needs within a framework that best suits their personal, professional and organizational needs. This is not to advocate the development of learning opportunities that are solely based upon experiential learning and the rejection of academic courses, but will allow practice nurses who have achieved specialist practice to develop in an individually negotiated manner. For a number of practice nurses this may already be an example of their practice, yet it also provides a greater opportunity for the majority.

The development of higher practice through a non-prescriptive approach affords the opportunity for freedom of practice and the exploration of new learning opportunities. This is particularly important given the development of medical education away from a systems-focused towards a client-focused approach to learning – this has been an important consideration in moving health care practitioners forward because it offers a real opportunity for practice nurses to be involved in and share learning with other health professionals. The breaking down of education barriers offers one of the most significant opportunities for practice nurses to influence other health care professionals' perspectives of the discipline and as such to realize their potential as health care providers.

Similarly, the changes in monitoring and evaluating medical practice will open opportunities for greater collaboration and shared learning with existing practitioners. For a realistic impact upon care provision it will be important for all concerned that learning meets both their professional development and service needs. The development of service and professional development are highlighted by Yerrell (1998) as effective means by which nurses can shape practice with support from the organizations within which they work. This model facilitates the development of nursing practice while enabling the practitioner to demonstrate innovation and impact upon the standard of and services offered to the population. It is through such an approach that the potential of the practice nurse will be truly identified. The challenge for nurse education will be to develop a new approach to learning that allows practice nurses to fulfil their potential in improving practice. This change can only be achieved if both education and nurses seize the opportunities.

Clinical Leadership

As community nursing changes, to meet the needs of the emerging health service, inevitably there will be a change in who and what groups will lead practice. Yet, who will emerge as the new leaders of practice? Can it realistically be the practice nurse? This is particularly interesting, because as the earlier chapters suggest, there remains a degree of uncertainty about what is the actual role of practice nurses, and therefore are they really in a position to lead community nursing? Yet the potential for clinical leadership is an important consideration for all practice nurses as we face the challenges of the 21st century.

Practice nurses as specialist practitioners are expected as part of their role to lead clinical practice, although as earlier chapters highlight this has not always been achievable. Even though practice nurses have adopted a predominantly medical focus to care provision, they have been significant in changing the access to nursing care within the primary care setting. The creativity and the developing nature of nursing care in general practice has demonstrated that practice nurses have led the way in forming new areas of practice, particularly in the development of direct access and health education to a wider proportion of the population. Practice nurses as a group and individual nurses clearly demonstrate the scope of clinical leadership.

However, for the future emerging role of the practice nurse it is important that practice nurses not only take responsibility for the development of clinical leadership, but also seize the opportunity to use their experiences to lead the profession in a wider context. The changing structure of health care provision has provided a small, but significant, opportunity for community-based nurses and midwives to influence care provision as members of primary care groups. The representation of practice nurses on these boards is variable, and can be in part be seen as the continued divisiveness within nursing, and the failure of practice nurses to identify themselves as leaders of practice. Girvin (1998) argues that this is not unsurprising because the underlying tradition and socialization that surround nursing have fundamentally inhibited the development of leadership. For practice nurses, the lack of a cohesive powerful leadership is also influenced by an employment structure that has excluded cooperation with other nurses and actively discouraged the practice nurses from forming a cohesive group.

The challenge for practice nurses is to recognize their leadership potential in the interests of the development of nursing and raising the quality of patient care. To realize their potential as leaders, practice nurses will be required to become both more politically aware and engage with other community nurses in the development of care provision. The development and actualization of political awareness are not impossible, but are difficult, given that they necessitate a widening of the practice nurse's network. This requires a positive concerted action that will demand a re-examination of wider issues, particularly those relating to employment issues. In particular, there is a need to bring practice nurses closer to other community nurses. Indeed, the closer working relationship with community nurses offers the best opportunity for practice nurses to define their own unique contribution to care provision. The closer working with community nurses will facilitate practice nurses to effectively identify potential leaders to both represent their interests and lead the profession forward.

Conclusion

Practice nursing has developed and grown within a political environment that has entrusted power with the GP as the principal instigator and influence upon health care delivery. Yet as we move onward in the new millennium it is questionable whether this power base will continue to be maintained, or whether the power will shift to other key players in the delivery of health care. The shifting agenda in health care delivery will offer a new challenge to practice nursing. The question, as posed by many others, centres upon whether we as practice nurses are ready to seize the potential opportunities

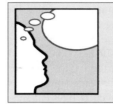

Reflection Points

■ What do need to do within your own area of practice to achieve your own potential?
■ How can you contribute to practice nursing as a whole in achieving its potential?

and thereby move practice forward, or will we sit back and wait to be directed? If practice nursing is to move forward it will require nurses to take risks, be creative and follow their nursing instincts.

In striving towards this, practice nurses must recognize that they have the 'power' to adapt and change nursing within the general practice setting. It is questionable whether practice nursing as a distinct group have the wider power base to influence nursing as a whole, although they are strong within this limited area. For this potential to be realized practice nurses as a group must articulate their vision for care and draw on their strengths. Practice nursing can no longer rely upon individual practice nurses who demonstrate the power to change, but become politically organized and move forward as a cohesive group working with and not competing with other nurses. As we re-examine the boundaries between nursing and medical practice, it is ever more important that we adopt a new nursing framework to ensure development of the practice nurse's role and thereby achieve professional status.

Further Reading

■ Freshwater D 1998 Transforming nursing through reflective practice. Blackwell Science, Oxford

References

Atkin K, Lunt N 1996 Negotiating the role of the practice nurse in general practice. Journal of Advanced Nursing 24:498–505

Atkin K, Lunt N, Parker G, Hirst M 1993 Nurses count: a national census of practice nurses. Social Policy Research Unit, The University of York, York

Bull J 1998 Integrated nursing: a review of the literature. British Journal of Community Nursing 3(3):124–129

Davies S 1999 Practice nurses' use of evidence based research. Nursing Times 95(4):57–60

Dent M, Burtney E 1997 Changes in practice nursing: professionalism, segmentation and sponsorship. Journal of Clinical Nursing 6:355–365

Department of Health 1990 General Medical Service Council – new GP contract. HMSO, London

Department of Health 1993 The challenges for nursing and midwifery in the 21st century. HMSO, London

Dolan B, Kitson A 1997 Future imperatives: developing health visiting in response to changing demands. Journal of Clinical Nursing 6(1):11–16

Freshwater D 1998 Transforming nursing through reflective practice. Blackwell Science, Oxford

Frier P 1989 The politics of education. In: Murphy P, Moon B (eds) Developments in learning and assessment. Hodder & Stoughton, London

Girvin J 1998 Leadership in nursing: essentials of management series. Macmillan, London

Henderson A 1994 Power and knowledge in nursing practice: the contribution of Foucault. Journal of Advanced Nursing 20:935–939

Jeffree P 1998 Practice nursing: its emergence as a high profile career opportunity. Practice Nurse 15(8):461–462

Jenkins-Clarke S, Carr-Hill R, Dixon P 1998 Teams and seams: skill mix in primary care. Journal of Advanced Nursing 28(5):1120–1126

Jewell D 1994 What's happening to practice nursing? British Medical Journal 308:735–736

Jones D 1997 The changing role of the practice nurse. Health and Social Care in the Community 5(2):77–83

Kitson A 1997 Developing excellence in nursing practice and care. Nursing Standard 12(2):33–37

Kitson A, Ahmed LB, Harvey G, Seers K, Thompson DR 1996 From research to practice: one organisational model for promoting research-based practice. Journal of Advanced Nursing 23:430–440

Mallik M 1998 Advocacy in nursing: perceptions and attitudes of the nursing elite in the United Kingdom. Journal of Advanced Nursing 28(5):1001–1011

Mason C 1997 Achieving quality in community health care nursing. Macmillan, London

OXCHECK 1994 Effectiveness of health checks conducted by nurses in primary care: results of the OXCHECK study after 1 year. British Medical Journal 308(6294):308–312

Piper S 1997 The limitations of well men clinics for health education. Nursing Standard 11(30):47–49

Quinney D, Pearson M, Pursey A 1997 'Care' in primary health care nursing. In: Hugman R, Peelo M, Soothill K (eds) Concepts of care: developments in health and social welfare. Arnold, London

Raatikainon R 1994 Power or lack of it in nursing care. Journal of Advanced Nursing 19:424–432

RCN 1997 Nurse practitioners – your questions answered Royal College of Nursing, London

Rees M 1996 Nurse-led management of minor illness in a GP surgery. Nursing Times 92(6):32–38

Reveley S 1998 The role of the triage nurse practitioner in general medical practice, an analysis of the role. Journal of Advanced Nursing 28(3):584–591

Rhead M, Strange F 1996 Nursing lecturer/practitioners: can lecturer/practitioners be music to our ears. Journal of Advanced Nursing 24:1265–1272

Rowe A, Billingham K, Plews C 1998 Missing links. Nursing Times 94(41):32–36

Salvage J 1988 Take me to your leader … the need for leadership in nursing. Nursing Times 84(40):24

Stilwell B 1988 Patients' attitudes to the availability of the nurse practitioner in general practice. In: Bowling A, Stilwell B (eds) The nurse in family practice. Scutari Press, London

Stilwell B, Restall D, Burke-Masters B 1988 Nurse practitioners in British general practice. In: Bowling A, Stilwell B (eds) The nurse in family practice. Scutari Press, London

Thomas LH, Bond S 1996 Measuring patients' satisfaction with nursing: 1990–1994. Journal of Advanced Nursing 23:747–756

Trnobranski PH 1994 Nurse practitioner: redefining the role of the community nurse. Journal of Advanced Nursing 19:134–139

UKCC 1990 The report of the post-registration and practice project. United Kingdom Central Council for Nursing, Midwifery and Health Visiting, London

UKCC 1996 Standards for education and practice following registration: specialist practice transitional arrangements, Registrar's letter 14/199b. United Kingdom Central Council for Nursing, Midwifery and Health Visiting, London

UKCC 1998 A higher level of practice: consultation document. United Kingdom Central Council for Nursing, Midwifery and Health Visiting, London

Williams SJ, Calnan M 1994 Perspective on prevention: the views of GPs. Sociology of Health and Illness 16(3):372–393

Witz A 1994 The challenge of nursing. In: Gabe J, Kelleher D, Williams G (eds) Challenging medicine. Routledge, London

Yerrell P 1998 The clinimed report – the organisation and management of nurses in general practice project. Buckinghamshire College, Buckinghamshire.

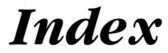

Index

Profiles, 34–37, 264
Protocols, 67–70, 272
  evidence-based practice, 68
  legal issues, 68–69, 272, 273
  nurse prescribing, 236, 237, 248–249
Psychotherapy, 182
Public health, 27, 87–89, 152–165
  approach to health care, 157–158
  collaborative working, 162–164
  community development, 162
  epidemiology, 264
  health strategy, 155–157
  historical perspective, 152–153
  nurse's role, 158–165
  nurse-led initiatives, 275–276
  partnerships, 162–164
  population-based approaches, 157–158, 160–161
  and poverty, 152–155, 161
  user involvement, 162–164
Public Health Alliance, 157–158, 165
Purchasers
  GPs, 74–75, 78–79
  user involvement, 146

Q
Qualifications, 4, 20–21, 24, 250, 295, 297–298
  specialist practitioners, 21, 22, 250, 261–263, 266, 280
Quality of care, 324
  quality assurance, 142
  quality measuring packages, 47
  quality standards, 146, 185, 272
Questionnaire surveys, 150

R
Receptionists, 274–275
Record keeping *see* Patient records
Reflective practice, 222–223, 226, 268–269, 316, 317
Registered mental nurses, 166–167
Relaxation strategies, 182
Research, 38
  and evidence-based practice, 46, 68, 200, 267, 272, 273–274, 316–317
  mental health, 166
  participation in, 316
  relevant to practice, 56
  and role development, 3–4, 273–274
Resource management, 37–42
Review of Prescribing, Supply and Administration of Medicines – Final Report (1999), 251–254
Role development, 3–25
  areas for development, 323
  characteristics of practice nurses, 310–311
  future, 308–329
  generalist role, 320
  government policy, 8–16
  health promotion, 129–131, 318–320
  health visitors, 313
  historical, 6–8, 232–234, 291
  impact of new GP contract, 12–13

  integrated nursing teams, 22–24, 325–326
  lack of clearly defined role, 312–313
  legal issues, 52–71, 272, 273
  mental health, 174–176, 181–184, 199, 200–201
  nurse education, 17–22, 109, 313–316
  nurse prescribing *see* Nurse prescribing
  opportunities, 317–324
  professional development, 58, 326–327
  public health, 158–165
  and relationships, 29–30
  research, 3–4, 273–274
  separatist approach, 311–312
  and skills, 40
  specialist practitioners, 261–263, 267–278
  threats, 309–310
  user involvement, 150–151
Roles, 30
Roy's adaptation model, 114–116
Royal College of General Practitioners (RCGP), 19
Royal College of Nursing
  group prescribing protocols, 249
  nurse prescribing, 233–237, 240–244, 245, 249–250, 253
  Parliamentary Panel, 241
  Practice Nurse Association, 5–6, 18, 22
  specialist practitioners, 250–251
Royal Pharmaceutical Society of Great Britain (RPSoGB), 236

S
SANE, 173
Schizophrenia, 171, 172–173
  physical health needs, 184–185
  relapse prevention, 180–181
  stigma, 191
Scope of Professional Practice (1992), 207, 251, 267, 291
Screening
  mental health, 176–181
  outreach, 177–178
  relapse prevention, 180–181
  suicide risk, 179–180
Secondary care, 72–74
Seedhouse's philosophy of need, 33–34
Self-care
  Orem's model, 110–111
  promoting philosophy of, 129–131
Self-employment, 4–5
Self-help groups, 138
Sexual health
  education, 276–277
  Health of the Nation targets, 15
Shaping the Future (ENB 1996), 27
Shared care, 194
Skill mix, 40, 109, 266, 274–275
Skills, 39–40
  clinical supervision, 213–214
  communication *see* Communication skills
Smoking, 129, 161
Social class, 125, 154
Social deprivation *see* Poverty
Social functioning scale (SFS), 178, 180
Social profiles, 34